Steven L. Cohn
(Editor)

Perioperative Medicine

Springer

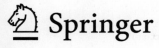

Editor
Steven L. Cohn
Director – Medical Consultation Service
Kings County Hospital Center
Clinical Professor of Medicine
SUNY Downstate
Brooklyn, NY

ISBN 978-0-85729-497-5 e-ISBN 978-0-85729-498-2
DOI 10.1007/978-0-85729-498-2
Springer London Dordrecht Heidelberg New York

British Library Cataloguing in Publication Data
A catalogue record for this book is available from the British Library

Library of Congress Control Number: 2011931531

Cover design: eStudioCalamar, Figueres/Berlin

Printed on acid-free paper

Springer is part of Springer Science+Business Media (www.springer.com)

Preface

Preoperative risk assessment and perioperative management are important aspects of clinical practice in internal medicine. Whereas surgeons and anesthesiologists spend most of their time caring for patients in the perioperative period, many primary-care physicians and hospitalists may feel inadequately trained or uncomfortable in this setting.

The goal of this book is to provide a streamlined approach to the medical aspects of perioperative care, limiting content to make it an easily readable and clinically useful guide. It is intended for use by hospitalists, general internists and specialists, anesthesiologists, surgeons, and residents in training who are involved in the care of patients before and after surgery.

The book is divided into four parts. The first part addresses general aspects of perioperative care, preoperative testing, medication management, and prophylaxis (surgical site infection, venous thromboembolism, endocarditis). The second part highlights aspects specific to various types of surgery, including patient- and surgery-specific risk factors and procedural complications. The third part reviews preoperative evaluation and perioperative management of coexisting medical conditions that affect surgical risk. The last part covers evaluation and management of some of the more frequently encountered postoperative complications.

Because medicine is a constantly changing field, new information may affect some of the recommendations in this book. The information contained in this book is based on what the authors felt was the best available evidence at the time. Additionally, errors, inaccuracies, and omissions may inadvertently occur despite the care that has been taken to avoid them. The reader is advised to use sound clinical judgment and to confirm all doses of medications before prescribing them.

I hope that you will find this information useful in your clinical practice and hope that it will lead to improved perioperative patient care.

Steven L. Cohn, M.D., FACP

Acknowledgment

I would like to thank the authors, most of whom are practicing internists, hospitalists, or anesthesiologists and members of the Society of General Internal Medicine (SGIM) Perioperative Medical Consultation Interest Group (www.sgim.org) or the Society for Perioperative Assessment and Quality Improvement (www.spaqi.org), who have contributed chapters for this book.

I would also like to acknowledge my wife, Deborah, children, Alison and Jeffrey, and mother, Lynn, for their love, encouragement, and support in general and specifically during this project.

Steven L. Cohn, M.D., FACP

Contents

Contributors

Richard B. Brooks, MD, MPH
Director of Inpatient Medical Consultation
San Francisco General Hospital
Assistant Clinical Professor
University of California
San Francisco, CA

Michael P. Carson, MD
Director of Research Outcomes
Jersey Shore University Medical Center
Clinical Associate Professor of Medicine;
Clinical Assistant Professor of Obstetrics and Gynecology, UMDNJ-Robert Wood Johnson Medical School
New Brunswick, NJ

Steven L. Cohn, MD, FACP
Director – Medical Consultation Service
Kings County Hospital Center
Clinical Professor of Medicine
SUNY Downstate
Brooklyn, NY

Barbara A. Cooper, MD, FACP
Director METU, Inpatient Consults and Telemedicine, Walter Reed Army Medical Center, Assistant Professor of Medicine, F. Edward Hebert School of Medicine, Uniformed Services University of Health Sciences
Washington, DC

Darin J. Correll, MD
Director, Postoperative Pain Management Service, Brigham and Women's Hospital
Assistant Professor of Anaesthesia
Harvard Medical School
Boston, MA

Amish Ajit Dangodara, MD
Director – Inpatient General Internal Medicine Hospitalist Consultation & Hospitalist Preoperative Clinic
UCI Medical Center
Professor of Medicine
University of California
Irvine School of Medicine
Orange, CA

Victor Duval, MD
Inpatient Perioperative Service Chief, Ronald Reagan UCLA Medical Center
Assistant Clinical Professor of Anesthesiology
UCLA School of Medicine
Los Angeles, CA

Nadene C. Fair, MD
Director – Perioperative Medicine (MSM-IM); Director-Telemetry
Grady Memorial Hospital
Assistant Professor of Medicine
Morehouse School of Medicine
Atlanta, GA

Leonard S. Feldman, MD, SFHM, FACP, FAAP
Associate Program Director, Osler Medical Residency; Director, Comprehensive General Medical Consult Service, Johns Hopkins Hospital, Assistant Professor of Medicine and Pediatrics
Johns Hopkins University
Baltimore, MD

Joleen Elizabeth Fixley, MD, FACP
Medical Director -Preoperative
Medical Evaluation Unit
Nebraska – Western Iowa VAMC
Assistant Professor of Internal Medicine
Creighton University Medical School
Omaha, NE

Shuwei Gao, MD
Medical Director, Anticoagulation
Clinic, University of Texas
MD Anderson Cancer Center
Assistant Professor of Medicine
University of Texas
MD Anderson Cancer Center
Houston, TX

Brian Harte, MD, FACP, SFHM
Chief Operating Officer
Cleveland Clinic Hillcrest Hospital
Interim Chair – Cleveland
Clinic Medicine Institute
Medical Director – Enterprise
Business Intelligence
Cleveland, OH

Lane K. Jacobs, MD
Chief – Section of General
Internal Medicine
Carolinas Medical Center
Clinical Associate Professor
of Medicine, UNC-Chapel Hill
Charlotte, NC

Bruce E. Johnson, MD
Associate Dean for Faculty Affairs
Carilion Roanoke Memorial Hospital
Professor of Medicine
Virginia Tech Carilion
School of Medicine
Roanoke, VA

Scott Kaatz, DO, MSc, FACP
Associate Residency Program Director;
Medical Director, Anticoagulation Clinics
Henry Ford Hospital, Clinical Associate
Professor of Medicine, Wayne State
University School of Medicine
Detroit, MI

Alok Kapoor, MD, MSc
Medical Director of Quality for Internal
Medicine Preoperative Assessment Center
(IMPAC), Boston Medical Center
Assistant Professor of Medicine
Boston University School of Medicine
Boston, MA

Ross Kerridge, MBBS, FRCA, FANZCA
Director, Perioperative Service
John Hunter Hospital & Royal Newcastle
Centre, Conjoint Associate Professor of
Anaesthesia, University of Newcastle
Callaghan, NSW, Australia

Beth G. Lewis, MD, MPH
Director of Obstetric Medicine
Saint Peters University Hospital
Assistant Professor of Medicine
Drexel University Medical School
New Brunswick, NJ

Ronald MacKenzie, MD
Associate Attending Physician Hospital
for Special Surgery; New York Cornell
Weill Medical Center; Memorial Sloan
Kettering Hospital, Associate Professor
of Clinical Medicine, New York Cornell
Weill Medical Center
New York, NY

Brian F. Mandell, MD, PhD, FACP, FACR
Cleveland Clinic, Professor and Chair
Department of Medicine
CCF Lerner College of Medicine of CWRU
Cleveland, OH

Ellen F. Manzullo, MD, FACP
Deputy Department Chair of General
Internal Medicine, Chief-Section of
General Internal Medicine, Ambulatory
Treatment, and Emergency Care
Professor of Medicine
University of Texas
MD Anderson Cancer Center
Houston, TX

Vivek K. Moitra, MD
Assistant Medical Director – Surgical Intensive Care Unit
Columbia Presbyterian Hospital
Assistant Professor of Anesthesiology
Columbia University College of Physicians and Surgeons
New York, NY

Visala S. Muluk, MD
Director – Medical Preoperative Evaluation Clinic, VAPHCS
Assistant Professor of Medicine
University of Pittsburgh
Pittsburgh, PA

Ibironke Oduyebo, MD
Hospitalist, Johns Hopkins University Hospital, Instructor in Medicine
Johns Hopkins School of Medicine
Baltimore, MD

David G. Paje, MD, FACP, FHM
Associate Division Head – Detroit Campus
Director, Division of Hospitalist Medicine
Henry Ford Hospital, Clinical Assistant Professor, Wayne State University School of Medicine
Detroit, MI

L. Reuven Pasternak, MD, MPH, MBA
Chief Executive Officer and Executive Vice President for Academic Affairs
Inova Fairfax Hospital – Inova Health System, Professor of Anesthesiology
Virginia Commonwealth University School of Medicine
Falls Church, VA

Kurt Pfeifer, MD, FACP
Associate Program Director – General Internal Medicine Residency
Froedtert Hospital
Associate Professor of Medicine
Medical College of Wisconsin
Milwaukee, WI

Kalpana R. Prakasa, MD
Hospitalist, Johns Hopkins University Hospital, Assistant Professor of Medicine
Johns Hopkins School of Medicine
Baltimore, MD

Paul J. Primeaux, MD
Residency Program Director;
Director – Liver Transplant Anesthesia
Tulane Medical Center
Clinical Assistant Professor
Tulane University School of Medicine

Deborah C. Richman, MBChB, FFA (SA)
Director – Preoperative Services
Assistant Professor of Clinical Anesthesiology, SUNY Stony Brook
Stony Brook, NY

Sunil K. Sahai, MD, FAAP, FACP
Medical Director – Internal Medicine Perioperative Assessment Center (IMPAC)
Associate Professor of Medicine
University of Texas
MD Anderson Cancer Center
Houston, TX

Benjamin L. Sapers, MD
Chair – Division of Consultative Medicine
Rhode Island Hospital, Assistant Professor of Medicine, Brown University
Providence, RI

Adam C. Schaffer, MD
Director of General Medical Consultation – Hospitalist Service
Brigham and Women's Hospital
Instructor in Medicine
Harvard Medical School
Boston, MA

Barbara Slawski, MD, MS
Chief – Section of Consultative and Perioperative Medicine, Froedtert Memorial Lutheran Hospital
Assistant Professor – Internal Medicine and Orthopedic Surgery
Medical College of Wisconsin
Milwaukee, WI

Howard S. Smith, MD, FACP
Academic Director of Pain Management
Director of Perioperative Services
Associate Professor of Anesthesiology
Internal Medicine, and Physical
Medicine and Rehabilitation
Albany Medical College
Albany, NY

Mihaela S. Stefan, MD
Director – Medical Consultation Program
Baystate Medical Center
Assistant Professor of Medicine
Tufts University School of Medicine

Edwin P. Su, MD
Attending Orthopedic Surgeon
Hospital for Special Surgery
Weill Cornell Medical College
New York, NY

Meghan Collen Tadel, MD
Attending Anesthesiologist – Preoperative
Assessment Services, Northwestern
Memorial Hospital
Assistant Professor of Anesthesiology
Northwestern University Feinberg
School of Medicine
Chicago, IL

Nomi L. Traub, MD
Attending Physician – Graduate
Medical Education
Atlanta Medical Center
Emory University
Atlanta, GA

Rebecca S. Twersky, MD, MPH
Medical Director – Ambulatory Surgery
Unit, University Hospital of Brooklyn
Professor and Vice Chair for Research
Department of Anesthesiology
SUNY Downstate
Brooklyn, NY

Brian Woods, MD
Department of Anesthesia,
Columbia University College
of Physicians and Surgeons
New York, NY

Part I

Preoperative Evaluation

Role of the Medical Consultant 1

Steven L. Cohn

1.1 Introduction

- Preoperative medical consultation and perioperative management of the surgical patient have become important components of the clinical practice of internists, particularly hospitalists, as well as other primary care physicians and subspecialists.
- Previous surveys found that many primary care physicians[1] and hospitalists[2] felt inadequately trained in perioperative medicine, and as a result, this area has been receiving additional emphasis as part of the core competencies for hospital medicine.
- With the growth of the hospitalist movement, the role of the consultant has evolved from providing evaluation and advice to include co-management of the patient in various settings.
- This chapter reviews the roles and responsibilities of the medical consultant, focusing on the principles of consultation and techniques to improve effectiveness.

1.2 General Principles of Consultation

- Almost 30 years ago, Goldman[3] and colleagues described the basic concepts for performing medical consultations. His "Ten Commandments for Effective Consultations" included the following:

 1. Determine the question.
 2. Establish urgency.
 3. Look for yourself.

S.L. Cohn
Internal Medicine-Medical Consultation Service,
SUNY Downstate - Kings County Hospital Center,
450 Clarkson Ave, Box 68, Brooklyn, NY 11203, USA
e-mail: steven.cohn@downstate.edu

S.L. Cohn (ed.), *Perioperative Medicine*,
DOI: 10.1007/978-0-85729-498-2_1, © Springer-Verlag London Limited 2011

4. Be as brief as appropriate.
5. Be specific and concise.
6. Provide contingency plans.
7. Honor thy turf.
8. Teach with tact.
9. Talk is cheap and effective.
10. Follow-up.

- These important concepts incorporated many of the ethical principles described by the American Medical Association (AMA)[4] and remain valid for the traditional consultation. However, some modifications are needed to cover the emerging role of hospitalists as co-managers.

1.3 Types of Consultation (Table 1.1)

- The consultant may be asked by the requesting physician to assume a variety of roles: consult only, consult and write orders, consult and follow with me, or consult and transfer to your service.
- The traditional or standard medical consultation consisted of a formal request from the patient's attending physician to evaluate the patient and answer a specific question.
  - The consultant was expected to address the question and to provide advice and recommendations, but not to write orders, bring in other consultants, or assume care – the requesting physician remained in control and responsible for the patient's overall care and treatment.

Table 1.1 Roles and responsibilities of different types of consultations

Role/responsibility	Traditional	Co-management	Curbside
MD in charge overall	Requesting physician	Shared responsibility	Requesting physician
Primary care of medical problems	Requesting physician	Medical – consultant Surgical – requesting physician	Requesting physician
Question addressed	Specific	Broader issues – other medical problems	Should not address either but offer to do formal consult or give only general advice
Order writing	No	Yes	No
Follow-up	Limited – as needed	Daily until discharge	No – no formal relationship

- The consultant also focused on the specific problem rather than looking for and addressing other issues.
- Consultations were requested only when necessary and not for routine management.
- There would be a brief follow-up period but not daily visits for the duration of hospitalization.

- This traditional consultant role has been changing over the past 10 years. A survey by Salerno[5] and colleagues revealed that many surgeons wanted the medical consultant to assume more of a co-management role. Specifically they wanted the consultant to have a more global approach, addressing all necessary medical issues as well as writing orders and providing ongoing follow-up.

  - Co-management arrangements have typically been with orthopedic surgeons but more recently are occurring with neurosurgeons.
  - Co-management has potential advantages of decreasing length of stay and possibly reducing complications although the few published studies to date have shown minimal benefits.
  - Surgeons and nurses often prefer co-management, but a possible disadvantage is that the co-managing consultant may feel subservient to the surgeon. He may be asked to assume responsibilities outside his area of training or to perform more mundane and trivial tasks.

- Yet another type of consultation is the so-called "curbside" [6]or informal consult in which the consultant is asked to provide an opinion or advice without personally seeing the patient. Although theoretically these should be avoided from a medicolegal standpoint, they occur frequently although there is no actual doctor–patient relationship.

  - Ideally the consultant should offer to perform a formal consult, but if any advice is given, it should be generic and simple.
  - The requesting physician should not make reference to the consultant in the medical record if he has not seen the patient; however, if the consultant has had any contact with the patient, he should write a note in the chart.

1.4 Determining the Question

- Because of the multiple types of consultations, it is incumbent upon the requesting physician to specify exactly what is being requested. If there is any uncertainty, the consultant should clarify this question by communicating directly with the requesting physician.
- A request for preoperative consultation may be to assess surgical risk, to provide a "green light" to proceed with anesthesia and surgery, to evaluate and answer a diagnostic or management issue, to reassure the requesting physician, or to document an opinion or findings for medicolegal purposes. Although the reason for a medical consult may be obvious, disagreement regarding the primary purpose for the consult still occurs between the requesting physician and the consultant.

- In many cases, consult requests are vague, non-specific (e.g., clearance or evaluation), or do not even ask a question. Without understanding the reason for the consult, the consultant's response may fail to answer the question being asked by the requesting physician.

1.5 Answering the Question

- Traditionally, the consultant restricted advice to the specific problem or question; however, more often the consultant is now addressing other issues noted during the evaluation. If these other findings and recommendations are relevant and important, many surgeons may prefer this approach. However, the requesting physician does not want a long "to-do" list for minor problems or issues that are not relevant and do not need to be addressed during the current hospitalization.
- If the reason for consultation is preoperative evaluation, the consultant needs to:
  1. Assess the patient's medical problems, including the severity and degree of control.
  2. Estimate surgical risk.
  3. Determine if the patient is in his or her optimal (or acceptable) medical condition for the planned procedure.
  4. Decide whether further tests or interventions are indicated.
  5. Make management recommendations regarding the patient's current medications and any necessary prophylaxis.
- Consultants often tell anesthesiologists and surgeons what they already know, but instead should focus on what they do not know but need to know. This includes "what they know they don't know" (which is hopefully why they requested the consult) and "what they don't know they don't know"!
- The consultant should avoid making recommendations about the type of anesthesia and other areas outside his area of expertise. Also, the term "cleared for surgery" should not be used, even if that was listed as the reason for the consultation, as this implies a guarantee that the patient will not have a complication.[7]

1.6 The Consultation Report (Table 1.2)

- Include specific information regarding demographics, medical problems, current medications, allergies, other relevant history, pertinent physical findings, and test results.
- Assess the patient's fitness for surgery ("optimal medical condition") and make specific recommendations for perioperative management including medication management and prophylactic measures to reduce surgical risk.

Table 1.2 The consultation report "checklist"

Demographics	Patient information Reason for consult Referring physician/service Surgery: procedure planned/date
Pertinent medical problems	Cardiopulmonary disease, DM, HTN, thyroid disease, bleeding disorder, stroke, seizures
Past surgical history	Operation, type of anesthesia, date, complications
Social history	Tobacco, alcohol, drug use
Medications (home and hospital); allergies	Name, dose, frequency, compliance; description of allergic reaction
Family history	Genetically related diseases: malignant hyperthermia, bleeding disorders
Review of systems	Cardiopulmonary focus (chest pain, dyspnea), exercise capacity, bleeding/bruising
Physical exam	Vital signs, usual exam with focus on airway, murmur/gallop, adventitious sounds, neurologic deficit, mental status
Lab tests	Depends on risk factors and procedure (CBC, BMP, ECG); other blood tests (PT/PTT, drug levels, TFTs); specific results of stress test, echocardiogram, PFTs, etc.
Impression	Patient is/is not in his/her optimal (acceptable) medical condition for the planned procedure.
Recommendations	Current meds (continue, stop, change dose), new meds, prophylaxis (SSI, VTE, IE, ischemia, aspiration), postop. monitoring (ECG, cardiac enzymes, telemetry, pulse oximetry)
Discussion	Discuss specifics of pertinent problems (severity, stability, degree of control), assess level of risk, and summarize

DM diabetes mellitus, *HTN* hypertension, *CBC* complete blood count, *BMP* basic metabolic panel, *ECG* electrocardiogram, *PT* prothrombin time, *PTT* partial thromboplastin time, *TFT* thyroid function test, *PFT* pulmonary function test, *SSI* surgical site infection, *VTE* venous thromboembolism, *IE* infective endocarditis

1.7 Optimizing Effectiveness

1.7.1 Factors Influencing or Improving Compliance[8] (Table 1.3)

- A number of factors have been associated with improved compliance with the consultant's recommendations. In general, following Goldman's Ten Commandments or Salerno's modification (see Table 1.4) will result in effective consultation.

Table 1.3 Factors that influence or improve compliance with consultant recommendations

Prompt response (within 24 h)
Limit number of recommendations (≤5)
Identify crucial or critical recommendations (versus routine)
Focus on central issues
Make specific relevant recommendations
Use definitive language
Specify drug dosage, route, frequency, duration
Frequent follow-up including progress notes
Direct verbal contact
Therapeutic (versus diagnostic) recommendations
Severity of illness

Reproduced with permission from Cohn and Macpherson[8]. For more information visit www.uptodate.com

- Determine and clarify the question: As noted, the reason for the consultation needs to be clearly defined by the requesting physician and understood and addressed by the consultant.
- Punctual response: The consultant needs to be available and able to respond in a timely fashion, depending on the urgency of the consultation.
  - True "stat" consults should be answered by phone within 10 min and in person in less than 30 min, and in general, elective consults should be answered within 24 h, preferably the same day they were requested.
- Recommendations:
  Prioritize and limit: The consultant should make specific, precise recommendations and list them in order of importance. Crucial or critical recommendations are more likely to be followed, as are those at the top of the list.
  - It was previously felt that the number of recommendations should be limited to no more than five. However, the more recent trend has been to leave as many recommendations as needed to answer the consult and to offer to help with writing and implementing them (co-management).
  - Recommendations for specific therapy are more likely to be followed than those for diagnostic tests.
- *Language*: The consultant should use definitive language, be specific with his recommendations, and provide contingency plans.
  - Specify the drug name, dose, frequency, route of administration, and duration of therapy when making recommendations for medications.

Table 1.4 Original and modified 10 commandments for effective consultations

1983 Commandments		2006 Modifications	
Commandment	Meaning	Commandment	Meaning
1. Determine the question	The consultant should call the primary physician if the specific question is not obvious	1. Determine your customer	Ask the requesting physician how you can best help them if a specific question is not obvious; they may want co-management
2. Establish urgency	The consultant must determine whether the consultation is emergent, urgent, or elective	2. Establish urgency	The consultant must determine whether the consultation is emergent, urgent, or elective
3. Look for yourself	Consultants are most effective when they are willing to gather data on their own	3. Look for yourself	Consultants are most effective when they are willing to gather data on their own
4. Be brief as appropriate	The consultant need not repeat in full detail the data that were already recorded	4. Be brief as appropriate	The consultant need not repeat in full detail the data that were already recorded
5. Be specific	Leaving a long list of suggestions may decrease the likelihood that any of them will be followed, including the critical ones	5. Be specific, thorough, and descend from thy ivory tower to help when requested	Leave as many specific recommendations as needed to answer the consult but ask the requesting physician if they need help with order writing
6. Provide contingency plans	Consultants should anticipate potential problems; a brief description of therapeutic options may save time later	6. Provide contingency plans and discuss their execution	Consultants should anticipate potential problems, document contingency plans, and provide a 24-h point of contact to help execute the plans if requested
7. Thou shalt not covet thy neighbor's turf	In most cases, consultants should play a subsidiary role	7. Thou may negotiate joint title to thy neighbor's turf	Consultants can and should co-manage any facet of patient care that the requesting physician desires; a frank discussion defining which specialty is responsible for what aspects of patient care is needed

(continued)

Table 1.4 (continued)

1983 Commandments		2006 Modifications	
Commandment	Meaning	Commandment	Meaning
8. Teach with tact	Requesting physicians appreciate consultants who make an active effort to share their expertise	8. Teach with tact and pragmatism	Judgments on leaving references should be tailored to the requesting physician's specialty, level of training, and urgency of the consult
9. Talk is cheap and effective	There is no substitute for direct personal contact with the primary physician	9. Talk is essential	There is no substitute for direct personal contact with the primary physician
10. Provide appropriate follow-up	Consultants should recognize the appropriate time to fade into a background role, but that time is almost never the same day the consultation note is signed	10. Follow-up daily	Daily written follow-up is desirable; when the patient's problems are not active, the consultant should discuss signing-off with the requesting physician beforehand

From Salerno et al.[5],

  - Tell the requesting physician what response to expect, how long it will take, and how and when to adjust the medication dose if necessary.

- Communication: Direct verbal communication with the requesting physician is crucial and is preferable to just leaving a note in the chart.
  - After completing the consultation, to expedite implementation of the care plan, contact the requesting physician to let him know that the consult has been answered, what the recommendations are, and what needs to be done. It is also important to communicate with other members of the healthcare team to coordinate care.
- Follow-up: Make appropriate follow-up visits to reassess the patient's condition and ensure that the recommendations were followed. Document your findings and update recommendations in the medical record.
  - There is no standard regarding how often the consultant needs to see the patient. This is determined by the patient's medical condition, type of surgery, and whether or not co-management was requested.
  - When the patient is medically stable and there is no longer a need for the medical consultant, sign off and document this in the chart. Also note recommendations and arrangements for long-term follow-up at this time.

1.8 Summary

- Perioperative medical consultation is a combination of art, science, and politics.
- A description of the ideal medical consultant is someone who will "render a report that informs without patronizing, educate without lecturing, direct without ordering, and solve the problem without making the referring physician appear to be stupid."[9]
- Hopefully by following these principles, the medical consultant will be effective in providing useful information and recommendations to the requesting physician who will then implement them in an attempt to improve patient outcome.

References

1. Devor M, Renvall M, Ramsdell J. Practice patterns and the adequacy of residency training in consultation medicine. *J Gen Intern Med.* 1993;8(10):554-560.
2. Plauth WH III, Pantilat SZ, Wachter RM, Fenton CL. Hospitalists' perceptions of their residency training needs: results of a national survey. *Am J Med.* 2001;111(3):247-254.
3. Goldman L, Lee T, Rudd P. Ten commandments for effective consultations. *Arch Intern Med.* 1983;143(9):1753-1755.
4. Opinions and reports of the judicial council. In: Gross RJ CG, Kammerer WS, eds. *Kammerer and Gross' medical consultation: the internist on the surgical, obstetric, and psychiatric services.* Philadelphia, PA: Williams & Wilkins; 1998:8.
5. Salerno SM, Hurst FP, Halvorson S, Mercado DL. Principles of effective consultation: an update for the 21st-century consultant. *Arch Intern Med.* 2007;167(3):271-275.
6. Kuo D, Gifford DR, Stein MD. Curbside consultation practices and attitudes among primary care physicians and medical subspecialists. *JAMA.* 1998;280(10):905-909.
7. Choi JJ. An anesthesiologist's philosophy on "medical clearance" for surgical patients. *Arch Intern Med.* 1987;147(12):2090-2092.
8. Cohn SL. Overview of the principles of medical consultation. In: Basow D, ed. *UpToDate.* Waltham, MA: UpToDate; 2009.
9. Bates R. The two sides of every successful consultation. *Med Econ.* 1979;7:173-180.

Preoperative Testing

2

L. Reuven Pasternak

2.1 Introduction

2.1.1 The Purpose of the Preoperative Assessment

- The preoperative assessment is designed to assess risks relevant to the perioperative period, including anesthesia, surgery and the recovery period.
- This process should not be expected to be a way to manage chronic health problems or new acute problems – these should be managed by the patient's primary care provider or referred to the appropriate specialist.
- The risk to the patient for surgery and anesthesia is a combination of their preoperative medical status (Table 2.1) and the intensity/invasiveness of their surgery.
- All testing and associated assessment and consultations are done on the basis of a reasonable expectation that the patient has a medical condition or risk factor and that its value will have an impact on perioperative management.

2.2 Preoperative Testing: When, Where, and Who?

- The preoperative assessment should be done prior to the day of surgery and the results made available for review by anesthesia directed staff prior to the morning of the day of surgery.
- The assessment may be done by primary care providers for individuals with table medical status and for whom major surgery is not anticipated. Others will require assessment by anesthesia staff or their extenders (Fig. 2.1).

L.R. Pasternak
Inova Fairfax Hospital – Inova Health System,
3300 Gallows Road, Falls Church, VA 22042, USA
e-mail: reuven.pasternak@inova.org

S.L. Cohn (ed.), *Perioperative Medicine*,
DOI: 10.1007/978-0-85729-498-2_2, © Springer-Verlag London Limited 2011

Table 2.1 American Society of Anesthesiologists classification

ASA status	Description	Example
P1	A normal, healthy patient	Healthy adult with no medical problems, no medications
P2	Patient with mild systemic disease	Well-controlled hypertension
P3	Patient with severe systemic disease	Angina pectoris without congestive heart failure, reactive airway disease regularly requiring inhalers
P4	Patient with severe systemic disease that is a constant threat to life	Severe congestive heart failure
P5	A moribund patient who is not expected to survive without the operation	Severe trauma, end stage terminally ill

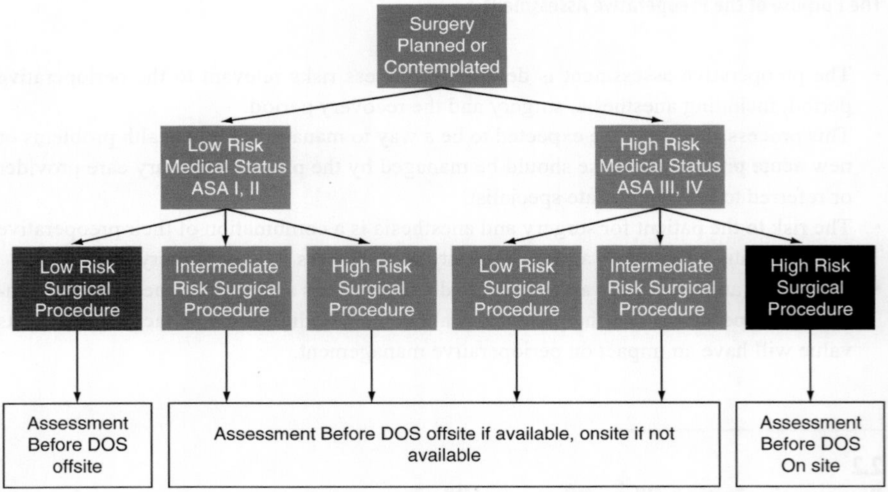

Fig. 2.1 Timing of the assessment

- Well-developed preoperative systems usually require only 25–33% of patients to actually visit the facility prior to the day of surgery; in other instances, information gathered by the preoperative system is sufficient to determine the relative risk for surgery.
- An assessment by non-anesthesia providers does not necessarily address all issues relevant for surgery and anesthesia. Anesthesia personnel may make a preliminary judgment on the basis of data provided by these sources.
- Absence of a system for preoperative assessment may result in delays of surgery, unnecessary cancellation and/or unnecessary testing to accommodate urgent needs.

2.3 Preoperative Testing

2.3.1 Guidelines

- Several standardized guidelines exist for determining the appropriateness of testing. These include the American Heart Association/American College of Cardiology guidelines as well as those of the American Society of Anesthesiology.
- The guidelines provide reasonable courses of action to pursue and should be balanced with an individual assessment.
- The group, institution, or system within which the perioperative system resides should have explicit guidelines for testing and process. This provides protection against the oft-feared and much-exaggerated concerns of medical liability.

2.3.2 The Value of Testing

- Testing is often done on the basis of custom or longstanding routine without rationale based on best available evidence or the patient's medical condition.
- Testing without specific indication has been shown not to have any positive effect on patient outcome. In one study the performance of 2,236 tests found that 1,828 did not have any indication, of which only 10 were abnormal and, of these, 4 with results of clinical significance. All four of these patients had their surgery without problem.[1] Another found that medical status and type of surgery were most predictive of the need for tests[2] while the most recent demonstrated no adverse events in a patient population undergoing ambulatory surgery without major medical risk factors who had no preoperative testing.[3]
- The ordering of large numbers of tests without indication increases the likelihood that a false positive test will lead to further, unnecessary testing and potential delays and cancellations.

2.4 Preoperative Tests

2.4.1 Physical Examination

- The extent of the physical examination should be guided by the nature of the medical issues associated with the patient and anticipated for surgery. Basic assessment of the airway and auscultation of cardiac and respiratory sounds are useful, but perhaps

secondary in importance to the obtaining of a history specific for issues to guide appropriate assessment.
- The preoperative assessment is not the optimal or appropriate time to engage in assessments not focused on perioperative care unless the provider is prepared to direct the patient to appropriate continuing care or consultation.
- New or unresolved issues should be referred to providers capable of providing continuing care after the perioperative period.
- The critical issue is whether the patient is as stable as reasonably possible or whether further assessment or management will minimize the risk associated with perioperative management.

2.4.2 Electrocardiogram (ECG)

- There is little evidence to support routine electrocardiograms on the basis of age >40, 50, or 60 alone, as is common in some recommendations.
- An abnormal ECG alone is not correlated with adverse outcomes. Studies have demonstrated that relying on ECGs alone is not predictive of adverse events.[4]
- The likelihood of an abnormal ECG is associated with age >65 and/or history of heart failure, angina, myocardial infarction, severe valvular disease or high cholesterol.[5] It is likely prudent to add diabetes mellitus and chronic renal and hepatic disease to these indications.

2.4.3 Additional Cardiac Testing (See Chap. 20)

- Testing for cardiac patients having non-cardiac surgery is best done in association with the recommendations of the American Heart Association/American College of Cardiology Task Force.[6]
- The basis of the additional cardiac assessment is to determine whether the patient is as stable as reasonably possible for surgery.

2.4.4 Chest Radiograph

- Though one of the most common of tests, chest X-rays have been found to be of little value in patients without specific indication. Charpak and colleagues, reporting on the utility of routine chest X-rays on 1,101 patients, found that only 5% had an impact on perioperative management.[7] In another review of 905 patients, 504 (22%) had risk factors of whom 22% had abnormalities, none of which were new or added to the clinical assessment of the patient.
- There is no indication for chest X-rays on the basis of age.
- X-rays should be obtained only in those cases where there is an acute or a chronic process that has changed within the past 6 months, or for planned thoracic surgery.

- The use of this information to guide management must be correlated with clinical information about the patient and a determination that the patient is as stable as reasonably possible for the planned procedure.

2.4.5 Hematocrit

- There is no indication for routine measuring the hematocrit in patients who do not have a medical history associated with anemia or a condition for which anemia may be a complication.
- Hematocrit should be measured in patients for whom significant blood loss is anticipated and/or who have a history consistent with cancer, kidney disease and liver disease, or signs of anemia on assessment.

2.4.6 White Blood Cell Count

- There is no evidence to support obtaining white cell counts in patients without an associated history of myeloproliferative disorder (e.g., solid tissue tumors, hematologic neoplasms, petechiae, purpura, splenomegaly or lymphadenopathy) and in those who are taking medications that might affect white blood status.
- Clinicians should not routinely obtain white blood cell counts before surgery.
- If an infection is suspected on the basis of symptoms and/or physical examination a white cell count may be obtained to assist in diagnosis. However, in these circumstances, it is better to defer elective surgery until the issue is resolved rather than trying to do an elective assessment on the day of surgery.

2.4.7 Platelet Count

- Obtain platelet counts in patients with a history of platelet abnormalities, symptoms or signs of impaired hemostasis on history and physical examination, myeloproliferative disorders, and in those receiving medications known to commonly alter platelet counts (e.g., chemotherapy, heparin).

2.4.8 Tests for Coagulation and Bleeding

- Tests for coagulation and bleeding should be reserved for those patients who are at risk on the basis of their medical history.
- These patients can be identified on the basis of medications and/or a history of liver disease, nutritional disorders or any history of bleeding tendency.

2.4.9
Prothrombin Time (PT)/International Normalized Ratio (INR)

- A potential rationale for obtaining a PT/INR before surgery would be to identify patients at risk for postoperative bleeding.
- The PT/INR is one of the least helpful tests in the preoperative armamentarium. In a recent review, it was the perfect unhelpful test.[8] Abnormal results occurred in 0.3% of patients and, among a subset of studies that evaluated outcomes, abnormal test results did not affect management and were not associated with increased postoperative bleeding rates in any patients.
- Clinicians can predict most patients with an elevated PT/INR based on clinical evaluation. For example, patients with known chronic liver disease, malnutrition or a history of bleeding tendencies are more likely to have an abnormal PT/INR than are unselected patients.
- Also obtain a preoperative PT/INR for all patients who are taking warfarin to help guide warfarin management.

2.4.10
Partial Thromboplastin Time

- While an abnormal partial thromboplastin time (PTT) is more common than an abnormal PT/INR, the test is equally unhelpful.
- In one review, 6.5% of all PTT values were abnormal, but only 0.1% of all tests influenced management.[8]
- Do not use the PTT as a screening preoperative test.

2.4.11
Bleeding Time

- The bleeding time was commonly used in the past to assess perioperative bleeding risk, especially in patients taking aspirin or non-steroidal anti-inflammatory agents.
- However, a normal bleeding time does not predict a low risk for surgical hemorrhage, and an abnormal bleeding time does not increase the risk of hemorrhage.
- Do not routinely obtain a bleeding time before surgery.
- For a patient whose history and physical examination suggest impaired hemostasis and whose PT/INR, PTT and platelet count are normal, a bleeding time may be an appropriate part of a more thorough hemostasis evaluation that includes consultation with a coagulation specialist.

2.4.12
Electrolytes

- There is no indication for routine ordering of serum electrolytes.[9]
- Electrolytes should be ordered based on the presence of medical conditions for which electrolyte disturbances are common (e.g., cardiac disease, renal disease,

hepatic disorders, diabetes mellitus) or where medications may cause electrolyte imbalance (e.g., diuretics, digoxin, ACE, ARB).
- The nature of current testing procedures makes it more likely that it is more efficient and no more expensive to order an electrolyte panel versus isolated values.

2.4.13 Renal Function Tests

- In contrast to the limited value of many commonly ordered preoperative tests, serum creatinine has value in identifying patients at risk for perioperative cardiac complications.
- In the revised cardiac risk index, serum creatinine >2.0 mg/dL was one of the six independent risk factors for cardiac complications.[11] It predicted cardiac risk as well as established risk factors including coronary artery disease, congestive heart failure and high risk surgical procedure. Other studies have demonstrated the value of chronic renal insufficiency as a predictor for adverse outcomes after cardiac and vascular surgery.
- Renal insufficiency is often unsuspected by clinical evaluation. In a recent review, 2.6% of routine preoperative serum creatinine measurements were abnormal and influenced perioperative management.[8]
- Measure serum creatinine in patients more than 50 years old, in those with diabetes, hypertension, renal insufficiency, cardiovascular disease or undergoing major surgery, and in those who are taking medications that affect renal function.

2.4.14 Glucose

- Most abnormal preoperative serum glucose results are in those with known diabetes; the incidence of an unexpected abnormal blood glucose concentration that might influence perioperative management is 0.5%.[8]
- Do not obtain serum glucose as a screening preoperative test in unselected patients. Serum glucose measurement is appropriate to screen patients with risk factors for diabetes such as obesity, and to assess glucose control in patients known to have diabetes or symptoms suggestive of diabetes.

2.4.15 Liver Function Tests

- The most commonly obtained preoperative liver function tests are the serum transaminases. Alkaline phosphatase is not commonly obtained and should not be part of routine preoperative testing.
- Patients with hepatic cirrhosis have markedly increased perioperative morbidity and mortality. The risk is proportional to the severity of the cirrhosis, as measured by the Childs–Pugh classification.

- In contrast, no evidence suggests that asymptomatic liver function test abnormalities predict postoperative complications; the rate of unexpected abnormalities that influence management is 0.1%.[8]
- Clinicians should not obtain screening liver function tests on unselected patients as part of preoperative testing.

2.4.16 Albumin

- Serum albumin concentration is a robust laboratory predictor of postoperative morbidity and mortality.
- In a study of 54,215 veterans, low serum albumin was the single strongest predictor of 30-day postoperative mortality among patients undergoing major non-cardiac surgery.[10] A linear relationship existed; the risk of mortality began to increase with serum albumin concentrations <3.5 g/dL. For patients with serum albumin concentrations <2.1 g/dL, the perioperative mortality rate was 28%. In other studies, low serum albumin concentrations have also predicted postoperative pulmonary complications.
- Although conditions such as recent severe blood loss and nephropathy can cause hypoalbuminemia, it is most often an indication of malnutrition. A few studies have shown a benefit of delaying surgery to allow time for vigorous nutrition to increase serum albumin, but most studies have not suggested benefit. Therefore, while a preoperative serum albumin concentration may have prognostic value, it usually does not affect patient management.
- Measure serum albumin concentration if it is likely to be low (e.g., in patients with liver disease, nephropathy, enteropathy, recent severe illness, blood loss or cachexia) and if the prognostic information is likely to affect the patient's care plan.

2.4.17 Urinalysis

- Urinalysis has been required in the past by state law for preoperative screening. This was on the basis of a belief that major abnormalities were present that could not be determined on the basis of a history. This was principally associated with detecting diabetes mellitus.
- One study[3] found that in a study of 3,666 patients only 1.4% were abnormal and had an impact on care.
- In practice, there is no indication for routine urinalysis for preoperative assessment.
- Urinalysis should be reserved for patients with acute urinary tract symptoms or for whom surgeons may want a baseline prior to genitourinary and joint replacement surgery.

2.4.18 Pregnancy Testing

- Pregnancy testing is one of the most controversial areas of testing for elective surgical procedures.
- Complications associated with surgery and anesthesia for pregnant patients are principally associated with site of surgery (abdomen, perineal area) and type of anesthesia (general).

- Commercial testing kits are highly sensitive and, in cases where testing are to be done, are a reasonable first step to test for pregnancy.
- Patients who are menopausal or who have had surgery rendering pregnancy virtually impossible (hysterectomy, bilateral oopherectomy) need not be tested.
- Patients who are fertile should be tested on the basis of their history and advice that surgery may pose a risk to their pregnancy if they are pregnant.

2.5 Summary Recommendations

- Table 2.2 summarizes recommendations for the use of preoperative laboratory tests, and includes an estimate of the incidence of abnormalities that affect perioperative management and the positive and negative likelihood ratios for postoperative complications.

Table 2.2 Summary: preoperative laboratory testing

Test	Indication
Health patient <65	• No testing except as need for postoperative management
ECG	• Age>65 • Presence of history of significant cardiovascular disease, hypertension • Thoracic/major vascular procedure
Chest X-ray	• None based on age • History of chronic pulmonary condition (e.g., asthma) that has changed within the past 6 months or which significant impair respiratory function • Thoracic procedure
Hematocrit	• History of anemia • Procedure with anticipated significant blood loss
CBC (Hct, WBC, platelet count)	• History of bleeding disorder, myeloproliferative disease, medications affecting blood formation • Procedure with anticipated significant blood loss
Glucose	• Diabetes mellitus or risk factors/symptoms (obesity, polyuria, polydipsia)
Serum electrolytes	• Diabetes mellitus and other endocrine disorders, renal disease, hepatic disorders • Medications affecting or affected by electrolytes, including those for cardiac disease, treatment for oncology
Liver function tests	• Cirrhosis or history of liver disease
Coagulation tests (PT/PTT)	• History of bleeding disorder, liver disease, or malnutrition • Patients on anticoagulants (warfarin, heparin)
Urinalysis	• Urologic procedure • History of recent/chronic urinary tract infection
Pregnancy test	• None in patient in whom menopausal or post-surgical procedure precluding pregnancy • Explicit patient history precluding risk for pregnancy

References

1. Kaplan EB, Sheiner LB, Boeckmann AJ, et al. The usefulness of preoperative laboratory screening. *JAMA*. 1985;253:3576.
2. Kitz DJ, Slusarz-Ladden C, Lecky JH. Hospital resources used for inpatient and ambulatory surgery. *Anesthesiology*. 1988;96:485-496.
3. Chung F, Yuan H, Yin L, Vairavanathan S, Wong DT. Elimination of preoperative testing in ambulatory surgery. *Anesth Analg*. 2009;108:467-475.
4. Tait AR, Parr HG, Tremper KK. Evaluation of the efficacy of routine preoperative electrocardiograms. *J Cardiothorac Vasc Anesth*. 1997;11:752.
5. Correll DJ, Hepner DL, Chang C, et al. Preoperative electrocardiograms – patient factors predictive of abnormalities. *Anesthesiology*. 2009;110:1217-1222.
6. Eagle KA, Berger PH, Calkins H, et al. ACC/AHA guideline update for perioperative cardiovascular evaluation for noncardiac surgery. *Circulation*. 2002;105:1257-1267.
7. Charpak Y, Blery C, Chastang C, et al. Prospective assessment of a protocol for selective ordering of chest x-rays. *Can J Anesth*. 1988;35(3):259-264.
8. Dzankik S, Pastor D, Gonzalez C, et al. The prevalence and predictive value of abnormal preoperative laboratory tests in elderly surgical patients. *Anesth Analg*. 2001;93:301.
9. Hirsh IA, Tomlinson DL, Slogoff S, et al. The overstated risk of preoperative hypokalemia. *Anesth Analg*. 1988;67:131.
10. Gibbs J, Cull W, Henderson W, Daley J, et al. Preoperative serum albumin level as a predictor of operative mortality and morbidity: results from the National VA Surgical Risk Study. *Arch Surg*. 1999;134:36.
11. Lee TH, Marcantonio ER, Mangione CM, et al. Derivation and prospective validation of a simple index for prediction of cardiac risk of major noncardiac surgery. *Circulation*. 1999; 100:1043.

Suggested Reading

American Society of Anesthesiology. Practice advisory for preanesthesia evaluation. *Anesthesiology*. 2002;96(2):485-496.

Hoeks SE, Scholte WJM, Lenzen MJ, et al. Guidelines for cardiac management in noncardiac surgery are poorly implemented in clinical practice. *Anesthesiology*. 2007;107:537-544.

Narr BJ, Warner ME, Schroeder DR, et al. Outcomes of patients with no laboratory assessment before anesthesia and a surgical procedure. *Mayo Clin Proc*. 1997;72:505.

Schein O, Katz J, Bass E, et al. The value of routine preoperative testing before cataract surgery. *N Eng J Med*. 2000;342:168.

Smetana GW, Macpherson DS. The case against routine preoperative laboratory testing. *Med Clin N Am*. 2003;87:7.

Perioperative Medication Management 3

Steven L. Cohn

3.1 Introduction

- Every year millions of patients undergo surgery, and most of them take one or more prescriptions or over-the-counter medications. The number of medications increases with age and in patients undergoing major surgical procedures.
- Medication errors are a major safety problem in hospitalized patients, and inappropriate withdrawal or continuation of medication in the perioperative period is associated with an increased risk for adverse events. In order to minimize these problems, the physician must understand the risks and benefits of these medications in the perioperative setting.
- Unfortunately, the published literature in this field is limited with few randomized controlled trials or conflicting results, so there is substantial variation in management from physician to physician.
- The following recommendations covering the major drug classes encountered in the perioperative period are based on a review of the literature, theoretical concerns, clinical experience, and expert opinion. It is beyond the scope of this chapter to discuss all medications, and the reader is referred to other online references and reviews for detailed information and supporting evidence.

3.2 Principles

- The first step is for the physician to obtain an accurate and complete list of all medications taken by the patient, both prescription and over the counter, and to determine the patient's compliance with that regimen.

S.L. Cohn
Internal Medicine-Medical Consultation Service,
SUNY Downstate - Kings County Hospital Center,
450 Clarkson Ave, Box 68, Brooklyn, NY 11203, USA
e-mail: steven.cohn@downstate.edu

S.L. Cohn (ed.), *Perioperative Medicine*,
DOI: 10.1007/978-0-85729-498-2_3, © Springer-Verlag London Limited 2011

- In deciding whether or not to continue a medication perioperatively, consider the following questions:
  - What is the indication and need for the medication?
  - What is the effect of stopping the drug on the primary disease?

    Will there be a rebound effect, clinical deterioration, or withdrawal symptoms?
  - What are the drug pharmacokinetics and how will they change in the perioperative setting?

    Consider absorption, half-life, route of administration, metabolism, and elimination.
  - Are there potential adverse effects of the medication, such as bleeding or hypoglycemia, on perioperative risk? Are there potential drug interactions with anesthetic agents?
  - Are there potential benefits of starting a drug prophylactically such as to prevent ischemia, thrombosis, infection, or aspiration?
- Based on these principles and a risk–benefit analysis, decide whether to continue, discontinue, or modify the regimen for each medication.
- Oral medications that need to be continued perioperatively should be given with a sip of water on the morning of surgery.
  - Although there may be an order for "NPO after midnight", it should read "NPO except for medications".
  - Also, if the medication would not ordinarily be administered before 10 AM and surgery is scheduled earlier, be sure to specify that it is given "on call to the OR".

3.3 Recommendations by Drug Category

3.3.1 Cardiovascular Medications

In general most cardiovascular drugs should be continued perioperatively. This includes antihypertensives, antiarrhythmics, and anti-anginal medications. Consider obtaining drug levels for antiarrhythmics if you suspect toxicity or noncompliance.

3.3.1.1 Antihypertensives

Patients with stable, controlled blood pressure preoperatively are less likely to experience wide swings in blood pressure intra- or postoperatively than patients with untreated or uncontrolled hypertension.

Alpha$_2$ Agonists (Clonidine)

- May reduce perioperative cardiac ischemia (possibly nonfatal MI and cardiac death), awaiting results of POISE-2.

- May decrease BP lability, preoperative anxiety, and amount of anesthesia required for maintenance.
- Abrupt discontinuation is associated with a classic withdrawal syndrome (hypertension, tachycardia, tremors, anxiety).

Recommendations

- Continue usual dose perioperatively including dose on AM of surgery; if prolonged NPO status is expected, can start transdermal preparation 24–48 h preop.
- Watch for hypotension and bradycardia.

Beta-Blockers

- Decrease heart rate and myocardial oxygen demand.
- Can decrease perioperative ischemia, nonfatal MI (and possibly cardiac death) in high-risk cardiac patients; may be harmful for low-risk patients and other subgroups, especially if a high dose is started shortly before surgery without time for dose titration (increased incidence of symptomatic bradycardia, hypotension, stroke, and total mortality in POISE).
- Abrupt discontinuation is associated with rebound ischemia, hypertension, and tachycardia.

Recommendations

- Continue perioperatively.
- Consider starting prophylactically before major vascular surgery or other intermediate–high risk surgery in high-risk patients with ischemia on stress testing or those with coronary heart disease or multiple risk factors (see Chap. 20). In this setting, beta-blockers should be started several weeks before surgery whenever possible and titrated to a resting heart rate between 55 and 70 per minute. (Contraindications include bronchospasm, pulmonary edema, and high-grade AV block.)
- Administer intravenously if unable to take orally. Esmolol, an intravenously administered short-acting beta-blocker, is often used intraoperatively for blood pressure and heart rate control.

Alpha and Alpha-Beta Blockers

- Alpha-blockers are used to treat benign prostatic hypertrophy and pheochromocytoma. The latter are used to treat heart failure, hypertension, and pheochromocytoma.

Recommendations

- Continue perioperatively except for tamsulosin which should be stopped several days before cataract surgery (associated with floppy iris syndrome).
- If treating pheochromocytoma, begin at least a week prior to surgery.
- Intravenous labetalol is often used for perioperative blood pressure control.

Calcium Channel Blockers

- Diltiazem may reduce perioperative ischemia and postoperative supraventricular tachyarrhythmias (based on limited data).

Recommendations

- Continue perioperatively.

Diuretics

- May cause hypovolemia and hypokalemia acutely; however, if the patient has been on a diuretic for several weeks, a steady state has probably been reached.

Recommendations

- Usually withheld on the morning of surgery (in theory, to prevent intravascular volume depletion; also, for patient comfort if awake during ambulatory surgery), but can be continued in patients with heart failure.
- Stop diuretics if blood pressure is on the low side on the morning of surgery, the patient appears volume depleted, or the BUN/creatinine ratio suggests a "prerenal picture".
- Can administer IV if necessary.
- Monitor potassium levels.

Nitrates

- Prophylactic use has not been shown to reduce perioperative coronary events.

Recommendations

- Continue perioperatively.
- Can apply nitropaste to substitute for oral nitrates if patient is NPO.

ACEI/ARB

- May be associated with increased incidence of hypotension with induction of anesthesia requiring fluid or pressor administration; however, they were not associated with an increase in perioperative MI.

Recommendations

- Controversial; while some recommend withholding the dose on the morning of surgery, I usually continue them cautiously as the potential benefit of the drug may outweigh the possible development of hypotension.
- Withhold if baseline BP is low on the morning of surgery.

3.3.1.2 Antiarrhythmics (Digoxin, Sotalol, Amiodarone)

Recommendations

- Continue perioperatively. Consider obtaining serum levels when indicated.

3.3.2 Lipid Lowering Agents

3.3.2.1 HMG Co-A Reductase Inhibitors ("Statins")

- In addition to their lipid lowering effect and long-term benefit to prevent atherosclerosis, these agents appear to prevent vascular plaque rupture.
- A number of large observational studies and two smaller RCTs have shown that statins are associated with a reduction in cardiac events and mortality, particularly for patients undergoing vascular surgery (see Chap. 20).
- However, presumably because of fear of rhabdomyolysis perioperatively, the pharmaceutical manufacturers recommend that statins be stopped before major surgery.

Recommendations

- Continue statins in the perioperative period as per ACC guidelines despite recommendations in the PDR to discontinue them.
- Consider starting prophylactically in high cardiac risk patients undergoing vascular or high-risk surgery, especially if the patient has an indication for statin therapy but is not on it.

3.3.2.2 Other Agents for Lipid Control

- Bile acid sequestrants (cholestyramine, colestipol), fibric acid derivatives (gemfibrozil), niacin, and ezetimibe reduce LDL cholesterol levels but have no definite short-term benefit in the perioperative period and may affect absorption of other medications.

Recommendations

- Discontinue bile acid sequestrants, niacin, fibric acid derivatives, and ezetimibe the day before surgery.

3.3.3
Medications Affecting Hemostasis

3.3.3.1
Antiplatelet Agents

Aspirin

- Aspirin irreversibly inhibits cyclooxygenase; so the patient will need 5–10 days after the last dose to replenish the entire population of platelets. However, only 50,000–100,000 platelets are necessary for adequate hemostasis for most surgeries.
- If aspirin is continued, some studies noted increased perioperative bleeding and need for transfusions while others did not.
  - Although aspirin may increase perioperative blood loss, it may be beneficial in patients undergoing carotid endarterectomy after TIA, may improve graft patency after peripheral vascular surgery, decreases mortality if given within 48 h after CABG, and may decrease perioperative cardiovascular events in patients at high risk.
- Case reports noted an increase in thromboembolic events within 30 days of discontinuing aspirin.
- Addition of aspirin to an appropriate DVT prophylaxis regimen may decrease postoperative pulmonary embolism in orthopedic patients.

Recommendations

- Consider the indication for therapy and risk of bleeding, and discuss with the surgeon.
- Often discontinued 5–7 days before surgery due to fear of increased bleeding, but this time interval may be longer than necessary.
- Continue in certain cases (vascular surgery or those at high risk for perioperative vascular events) as noted above, and start postoperatively after CABG.

Thienopyridines: Clopidogrel, Prasugrel, and Ticlopidine

- Irreversibly inhibit P2Y12 ADP-induced platelet aggregation.
- Associated with increased bleeding, especially when combined with aspirin.

Recommendations

- Discontinue clopidogrel 5–7 days prior to surgery, prasugrel 7 days before surgery, and ticlopidine 10–14 days before surgery.
- Postpone noncardiac surgery for at least 4 weeks after PCI with bare metal stenting (BMS) and 12 months after placement of a drug-eluting stent (DES) to allow continuation of dual antiplatelet therapy. If surgery is necessary sooner, continue aspirin if possible and stop the thienopyridine approximately 1 week before surgery and restart it as soon as is feasible postoperatively (see Chap. 20).

Dipyridamole

- Dipyridamole is reversible platelet adhesion inhibitor with a half-life of 10 h and inhibits activity of adenosine deaminase and phosphodiesterase leading to accumulation of adenosine and CAMP and inhibiting platelet aggregation.

Recommendations

- Uncertain – minimal data to advise whether to stop or continue. Need to balance risk of bleeding with any potential benefit of continuing it. If discontinued, should probably be done 2–3 days before surgery (five half-lives).

Cilostazol

- Reversible cAMP PDE-3 inhibitor with a half-life of 12 h.

Recommendations

- Discontinue 3–5 days before surgery.

Pentoxifylline

- Competitive nonselective phosphodiesterase inhibitor and a nonselective adenosine receptor antagonist with a half-life between 1 and 1.5 h. Lowers blood viscosity and improves erythrocyte flexibility.
- Associated with increased risk for bleeding with or without other anticoagulants or antiplatelet agents.

Recommendations

- Stop at least 8 h before surgery (AM of surgery)

3.3.3.2 Non-steroidal Anti-Inflammatory Drugs

Cox-1 Inhibitors

Although these drugs may increase the risk of perioperative bleeding and possibly renal insufficiency, they also may decrease postoperative pain and the use of opioid analgesics.

Recommendations

- Controversial. Typically these drugs are discontinued 1–3 days before surgery, depending on the half-life and potency of the drug, but they can be given postoperatively for analgesia.

Cox-2 Inhibitors

- Rofecoxib and valdecoxib have been withdrawn from the US market.
- Celecoxib has not been shown to affect platelet activity at usual doses (up to 400 mg/day) although theoretical concerns exist for potentiating renal insufficiency.

Recommendations

- Discontinue 1–3 days prior to surgery.

3.3.3.3 Anticoagulants

Perioperative management of anticoagulation therapy is discussed in detail in Chap. 4. Some general guidelines are listed below.

Warfarin

- The risk of bleeding with continuation of an anticoagulant needs to be balanced with the risk of a thromboembolic event if the drug is stopped. This latter risk is based on the indication for anticoagulation and the periprocedural risk.
- Various regimens have been described for discontinuing warfarin before surgery and for "bridging" therapy with unfractionated or low molecular weight heparin, if indicated.

Recommendations – options include

- Continuing anticoagulation for minor procedures where the bleeding risk is low
- Discontinuing or decreasing the dose of warfarin 5 days prior to surgery where the risk of bleeding is higher, but the risk of thromboembolism is modest; INR should be <1.5 on the morning of surgery

- Bridging therapy with heparin (UFH or LMWH) for patients at high risk for thromboembolism in the absence of anticoagulation
- Starting warfarin preoperatively on the evening before or night of surgery if indicated for DVT prophylaxis in orthopedic surgery (TKR, THR, hip fracture)

Unfractionated Heparin (UFH)

Recommendations

- Discontinue full-dose anticoagulation 4–6 h before surgery and restart postoperatively as soon as deemed safe by the surgeon (usually not before 12–24 h postoperatively after procedures with secured hemostasis and low risk of bleeding or not before 48–72 h after high bleeding risk procedures). Monitor PTT and platelet count (for HIT).
- Continue or start subcutaneous heparin if indicated for DVT prophylaxis (5,000 IU sc q8-12 h depending on the level of risk) (see Chap. 5).

Low Molecular Weight Heparin (LMWH)

- In general no monitoring is necessary regarding the level of anticoagulation; however, anti-Xa activity can be checked if it is of concern in special populations (morbidly obese, severely underweight, renal impairment).
- Different LMWHs have different indications, contraindications, and warnings. Consult the manufacturer's labeling.
- Anticoagulant effects are only partly reversible with protamine sulfate.

Recommendations

- Discontinue full-dose anticoagulation 24 h preoperatively and restart postoperatively when deemed safe by the surgeon.
- If neuraxial anesthesia is planned, discontinue full dose LMWH 24 h before and prophylactic dose LMWH 12 h before spinal or epidural needle insertion. Allow at least 2 h after the needle or epidural catheter have been removed before starting or restarting LMWH.
- Continue or start if indicated for DVT prophylaxis (see Chap. 5).

Synthetic Pentasaccharides (Fondaparinux)

- Selectively inhibits factor Xa, has a long half-life (17 h), renal elimination, fixed dose, no monitoring for anticoagulant effect, and is partially reversible with recombinant factor VIIa. Contraindicated with creatinine clearance <30. Used primarily for VTE prophylaxis in orthopedic surgery patients and for the treatment of VTE.
- New oral Xa inhibitors (rivaroxaban, apixaban) are awaiting FDA approval.

Recommendations

- Start 6 h postoperatively for DVT prophylaxis in orthopedic surgery patients (see Chap. 5).
- Similar precautions as LMWH regarding neuraxial anesthesia and epidural catheters, but needs to be stopped even sooner (in general, neuraxial anesthesia is contraindicated in these patients).

Dabigatran

- This is an oral competetive, direct thrombin inhibitor recently approved to reduce stroke and systemic embolism in patients with non-valvular atrial fibrillation.

Recommendations

- If possible, discontinue dabigatran 1–2 days (CrCl ≥ 50 mL/min) or 3–5 days (CrCl < 50 mL/min) before invasive or surgical procedures because of the increased risk of bleeding.
- Consider longer times for patients undergoing major surgery, spinal puncture, or placement of a spinal or epidural catheter or port, in whom complete hemostasis may be required.

3.3.4 Pulmonary Medications

- The goal of preoperative pulmonary management in patients with COPD or asthma is to optimize their pulmonary function, usually by means of beta-agonist and steroid inhalers.

3.3.4.1 Inhaled Agents: Beta-Agonists, Ipratropium, Steroids

Recommendations

- Continue via metered-dose inhalers or via nebulizers.

3.3.4.2 Theophylline

- There are no studies of theophylline in the perioperative period, but toxic levels may be associated with arrhythmias —consider checking drug levels.

Recommendations

- Can either continue on the morning of surgery or stop it the night before.

3.3.4.3
Leukotriene Inhibitors

- Despite a short half-life, these agents have continued effect for up to 3 weeks after discontinuation.

Recommendations

- Continue perioperatively.

3.3.4.4
Systemic Corticosteroids

Recommendations

- Continue or increase the dose (see Sect. 3.3.5.3, Sect. 22.2, and Table 22.5).

3.3.5
Endocrine

3.3.5.1
Diabetic Agents

Tight perioperative glucose control is important to reduce the incidence of infections and possibly improve outcome in critically ill patients. Frequently sample blood glucose to determine insulin requirements and minimize hypoglycemia (see Chap. 22).

Oral hypoglycemics

Recommendations

- **Sulfonylureas/glitazones**: Withhold on the morning of surgery.
- **Metformin**: usually stop the day before surgery (some recommend 48 h before) and delay reinitiation postoperatively if the surgery is complicated by hypotension, renal insufficiency, or congestive heart failure.
  - Can restart oral agents when patient is able to eat normally; however, current practice favors use of insulin for in-hospital glycemic management.

Insulins

- Individualize insulin management based on the type of insulin, degree of control, the patient, and the procedure.

Recommendations

NPH (Intermediate Acting Insulins)

- Can usually continue evening dose unless very tightly controlled. In those cases, consider reducing the dose the night before surgery.
- Administer one half to two-thirds of the usual morning dose on the AM of surgery.
  - For prolonged surgical procedures, use regular insulin boluses or an insulin drip at 1–2 Units per hour.

Mixed insulin (70/30):

- Can give one half to two-thirds of equivalent dose of the NPH portion.

Long-acting basal insulin (glargine)

- Depending on degree of glucose control and type of procedure, can continue usual dose or decrease it the night before surgery.

Intravenous insulin drip

- For critical care patients, diabetic ketoacidosis, or lengthy, complex procedures, continuous insulin infusions should be used to avoid the known perioperative variability in insulin absorption with subcutaneous administration.

3.3.5.2 Thyroid Agents

- Postpone elective procedures in patients who are hyperthyroid until the hyperthyroidism is well controlled (see Chap. 22).
- Mild hypothyroidism is not associated with serious perioperative complications.
- Levothyroxine persists in the circulation for many days; so missing several doses of oral thyroid replacement in the perioperative period is inconsequential.

Recommendations

- Continue antithyroid medication, including beta-blockers, perioperatively.
- Continue thyroid replacement medication perioperatively.

3.3.5.3
Corticosteroids

- Evaluate the possibility of suppression of hypothalamic-pituitary-adrenal axis (see Chap. 22).
- If history of steroid use at a physiologic dose or greater for at least 3 weeks in the past 6 months, the hypothalamic-pituitary-adrenal axis may be suppressed, and the patient may not be able to generate the appropriate adrenocortical response to the stress of surgery.

Recommendations

- Continue or increase the dose of corticosteroids (hydrocortisone or its equivalent) based on the history, usual dose and duration of therapy, and anticipated stress of surgery.
- Can give a bolus of 50–100 mg of hydrocortisone followed by 25–50 mg q8h, adjusting dose and duration to ongoing stress of surgery. A maximum of 200 mg/day is more than adequate. Can taper or discontinue over 24–72 h based on the ongoing stress of surgery.

3.3.5.4
Oral Contraceptives, Hormone Replacement (HRT), and Selective Estrogen Receptor Modulators (SERM)

- These medications are associated with an increased risk of venous thrombosis.
- The decision to continue oral contraceptives before elective surgery should balance the risk of thrombosis and the risks of discontinuation (unintended pregnancy, estrogen withdrawal symptoms).

Recommendations

- Theoretically, patients undergoing elective surgery with a high risk for VTE should discontinue hormonal contraception 3 weeks prior to surgery and use alternative contraception; however, this is rarely done in actual clinical practice.
- Patients undergoing surgeries with a lower risk for venous thromboembolism can continue the medications but should receive DVT prophylaxis (possibly more intensive) perioperatively.

3.3.6
Gastrointestinal Medications

- H2 blockers and proton pump inhibitors prevent gastric acid production and help prevent stress ulcers. Stress ulcers are more common with prolonged postoperative mechanical ventilation or ICU stay.

Recommendations

- Continue H2 blockers or proton pump inhibitors perioperatively. Can substitute intravenous forms if the patient can take them orally.
- Consider prophylactic use to minimize risk of aspiration and prevent stress ulcers.

3.3.7 Psychotropic Medications

3.3.7.1 SSRIs

- Selective serotonin reuptake inhibitors (SSRIs) affect platelet aggregation and have been associated with an increase in gastrointestinal bleeding in non-surgical settings. It is unclear whether their use is associated with increased perioperative transfusions.
- Stopping SSRIs has been associated with a withdrawal syndrome and may worsen a patient's psychiatric problem.

Recommendation

- Continue SSRIs. There is insufficient evidence to recommend discontinuing these drugs to prevent potential perioperative bleeding; furthermore, the washout period may be several weeks.
  - Consider tapering and discontinuing 3 weeks before neurosurgical procedures where perioperative hemorrhage may have catastrophic consequences.

3.3.7.2 Tricyclic Antidepressants

- Tricyclic antidepressants inhibit synaptic uptake of norepinephrine and serotonin.
- These agents may be proarrhythmic but there is sparse clinical data in the perioperative setting.
- Abrupt withdrawal can lead to insomnia, headache, nausea, excess salivation, and diaphoresis.

Recommendation

- Continue tricyclic antidepressants perioperatively, especially for patients taking high doses (although some suggest tapering and stopping before surgery).

3.3.7.3
Anxiolytic Agents (Benzodiazepines and Buspirone)

- Benzodiazepines are commonly used in the perioperative period to reduce anxiety.
- Abrupt withdrawal of benzodiazepine from patients on chronic therapy can lead to an excitatory state including delirium and seizures.

Recommendations

- Continue benzodiazepines and buspirone in the perioperative period.
- Can substitute parenteral forms for patients unable to take oral medications.

3.3.7.4
Antipsychotic Agents

- Antipsychotics have antiemetic and sedative properties and have been used as part of anesthesia.
- Experience with the newer antipsychotics (olanzapine, quetiapine, risperidone, ziprasidone) during the perioperative period is limited.

Recommendations

- In general, continue antipsychotics perioperatively.
- If oral agents cannot be given, haloperidol and olanzapine can be given parenterally.

3.3.7.5
Monoamine Oxidase Inhibitors

- In the presence of MAO inhibitors, routine anesthetic care, such as the administration of a sympathomimetic agent such as ephedrine, can lead to massive accumulation of norepinephrine in the central and autonomic nervous system.
- When administered to patients on MAO inhibitors meperidine and dextromethorphan can cause the serotonin syndrome manifested as agitation, fever, seizures, coma, and even death.

Recommendations

- Usually discontinue 10–14 days before surgery.
- If the anesthesiologist is familiar with MAO-safe procedures, these agents can be continued throughout the perioperative period. The newer MAO inhibitors are often continued.
- If MAO inhibitors are continued, order a hospital diet that avoids tyramine-containing foods.

3.3.7.6
Mood Stabilizing Agents (Lithium, Valproic Acid)

- Lithium can prolong the effect of muscle relaxants, impair concentration of urine leading to volume depletion and hypernatremia (nephrogenic diabetes insipidus), and cause hypothyroidism.

Recommendations

- Continue lithium and valproic acid through the perioperative period. There is no parenteral substitute for lithium. Intravenous valproate sodium (Depacon) can be substituted for patients who usually take valproic acid and are NPO.
- Monitor fluid and electrolyte status, especially sodium.
- Check thyroid function preoperatively if not done recently.

3.3.8
Chronic Opioid Therapy

- Patients on opioids for treatment of chronic pain may need higher doses to treat surgery-related pain.
- Abrupt discontinuation of opioids can cause withdrawal and exacerbate chronic pain.

Recommendations

- Continue chronic opioids in the perioperative period.
- Intravenous, intramuscular, and topical preparations can be substituted.
- Equianalgesic doses of parenteral substitutes should be initiated with the realization that higher doses and rapid dose escalation may be needed temporarily to control surgery-related pain.
- Perioperative pain management is discussed in Chap. 45.

3.3.9
Rheumatologic Medications (see Chap. 28)

3.3.9.1
Disease Modifying Anti-Rheumatic Drugs (DMARDs)

- DMARDs include methotrexate, hydroxychloroquine, sulfasalazine, azathioprine, and leflunomide. Some may cause immunosuppression, impairing wound healing and increasing the risk of perioperative wound infection.

- One randomized trial in orthopedic patients found no increased rate of infection in patients who continued weekly methotrexate compared to those who held the agent 2 weeks before surgery.
- Withdrawal of DMARDs can lead to rheumatoid arthritis flares.
- Many DMARDs are excreted through the kidney and may accumulate if renal function is impaired.

Recommendations

- Continue methotrexate perioperatively as long as renal function is normal.
- Consider stopping leflunomide 2 weeks before surgery because of its long half-life and resuming it shortly after surgery.
- Continue sulfasalazine, azathioprine, and hydroxychloroquine perioperatively.

3.3.9.2 Anti-Cytokines

- Anti-cytokines, also known as biologic active agents, include etanercept, infliximab, adalimumab, anakinra, and rituximab.
- These agents impair tumor necrosis factor-alpha action or interleukin-1 receptors.

Recommendation

- Consult rheumatology.
- Consider discontinuing anti-cytokines 1–2 weeks before surgery and restarting them 1–2 weeks after surgery; however, infliximab appeared to be safe if continued perioperatively in studies in patients with inflammatory bowel disease.

3.3.9.3 Agents for Gout

- Surgery can lead to flares of gout possibly because of fluid and electrolyte shifts leading to abrupt changes in uric acid concentration.

Recommendations

- Continue uric acid lowering drugs such as allopurinol, probenecid, and oral colchicine perioperatively.
- Treat perioperative gout flares with NSAIDs or oral, systemic, or intra-articular corticosteroids.
- Avoid parenteral colchicine because of potential skin necrosis with inadvertent IV infiltration.

3.3.10
Neurologic Medications (see Chaps. 38–39)

3.3.10.1
Anti-Seizure Medications

- Certain anesthetic phases, metabolic derangements, ethanol withdrawal, and intracranial procedures can increase the risk of seizures.

Recommendations

- Continue antiepileptic drugs (AEDs) perioperatively, especially in patients with frequent, generalized, tonic-clonic seizures.
- Check drug levels.
- Intravenous phenytoin, phenobarbital, or valproate can be substituted if oral AEDs cannot be taken.

3.3.10.2
Anti-Parkinsonian Medications

- Perioperative morbidity related to swallowing difficulty, pulmonary insufficiency, and delirium are common.
- Although some anti-Parkinson's drugs can have deleterious hemodynamic effects such as arrhythmias in the perioperative period, withdrawal of these agents can increase Parkinson-related symptoms and can cause the neuroleptic malignant syndrome.

Recommendations

- Give levodopa/carbidopa the evening before surgery but withhold it until the patient can again take oral medications.
- Hold levodopa/carbidopa/entacapone preparations longer before surgery.
- Discontinue tolcapone, which prolongs the action of levodopa/carbidopa, 1 day before surgery.
- Hold bromocriptine and pergolide the evening before surgery and restart them when oral medications are resumed, as long as the patient is hemodynamically stable.
- To avoid precipitating the neuroleptic malignant syndrome, administer ropinirole and pramipexole on the morning of surgery and resume them when the patient is taking oral medications.
- Discontinue selegiline, a Type B MAO inhibitor, several days before surgery.
- Parenteral anticholinergic agents such as biperiden, benztropine, and diphenhydramine can be used in Parkinsonian patients who cannot take oral medications and in whom symptoms flare in the absence of usual therapy.

3.3.10.3
Medications for Myasthenia Gravis

- Patients with myasthenia gravis can have respiratory insufficiency related to myasthenic crisis during the perioperative period.
- Management of immunosuppressives such as corticosteroids is covered in Chap. 28.

Recommendations

- Pyridostigmine is optional on the morning of surgery.
  - Short-acting pyridostigmine should be substituted for the long-acting preparation the evening before surgery.
- Parenteral pyridostigmine can be substituted in patients unable to take oral medications for a prolonged period using one-tenth of the usual dose for intramuscular and 1/30th the usual dose for intravenous administration or a continuous infusion at 2 mg/h.

3.3.11
Herbal Medications

- Many patients use herbal medications and health supplements but may not reveal the use of these therapies during usual questioning—therefore inquire about them specifically.
- Some herbal preparations have been associated with excessive perioperative sedation (e.g., kava, valerian) and with bleeding complications (e.g., garlic, ginkgo, ginseng).

Recommendation

- Advise patients to discontinue herbal agents and other health supplements at least 1 week before surgery.

3.4
Summary

- Table 3.1 summarizes the recommendations discussed.
- Evidence regarding management of medications in the perioperative period is often limited.
- Consider a risk–benefit analysis in any decision to continue, discontinue, or modify the regimen for any medication.

Table 3.1 Summary of perioperative medication management

Medication class	Recommendation
Cardiovascular medications	• Continue most agents • Consider prophylactic beta-blockers in patients at high risk of perioperative cardiac morbidity • Withhold diuretics on the morning of surgery especially if signs of volume depletion • Caution with ACEI/ARBs
Lipid lowering agents	• Continue "statins" • Discontinue other agents
Anticoagulants and other drugs affecting hemostasis (antiplatelet, NSAIDs)	• Continue for minor surgery • Discontinue at appropriate interval before major surgery • Consider bridging anticoagulation for patients at high risk of interim thrombosis (see Chap. 4)
Pulmonary medications (inhalers)	• Continue
Corticosteroids	• Continue chronic corticosteroids. Increase dosage to account for surgical stress
Diabetic medications	• Withhold oral hypoglycemics on morning of surgery and resume when patient resumes eating • For type 1 diabetics, continue some form of insulin (long acting or intravenous) at all times • For type 2 diabetics, decrease dose of morning intermediate insulin depending on anticipated duration of NPO status and time of surgery • Continue basal insulin, usually at same dose
Thyroid medications	• Continue thyroid hormone replacement • Postpone surgery until hyperthyroidism controlled
Oral contraceptives, hormone replacement, and SERMs	• Consider discontinuing several weeks before surgery in patients at high risk for perioperative venous thromboembolism, otherwise continue
Gastrointestinal medications	• Continue • Substitute parenteral forms in patients who are NPO for prolonged periods or those at high risk for stress ulceration
Psychotropic medications	• Continue SSRIs for most patients. Consider stopping several weeks before surgery where perioperative hemorrhage could be catastrophic (CNS surgery) • Continue tricyclic antidepressants, benzodiazepines, lithium, and antipsychotics • For MAOs, continue or discontinue depending on anesthesiologist preference
Chronic opioids	• Continue. Substitute equianalgesic or higher doses to manage surgical pain

Table 3.1 (continued)

Medication class	Recommendation
Rheumatologic medications	• Continue methotrexate • Continue most DMARDs • Consider stopping anticytokines 1–2 weeks before. • Continue hypouricemic agents
Neurologic medications	• Continue anti-seizure medications • Hold anti-Parkinsonian agents briefly • Continue agents for myasthenia gravis
Herbal medications	• Discontinue all agents 1 week before surgery

Source: Modified with permission from Cohn and Macpherson.1 Copyright © 2006 The McGraw Hill Companies, Inc

Reference

1. Cohn SL, Macpherson DS. Perioperative medication management. In: Cohn SL, Smetana GW, Weed HG, eds. *Perioperative Medicine - Just the Facts*. New York: McGraw Hill; 2006.

Further Reading

Cohn SL. Perioperative medication management. http://pier.acponline.org/physicians/diseases/d835/d835.html [Date Accessed: 2010 June 20] In: PIER [online database]. Philadelphia: American College of Physicians; 2010.

Cygan R, Waitzkin H. Stopping and restarting medications in the perioperative period. *J Gen Intern Med*. 1987;2:270-283.

Kroenke K, Gooby-Toedt D, Jackson JL. Chronic medications in the perioperative period. *South Med J*. 1998;91:358-364.

Mercado DL, Petty BG. Perioperative medication management. *Med Clin North Am*. 2003;87:41-57.

Muluk V, Macpherson DS. Perioperative medication management. In: Rose BD, ed. *UpToDate*. Wellesley: UpToDate; 2010.

Smith MS, Muir H, Hall R. Perioperative management of drug therapy. *Drugs*. 1996;51:238-259.

Perioperative Management of Anticoagulation

4

Scott Kaatz and David G. Paje

4.1 Introduction

- Managing antithrombotic agents in patients undergoing surgery is a common clinical challenge, often requiring temporary interruption of treatment prior to the procedure. Antithrombotic agents can generally be grouped into anticoagulants and antiplatelet agents. Anticoagulants include warfarin, unfractionated heparin (UFH), low-molecular weight heparin (LMWH), fondaparinux, direct thrombin inhibitors (DTI) and direct Xa inhibitors. Antiplatelet agents include aspirin and other nonsteroidal anti-inflammatory drugs (NSAID), thienopyridines (e.g., clopidogrel, prasugrel, ticlopidine), phosphodiesterase inhibitors (e.g., dipyridamole, cilostazol) and glycoprotein IIb/IIIa receptor inhibitors (e.g., abciximab, eptifibatide, tirofiban).
- Approximately 250,000 patients in North America on warfarin therapy will undergo surgery or an invasive procedure each year.[1] Many of these patients will require cessation of warfarin during surgery and this period of time without anticoagulation puts them at risk for thromboembolic events.
  - Bridging this gap in anticoagulation with rapid-onset and shorter acting anticoagulants like UFH or LMWH has become common practice. In the past decade, LMWH has become an increasingly popular choice because of the practical benefit of subcutaneous administration which allows the "bridging therapy" to be done outside the hospital.
  - To date, no randomized trial has determined whether bridging anticoagulation is necessary during perioperative warfarin interruption. Two ongoing trials designed to answer this particular question are not expected to be completed until 2013.[2] Until then, the decision as to which patients should be bridged, and when to stop and restart warfarin and LMWH perioperatively depends on balancing the risk of thrombosis with the risk of bleeding attributed to bridging.

S. Kaatz (✉)
General Internal Medicine, Henry Ford Hospital,
2799 W. Grand Blvd., Detroit, MI 48098, USA
e-mail: skaatz1@hfhs.org

S.L. Cohn (ed.), *Perioperative Medicine*,
DOI: 10.1007/978-0-85729-498-2_4,

- Platelets have a circulating life span of 10 days, which means 10% of the platelet pool is replaced daily. Non-steroidal anti-inflammatory drugs and cilostazol have reversible antiplatelet effects, however, these drugs are typically not used as antithrombotics and will not be discussed. The antiplatelet drugs aspirin and clopidogrel cause irreversible inhibition of platelet function, and once discontinued, it takes approximately 7–10 days to replace the entire platelet pool. This is the physiologic basis for the recommendations regarding preoperative management of these agents.
  - There are no randomized trials comparing the risk of thromboembolic events if antiplatelets are withheld prior to surgery with the risk of perioperative bleeding if they are continued.[1] POISE-2 trial will attempt to evaluate the efficacy and safety of continuing or discontinuing antiplatelet therapy for noncardiac surgery.[2] Unlike LMWH bridging in patients on warfarin, there is no similar medication that has been studied to "bridge" the interruption of antiplatelet therapy.

4.2 Patient-Specific Risk Factors for Thromboembolism

4.2.1 Patients on Warfarin Requiring Surgery or an Invasive Procedure

- There are three main disease categories that are anticoagulated with warfarin: atrial fibrillation, mechanical heart valves and venous thromboembolic disease. Patients on warfarin for any of these indications should be individually risk stratified to determine whether LMWH bridging therapy is necessary for an elective surgery or invasive procedure. However, there is no well-validated method to estimate the risk of thrombosis during the perioperative period in patients who require ongoing anticoagulation therapy (Table 4.1).
- Atrial fibrillation

Table 4.1 Risk stratification in patients on warfarin for LMWH bridging

Classification	Bridging	Atrial fibrillation $CHADS_2$ score	Mechanical valves	Venous thromboembolism
High risk	Advised	5 or 6	Any mitral valve Recent stroke Ball-cage or single tilting disk aortic valve	VTE in past 3 months
Moderate risk	Case by case decision	3 or 4	Bileaflet aortic valve with other stroke risk factors	VTE in past 3–12 months
Low risk	Not recommended	1 or 2	Bileaflet aortic valve with no other stroke risk factors	VTE > 12 months ago

VTE venous thromboembolism

- The $CHADS_2$ score has been widely accepted as a validated risk stratification tool to predict stroke in patients with atrial fibrillation.[3] The $CHADS_2$ risk stratification scheme assigns one point each for a history of congestive heart failure, hypertension, age ≥ 75 and diabetes, and two points for a history of stroke or transient ischemic attack.[3]
- Simple mathematical proration of the $CHADS_2$ annualized risk of stroke to the brief period of time patients are off warfarin underestimates the perioperative risk of stroke. Moreover, patients with atrial fibrillation have about 1% absolute increase in the 30-day rate of stroke when compared to patients without atrial fibrillation undergoing similar surgeries.[4]
- Nevertheless, the $CHADS_2$ score has been adopted as a risk stratification tool to help decide which patients should undergo bridging therapy. It is a reasonable guide even though it has not been fully validated in the perioperative setting.[1]

• Mechanical heart valves

- Valve position, type of valve and additional stroke risk factors are all used to predict the risk of stroke during warfarin interruption.
- Patients with mechanical valves in the mitral position are felt to be at a higher risk of embolic stroke than those with aortic valves.
- Older valves like the ball-cage or single-tilting disk likely have a higher thromboembolic risk than newer bileaflet valves.
- Clinical reason dictates that patients with additional risk factors for stroke, especially a history of prior stroke, are at great risk of thromboembolic complications when warfarin therapy is interrupted.
- Combining the three elements of valve position, type of valve, and additional stroke risk factors forms the basis for risk stratification models to guide the decision to use bridging therapy.[1]

• Venous thromboembolic disease

- Deep vein thrombosis and pulmonary embolism can be considered different manifestations of venous thromboembolism (VTE). The following three factors must be considered when assessing the need for continued anticoagulation perioperatively[5]:

  The risk of recurrent VTE is highest in the first several months after diagnosis.

  The case-fatality rate or the risk of dying from recurrent VTE is highest during the initial 3–6 months of treatment.

  Patients who initially present with pulmonary embolism are at a greater risk of death (higher case fatality rate) than those who present with deep vein thrombosis.

4.2.2
Patients on Aspirin or Clopidogrel Requiring Surgery or an Invasive Procedure

• Aspirin is used for primary prevention of cardiovascular disease and as secondary prevention and treatment of myocardial infarction, stroke and peripheral vascular disease.
• Clopidogrel is typically used for the treatment of myocardial infarction and stroke, and in combination with aspirin, it is prescribed in patients with acute coronary syndrome (ACS) and coronary artery stents.

- Each of these indications has different risks of thromboembolic disease, and the situation that brings the most challenge in perioperative management is that of a patient with a recent coronary artery stent which is discussed in Chap. 20.

4.3 Surgery-Specific Risk Factors for Perioperative Bleeding

- There are no validated tools to predict bleeding complications in patients on warfarin therapy who require surgery or an invasive procedure. The largest cohort study using a single bridging protocol categorized procedures into high and non-high bleeding risk.[6] A pragmatic model is to classify procedures into low, moderate and high bleeding risk to help guide perioperative anticoagulation management.
  - Procedures with low risk of bleeding can be performed without warfarin interruption. These include minor dental (tooth extractions and root canals), ophthalmologic (cataract surgery) and minor dermatologic procedures. Warfarin need not be interrupted for these procedures, and hence there is no need for bridging therapy.[1]
  - High-risk surgery patients include those where hemostasis is difficult (transurethral prostatectomy) or where bleeding could be critical (neurosurgery) and warfarin needs to be discontinued.
  - Moderate risk surgery falls between these extremes.
- A similar approach is reasonable for patients on antiplatelet therapy. If the bleeding risk is low, antiplatelets may be continued, but if the bleeding risk is high, then aspirin and/or clopidogrel have to be stopped.
- For patients who are on aspirin for primary prevention, the risk of bleeding from minor procedures may outweigh the benefit of continuing aspirin perioperatively.

4.4 Preoperative Evaluation

4.4.1 For Patients on Warfarin

- Preoperative consultation should optimally be done approximately 2 weeks prior to a planned surgery or invasive procedure. This allows time for appropriate planning, especially if bridging with LMWH is indicated.
- For patients who require LMWH bridging therapy, several issues need to be addressed in the initial preoperative consultation.
  - Insurance preauthorization, if necessary, needs to be attained, and patients or their family members need to be taught LMWH injection techniques. Also, arrangements for disposal of needles must be addressed.

- An international normalized ratio of the prothrombin time (INR) should be done approximately 7 days prior to surgery and if high, the timing of warfarin interruption should be adjusted accordingly.

- For patients undergoing minor procedures, direct communication with the dentist or responsible physician can be very useful. This has been particularly useful in our practice for patients undergoing minor dental procedures, and we found sharing studies published in the *Journal of the American Dental Association*[7] can serve as a powerful educational tool to prevent unnecessary warfarin interruptions.

4.4.2 For Patients on Aspirin or Clopidogrel

- Preoperative consultation ideally should also be done approximately 2 weeks before surgery to allow adequate time for antiplatelet discontinuation. Guidelines recommend holding both aspirin and clopidogrel for 7–10 days prior to surgery[1] to allow new platelets to replace those that have undergone irreversible inhibition.

4.5 Perioperative Management

4.5.1 Patients on Warfarin

- Table 4.2 is a suggested bridging protocol that includes the timing of INR monitoring, warfarin interruption and reinitiation, and LMWH dosing. Issues that affect the scheduling of these steps include: pharmacodynamics of warfarin, time to offset the effect of LMWH, timing of postoperative LMWH and risk of bleeding, and when to stop postoperative LMWH.
- Warfarin is usually interrupted 5 days prior to the procedure, which is how long it takes to reconstitute clotting factors; however, there is considerable patient-to-patient variation. In a study of 22 patients with an INR range of 2–3, almost all patients had an INR of less than 1.5 after holding warfarin for 5 days.[8] Most patients can undergo surgery with an INR of less than 1.5. For those cases where a lower INR is necessary for surgery or where the therapeutic INR was kept at a higher range, more time is needed and warfarin should be interrupted for more than 5 days before the procedure. This emphasizes the importance of initial perioperative consultation approximately 2 weeks prior to surgery so that the immediate preoperative INR can be agreed upon and there is enough time to achieve this goal.

  - Most procedures can be done if the INR is <1.5 and if the INR is greater than anticipated on the day before surgery, 1–2 mg of oral vitamin K may be given.[1,9]

- LMWH has a peak onset of action of 3–5 h and an elimination half-life of 3–6 h,[10] unlike the slow onset and slow natural reversal of warfarin. When bridging, LMWH should be

Table 4.2 Bridging protocol for patients on warfarin

Pre-op day	Process
10–14	Initial consultation Determine need for bridging based on risk assessment Check creatinine clearance Begin insurance authorization for LMWH Begin LMWH teaching
7–10	Check INR Hold aspirin or clopidogrel
5–6	Hold warfarin
3–4	Begin LMWH bridging if indicated
1	Last dose of LMWH in morning • Omit evening dose if using twice daily dosing • Give 1/2 dose LMWH if using once daily dosing
	Check INR and give low dose vitamin K if necessary
Day of surgery	Restart warfarin evening of surgery if hemostasis secured
Post-op day	
1	Begin LMWH if hemostasis secure and low-moderate risk bleeding procedure
2–3	Begin LMWH if hemostasis secure and high risk bleeding procedure
5–7	Stop LMWH when first INR in therapeutic range

LMWH low molecular weight heparin, *INR* international normalized ratio of the prothrombin time

started approximately 3 days prior to surgery or 2 days after warfarin is held which is the time when its effect is starting to wane. The key questions are when to stop LMWH preoperatively and when to reinitiate postoperatively.

– LMWH should be stopped approximately 24 h before surgery (last dose given on the morning of preoperative day 1) if twice a day LMWH dosing is used. In a study of patients undergoing bridging therapy who were given their last dose of LMWH 12 h preoperatively, 30% of the patients had a residual anticoagulation effect (measured by anti-Xa activity) at the time of surgery when therapeutic doses of LMWH were used for bridging.[11] Therefore, guidelines recommend that only half of the daily dose of LMWH should be given on the day prior to surgery[1] (see Tables 4.2 and 4.3).

– LMWH bridging cannot be started until postoperative hemostasis is secure, and this requires close collaboration with the surgeon. The timing of postoperative LMWH has evolved over time and guidelines recommend delaying the start of postoperative LMWH until day 2–3 or even omitting LMWH for patients undergoing major or high bleeding risk surgery. A study that started once daily dose enoxaparin (1.5 mg/kg) on postoperative day 1 reported a 20% major bleeding rate in patients undergoing orthopedic surgery,[12] and

Table 4.3 Low molecular weight heparin perioperative dosing

	Dalteparin	Enoxaparin	Tinzaparin
Twice daily dose	100 u/kg	1 mg/kg	na
Once daily dose	200 u/kg	1.5 mg/kg	175 u/kg
Dose to be given 24 h preoperatively	100 u/kg	1 mg/kg	87.5 u/kg

postoperative bleeding has been shown to cause a paradoxical increase in thromboembolic events because reinitiating warfarin is subsequently delayed.[9] Some cohort studies have circumvented postoperative bleeding in major surgery by not using bridging LMWH after surgery[6] or by using prophylactic dose LMWH in high-risk patients.[9]

– LMWH can be stopped once the INR is in the therapeutic range and there is no need to have two consecutive INRs in range before discontinuing LMWH.[6,9]

- Spinal and Epidural Anesthesia

  – The Food and Drug Administration (FDA) mandates a boxed warning regarding the risk of spinal hematoma when using LMWH among patients who undergo spinal or epidural anesthesia.
  – In 2010, the American Society of Regional Anesthesia and Pain Medicine (ASRA) published updated guidelines (third edition) on the use of regional anesthesia in patients receiving antithrombotic or thrombolytic therapy.[13]
  – The last therapeutic dose (bridging dose) of preoperative LMWH should be given at least 24 h prior to needle insertion for regional anesthesia and the first dose of LMWH should be at least 24 h after needle insertion postoperatively[13]; see Table 4.2.

  The ASRA guidelines recommend removal of indwelling catheters prior to the postoperative initiation of therapeutic-dose LMWH and suggest a delay of at least 2 h between catheter removal and LMWH administration.

  – Warfarin should ideally be held for 4–5 days prior to regional anesthesia needle insertion, with a target preprocedure INR of less than 1.5. Caution should be used when concomitant antiplatelet medications are used. This is consistent with the timing of warfarin interruption, which is detailed in Table 4.2.

- Emergent surgery

  – Patients anticoagulated with warfarin who need urgent or emergent surgery require rapid reversal of anticoagulation. While there are no randomized trials addressing the most effective way to achieve this, the following options are commonly used:

  Vitamin K at doses of 2.5–5 mg will typically reverse an INR in the usual therapeutic range within 12–18 h.[1] While the oral route is preferred, intravenous vitamin K likely works faster but carries a risk of anaphylaxis.

  Fresh frozen plasma or prothrombin concentrates can rapidly reverse the INR temporarily. Fresh frozen plasma has a half-life of 4–6 h, thus vitamin K must also be given to neutralize warfarin once the effect of FFP has dissipated.[1]

4.5.2 For Patients on Antiplatelets

- There are no "bridging" agents to fill in the gap in therapy when aspirin or clopidogrel is discontinued prior to surgery, and there are no validated risk stratification schemes to guide the risks and benefits of withholding antiplatelet therapy.
- The use of antiplatelets in vascular surgery, cardiovascular surgery and in patients with recent coronary artery stents is discussed in Chaps. 11 and 20.
- Aspirin, clopidogrel and prasugrel (a new thienopyridine) should be stopped 7–10 days prior to surgical or invasive procedures and resumed once hemostasis is secured, which is usually on postoperative day 1.[1]

4.6 Conclusions

- Patients on chronic anticoagulation therapy frequently require surgery or an invasive procedure, and close communication between perioperative consultants and the physician performing the procedure is key to the effective and safe management of these patients.
- Patients undergoing procedures with low risk of bleeding do not require interruption of anticoagulation or antiplatelet therapy, especially if they have a high risk of thromboembolic events.
- Patients who have a high risk of thromboembolic complications may benefit from a perioperative bridging regimen with LMWH.
- Key points in LMWH bridging include stopping treatment 24 h before surgery and regional anesthesia and not resuming postoperatively until the day after the procedure.
- Patients undergoing major surgery should either have their LMWH reinitiation delayed until postoperative day 2 or 3, withheld or reduced to prophylactic dosing, depending on the risk of bleeding.
- Antiplatelet therapy should be stopped 7–10 days prior to surgery and then restarted once hemostasis is ensured, which is usually the day following the procedure.

References

1. Douketis JD, Berger PB, Dunn AS, et al. The perioperative management of antithrombotic therapy: American college of chest physicians evidence-based clinical practice guidelines (8th edition). *Chest*. 2008;133(6 suppl):299S-339S.
2. United States National Institute of Health. www.clinicaltrials.gov. July 7, 2010.
3. Gage BF, Waterman AD, Shannon W, Boechler M, Rich MW, Radford MJ. Validation of clinical classification schemes for predicting stroke: results from the national registry of atrial fibrillation. *JAMA*. 2001;285(22):2864-2870.
4. Kaatz S, Douketis JD, Zhou H, Gage BF, White RH. Risk of stroke after surgery in patients with and without chronic atrial fibrillation. *J Thromb Haemost*. 2010;8(5):884-890.

5. Carrier M, Le Gal G, Wells PS, Rodger MA. Systematic review: case-fatality rates of recurrent venous thromboembolism and major bleeding events among patients treated for venous thromboembolism. *Ann Intern Med.* 2010;152(9):578-589.
6. Douketis JD, Johnson JA, Turpie AG. Low-molecular-weight heparin as bridging anticoagulation during interruption of warfarin: assessment of a standardized periprocedural anticoagulation regimen. *Arch Intern Med.* 2004;164(12):1319-1326.
7. Jeske AH, Suchko GD. Lack of a scientific basis for routine discontinuation of oral anticoagulation therapy before dental treatment. *J Am Dent Assoc.* 2003;134(11):1492-1497.
8. White RH, McKittrick T, Hutchinson R, Twitchell J. Temporary discontinuation of warfarin therapy: changes in the international normalized ratio. *Ann Intern Med.* 1995;122(1):40-42.
9. Kovacs MJ, Kearon C, Rodger M, et al. Single-arm study of bridging therapy with low-molecular-weight heparin for patients at risk of arterial embolism who require temporary interruption of warfarin. *Circulation.* 2004;110(12):1658-1663.
10. Hirsh J, Bauer KA, Donati MB, Gould M, Samama MM, Weitz JI. Parenteral anticoagulants: American college of chest physicians evidence-based clinical practice guidelines (8th edition). *Chest.* 2008;133(6 suppl):141S-159S.
11. Douketis JD, Woods K, Foster GA, Crowther MA. Bridging anticoagulation with low-molecular-weight heparin after interruption of warfarin therapy is associated with a residual anticoagulant effect prior to surgery. *Thromb Haemost.* 2005;94(3):528-531.
12. Dunn AS, Spyropoulos AC, Turpie AG. Bridging therapy in patients on long-term oral anticoagulants who require surgery: the Prospective Peri-operative Enoxaparin Cohort Trial (PROSPECT). *J Thromb Haemost.* 2007;5(11):2211-2218.
13. Horlocker TT, Wedel DJ, Rowlingson JC, et al. Regional anesthesia in the patient receiving antithrombotic or thrombolytic therapy: American society of regional anesthesia and pain medicine evidence-based guidelines (third edition). *Reg Anesth Pain Med.* 2010;35(1): 64-101.

Venous Thromboembolism Prophylaxis 5

Steven L. Cohn

5.1 Introduction

- Venous thromboembolism (VTE) is a common complication after surgery. Deep vein thrombosis (DVT) and pulmonary embolism (PE) affect at least 350,000–600,000 Americans, contributing to 100,000–180,000 deaths each year. These numbers probably underestimate the true incidence which may be 2–3 times higher and are expected to increase as the US population ages. It is estimated that about half of these cases attributed to hospitalized patients occur in surgical patients, and it has become a national patient safety issue.
- The Surgeon General[1] issued a call to action to reduce the risk of VTE by being aware of the signs and symptoms of VTE, knowing the triggering factors, and employing effective methods of prevention during high-risk periods.
- The prevalence of postoperative VTE varies depending on the patient's risk factors for VTE (Table 5.1), the type of surgery (Table 5.2), and the type and duration of prophylaxis.
- Postoperative VTE is often silent as evidenced by clinical trials using routine venography to study the prevalence of postoperative DVT in the absence of prophylaxis.
- Most symptomatic postoperative DVTs occur after hospital discharge. Because the first manifestation of VTE may be a fatal PE, prevention is key. Reliance on signs and symptoms of early DVT and routine screening for postoperative DVT are unreliable, expensive, and not recommended.
- Because VTE has chronic sequelae, such as post-thrombotic syndrome, chronic pulmonary hypertension, and an increased risk for recurrent VTE, the best strategy is to prevent the initial event by providing VTE prophylaxis for almost all surgical patients.
- A collaborative effort with surgeons, anesthesiologists, nursing, and medical consultants is important to optimize universal implementation of risk assessment and perioperative VTE prophylaxis.

S.L. Cohn
Internal Medicine-Medical Consultation Service,
SUNY Downstate - Kings County Hospital Center,
450 Clarkson Ave, Box 68, Brooklyn, NY 11203, USA
e-mail: steven.cohn@downstate.edu

S.L. Cohn (ed.), *Perioperative Medicine*,
DOI: 10.1007/978-0-85729-498-2_5, © Springer-Verlag London Limited 2011

Table 5.1 Risk factors for VTE (with most common mechanism)[a]

Stasis	Endothelial injury	Hypercoagulability
Older age	Surgery	Cancer/chemotherapy
Immobility/bed rest	Previous VTE	High estrogen states (pregnancy/post-partum, OCP, HRT)
Stroke, paralysis, SCI	Central venous catheter	Acute infection/sepsis
CHF	Trauma	IBD
COPD/respiratory failure		Nephrotic syndrome
Anesthesia (general, spinal, or epidural)		Thrombophilia
Obesity		
Hyperviscosity, polycythemia		

[a]List is not all inclusive; some factors have multiple mechanisms

Table 5.2 VTE risk stratification and prophylaxis options

Level of risk	Examples	VTE risk without prophylaxis (%)	Prophylaxis optionsa
Low risk	Minor surgery, mobile patient	<10	No specific prophylaxis other than **early ambulation**
Moderate risk	Most general surgery, open gynecologic or urologic surgery	10–40	**LMWH** (enoxaparin 40 mg; dalteparin 2,500–5,000 Units) **LDUH** (5,000 Units q8–12 h) **Fondaparinux** (2.5 mg)
High risk	Hip or knee arthroplasty, HFS; major trauma, SCI	40–80	**LMWH** (enoxaparin 30 mg q12 h or 40 mg once daily; dalteparin 2,500–5,000 Units) **Fondaparinux** (2.5 mg) **Oral VKA** (warfarin: INR 2–3)
Moderate or high VTE risk ***plus*** high bleeding risk	Intracranial or spine surgery		***Mechanical*** (IPC, GCS)

Source: Adapted from Geerts[2]

VTE venous thromboembolism, *HFS* hip fracture surgery, *SCI* spinal cord injury, *LMWH* low molecular weight heparin, *LDUF* low dose unfractionated heparin, *VKA* vitamin K antagonist, *IPC* intermittent pneumatic compression, *GCS* graded compression stockings

[a]Assuming normal weight and renal function. Check with manufacturers' recommendations for specific dosing guidelines, including warning before neuraxial anesthesia, timing of administration, and postoperative dosing. Note: newer oral agents (direct thrombin inhibitors and Xa inhibitors) are currently available outside the US for thromboprophylaxis for orthopedic surgery

- Evidence-based guidelines from different societies support several methods of prophylaxis in a variety of surgical settings; therefore, one should respect individual practice preferences to avoid unwanted complications or conflicts in management. This chapter, however, will focus on recommendations from the 8th Edition of the American College of Chest Physician (ACCP) guidelines.[2]

5.2 Patient-Related Risk Factors

- Virchow's triad describes three underlying mechanisms for venous thrombosis: venous stasis, endothelial injury, and hypercoagulability.
- Important patient-related risk factors for VTE reflect these underlying pathophysiologic processes and include increasing age, immobility, malignancy, prior VTE, heart failure, and other factors (see Table 5.1).
- VTE risk increases in proportion to the number of predisposing factors.

5.3 Surgery-Related Risk Factors

- All three elements of Virchow's triad are present in the surgical setting. The supine position coupled with anesthesia leads to stasis, subsequent decreased clearing of the clotting factors leads to a hypercoagulable state, and the surgery itself may cause endothelial injury.
- The risk conferred by the surgery itself may sometimes be so high that it alone dictates the type of prophylaxis regardless of the patient's risk factors. For example, patients undergoing knee or hip replacement or hip fracture surgery are automatically in the highest risk category.
- Table 5.2 lists the various types of surgeries and the associated prevalence of DVT in these various patient groups in the absence of prophylaxis.

5.4 Preoperative Evaluation and Risk Stratification

- Preoperative VTE risk is estimated by considering both patient- and surgery-specific factors. Previous models defined risk categories based on the number of risk factors, various point totals based on scoring system, or used age and the type of surgery.
- The 8th ACCP Guidelines[2] took a different approach and looked at the risk of developing a VTE in the absence of prophylaxis. They defined three groups: low risk (<10%),

moderate risk (10–40%), and high risk (>40%), and made recommendations for prophylaxis in each group (Table 5.2).

- Because there are various modalities recommended for prophylaxis, and both pharmacologic and non-pharmacologic methods carry risk (e.g., bleeding, thrombocytopenia) or may be uncomfortable to patients (e.g., needle sticks, stockings, pneumatic devices), the prophylaxis chosen should incorporate patient- and procedure-related risk factors as well as patient and provider preferences.
  - If VTE prophylaxis is warranted, consider the risks associated with the recommended, evidence-based modality.
  - In consultation with surgical colleagues, consider the inherent surgery-specific bleeding risk and defer initiation of pharmacologic anticoagulation unless the benefit of VTE prophylaxis outweighs the bleeding risk.
  - In general, pharmacologic prophylaxis is recommended over mechanical prophylaxis unless there is a contraindication (e.g., active bleeding). The exceptions to this include patients undergoing neurosurgery (intracranial) or spine surgery where a little bleeding can result in significant morbidity.
  - In patients at high risk for bleeding, initiate VTE prophylaxis with non-pharmacologic methods (e.g., graded compression stockings (GCS), intermittent pneumatic compression (IPC) devices) initially, and add pharmacologic methods once the bleeding risk is minimized.
  - Avoid unfractionated or low-molecular weight heparin in patients with a known history of immune-mediated heparin-induced thrombocytopenia (HIT). If necessary (e.g., cardiac surgery), consider alternatives such as direct thrombin inhibitors or off pump surgery. Another option, although not FDA approved for this indication, for patients with a history of HIT is fondaparinux because it does not cross react with heparin or cause HIT.

5.5 Perioperative Management

Table 5.3 summarizes the ACCP recommendations for VTE prophylaxis[2] according to the type of surgery.

5.5.1 Pharmacologic Options

- <u>Aspirin</u> is not very effective for prophylaxis against VTE and the ACCP guidelines recommend <u>against</u> its use in any surgical group as a single prophylaxis agent. However, the American Academy of Orthopedic Surgeons (AAOS) issued their own consensus guidelines[3] in which they include aspirin as an option for prophylaxis (to prevent PE) in patients undergoing hip or knee replacement or hip fracture surgery. Their recommendations use

Table 5.3 Summary of VTE prophylaxis options for selected surgical patients (ACCP 2008)

Risk level		Recommended prophylaxis
General surgery		
Low risk		Recommend against specific thromboprophylaxis OTHER THAN early, frequent ambulation (1A)
Moderate risk – major surgery benign disease		LMWH, LDUH, or fondaparinux (1A)
Higher risk – major surgery for cancer		LMWH, LDUH tid, or fondaparinux (1A)
High risk with multiple risk factors		LMWH, LDUH tid, or fondaparinux (1A) combined with GCS and/or IPC (1C)
General surgery with high risk for bleeding		GCS and/or IPC (1A); add/substitute pharmacologic prophylaxis when bleeding risk decreases (1C)
Duration	After major general surgical procedures	Continue prophylaxis until discharge (1A)
	Selected high risk surgery patients (e.g., after cancer surgery or with prior VTE)	Continue prophylaxis with LMWH up to 28 days after discharge (2A)
Gynecologic surgery		
Low risk, minor procedures, no additional risk factors		Recommend against specific thromboprophylaxis OTHER THAN early, frequent ambulation (1A)
Laparoscopic procedures with additional risk factors		One or more of LMWH, LDUH, IPC or GCS (1C)
Major surgery – benign disease, no additional risk factors		Recommend routine use of prophylaxis (1A) using LMWH (1A), LDUH (1A), or IPC started just before surgery and used continuously while the patient is not ambulating (1B)
Extensive surgery – malignancy or additional risk factors		LMWH (1A), LDUH tid (1A), or IPC started just before surgery and used continuously while the patient is not ambulating (1A) alternatively – combination of LMWH or LDUH plus mechanical prophylaxis, or fondaparinux (1C)
Duration	Major gynecologic procedures	Continue prophylaxis until discharge from hospital (1A)
	For selected high-risk gyn patients, (e.g., after cancer surgery or with prior VTE)	Continue prophylaxis after hospital discharge with LMWH for up to 28 days (2C)
Laparoscopic surgery		
Entirely laparoscopic with no additional risk factors		Recommend against specific prophylaxis OTHER THAN early, frequent ambulation (1B)
With additional risk factors		One or more of LMWH, LDUH, fondaparinux, IPC, or GCS (1C)

(continued)

Table 5.3 (continued)

Risk level	Recommended prophylaxis
Urologic surgery	
Transurethral or low risk procedures	Recommend against specific thromboprophylaxis OTHER THAN early, frequent ambulation (1A)
Major open procedures	LDUH bid/tid (1B), GCS/IPC (1B), LMWH (1C), fondaparinux (1C), OR pharmacologic combined with mechanical (1C)
Urologic surgery with active bleeding or very high bleeding risk	GCS or IPC (1C)
Bariatric surgery	
In-patient bariatric surgery	LMWH, LDUH tid, or fondaparinux OR pharmacologic combined with GCS/IPC (1C) Suggest higher doses of LMWH or LDUH (2C)
Thoracic surgery	
Major thoracic surgery	LMWH, LDUH, or fondaparinux (1C)
Thoracic surgery with high risk of bleeding	GCS or IPC (1C)
Total hip replacement	
With no additional risk factors	Routine use of one of the following: (all grade 1A) 1. LMWH (at a usual high-risk dose, started 12 h before surgery or 12–24 h after surgery, or 4–6 h after surgery at half the usual high-risk dose and then increasing to the usual high-risk dose the following day) 2. Fondaparinux (2.5 mg started 6–24 h after surgery) 3. Adjusted-dose VKA started preoperatively or the evening of the surgical day (INR target 2.5; range 2–3) Do not use any of the following as the sole method of prophylaxis: aspirin, dextran, LDUH, GCS, or VFP (1A)
With high risk of bleeding	Optimal use of mechanical prophylaxis with VFP or IPC (1A) Add or substitute pharmacologic prophylaxis when bleeding risk decreases (1C)
Duration THR	Prophylaxis with one of the recommended options for at *least 10 days*. (1A) Extend beyond 10 days and up to 35 days after surgery (1B) using LMWH (1A), a VKA (1B), or fondaparinux (1C)

Table 5.3 (continued)

Risk level		Recommended prophylaxis
Total knee replacement		
With no additional risk factors		LMWH (at the usual high-risk dose), fondaparinux, or adjusted-dose VKA (INR target 2.5; INR range 2.0–3.0) (1A) Alternative – optimal use of IPC (1B) Do not use any of the following as the only method of thromboprophylaxis: aspirin (1A), LDUH (1A), or VFP (1B)
TKR with high risk of bleeding		Optimal use of mechanical prophylaxis with IPC (1A) or VFP (1B). Add or substitute pharmacologic thromboprophylaxis when bleeding risk decreases (1C)
Duration	TKR	Prophylaxis with one of the recommended options for at *least 10 days*. (1A) Extend beyond 10 days and up to 35 days after surgery (2B) using LMWH (1C), a VKA (1C), or fondaparinux (1C)
Hip fracture surgery		
With no additional risk factors		Routine prophylaxis with fondaparinux (1A), LMWH (1B), adjusted-dose VKA (INR target 2.5; range 2–3) (1B), or LDUH (1B); Do not use aspirin alone (1A) For patients receiving LMWH as prophylaxis, start either 12 hrs preoperatively or 12–24 hrs postoperatively (1A); For patients receiving fondaparinux, start 2.5 mg either 6–8 h after surgery or the next day (1A) For patients receiving *VKA*, start preoperatively or the evening of the surgical day (1A)
With high risk of bleeding		Optimal use of mechanical thromboprophylaxis (1A) Add or substitute pharmacologic thromboprophylaxis when bleeding risk decreases (1C)
Duration	For HFS	Prophylaxis with one of the recommended options for at *least 10 days*. (1A) Extend beyond 10 days and up to 35 days after surgery (1A) using fondaparinux (1A), LMWH (1C), or a VKA (1C)

(continued)

Table 5.3 (continued)

Risk level	Recommended prophylaxis
Isolated lower extremity injuries distal to the knee	
	Do not routinely use thromboprophylaxis (2A)
Knee arthroscopy	
With no additional risk factors	Recommend against specific thromboprophylaxis OTHER THAN early mobilization (2B)
With additional risk factors or complicated procedure	LMWH (1B)
Elective spine surgery	
With no additional risk factors	Recommend against specific thromboprophylaxis OTHER THAN early, frequent ambulation (2C)
With additional risk factors or anterior surgical approach	Postoperative LDUH (1B), LMWH (1B), or IPC (1B); Alternative is GCS (2B)
With multiple risk factors	Pharmacologic combined with mechanical (2C)

Source: Adapted from: Geerts[2]

Please refer to the full ACCP guidelines for a complete list of recommendations

LMWH low molecular weight heparin, *LDUH* low dose unfractionated heparin, *GCS* graduated compression stockings, *IPC* intermittent pneumatic compression, *INR* international normalized ratio, *VFP* venous foot pump, *VKA* vitamin K antagonist, *THR* total hip replacement, *TKR* total knee replacement, *HFS* hip fracture surgery

different methodology and are based on preventing symptomatic PE (rather than overall VTE) and minimizing bleeding risk.

- UFH is inexpensive, has a short half-life, and requires dosing two or three times daily. Its anticoagulant effect can be easily reversed with protamine if needed. There is a risk of heparin-induced thrombocytopenia (HIT) that may be as high as 5% in orthopedic patients.
- Warfarin has the advantage of oral administration and is relatively inexpensive. However, it requires monitoring with an INR, has multiple drug and food interactions, and has a narrow therapeutic range. In addition, its onset of action takes several days, and patients may be at increased risk for VTE while the INR is sub-therapeutic. It is reasonable to use LMWH and/or IPC devices until the INR becomes therapeutic. Pooled analysis of randomized clinical trials comparing LMWH to warfarin shows less VTE but a trend toward increased bleeding with LMWH.
- LMWHs are well absorbed from subcutaneous tissue, have a rapid onset of action, can be dosed once or twice daily, and cause less HIT compared to UFH. Although acquisition costs are higher for LMWH, it may be more cost-effective than warfarin as suggested by studies that included costs of monitoring and complications, and generic enoxaparin has recently been approved.

- LMWHs are metabolized by the kidneys and may accumulate in patients with renal insufficiency (creatinine clearance <30 cc/min). The options in these patients include monitoring with anti-Xa levels, reducing the dose, or using an alternative method. Enoxaparin is the only LMWH with a specific recommendation for renal insufficiency, which is to decrease the prophylactic dose from 40 to 30 mg SC once-daily.

- Fondaparinux is a synthetic pentasaccharide that inhibits factor X, has a long half-life (17–21 h), and is dosed once daily subcutaneously. It has a rapid onset of action, but its anticoagulant effect cannot adequately and routinely be reversed. Recombinant Factor VIIa (Novo-Seven) may be useful to reverse the anticoagulant effect of fondaparinux in case of serious bleeding complications or need for acute surgery during treatment with fondaparinux.
  - Fondaparinux is cleared renally and therefore contraindicated in patients with a creatinine clearance <30 ml/min. It may be more effective in preventing VTE compared to LMWHs after major joint replacement when dosed within 6–8 h after surgery but may cause more bleeding, particularly after knee replacement surgery.

- New oral agents: There are several drugs available outside the US that are awaiting FDA approval. These include oral direct Xa inhibitors (rivaroxaban, apixaban) and direct thrombin inhibitors (dabigatran, which was recently approved for stroke prevention in patients with atrial fibrillation). The potential advantages of these drugs are that they are administered in a fixed dose, require no monitoring (similar to LMWH), and are taken orally.

5.5.2 Non-Pharmacologic (Mechanical) Options

- Early ambulation should be recommended for all patients.
- GCS and IPCs can be used alone when bleeding risk is high or as an adjunct to pharmacologic prophylaxis in selected high-risk cases.
  - GCS need to be fitted correctly because if they are too tight, they may cause stasis and increase risk of VTE.
  - For IPCs to be beneficial, patients must wear them at least 15 h a day.

5.5.3 Neuraxial (Spinal and Epidural) Anesthesia

- Spinal hematoma may complicate spinal or epidural anesthesia in patients receiving pharmacologic VTE prophylaxis if special precautions are not exercised. Guidelines from the American Society of Regional Anesthesia (ASRA)[4] include the following recommendations:
- Delay the initiation of UFH for 1 h after needle placement and removal of epidural catheters until 2–4 h after the last prophylactic dose.

- LMWHs carry a boxed warning from the FDA regarding the risk of spinal hematoma.
  - Before inserting a spinal needle or epidural catheter, wait 24 h if patients received full dose LMWH prior to surgery and 12 h prior to insertion after a prophylactic dose of LMWH.
  - Wait a minimum of 2 h after catheter removal prior to dosing LMWH.
- Withhold warfarin for 4–5 days prior to catheter insertion, and remove the catheter only after ensuring that the INR is <1.5.
- Optimal management of neuraxial anesthesia is unknown for patients who receive fondaparinux for VTE prophylaxis. ASRA guidelines state that "until further clinical experience is available, performance of neuraxial techniques should occur under conditions used in clinical trials (single-needle pass, atraumatic needle placement, avoidance of indwelling neuraxial catheters). If this is not feasible, an alternate method of prophylaxis should be considered".

5.5.4 Post-Discharge or Extended Prophylaxis

- In general prophylaxis should be given for the duration of hospitalization, and most studies used a minimum of 7–10 days of prophylaxis. Since the length of stay has decreased significantly over the years, many patients are discharged before receiving this duration, and patients are not routinely given prophylaxis after discharge and therefore may still be at risk.
- Certain types of patient-related risks and surgeries are known to confer a high risk for VTE even after discharge from the hospital. Patients for whom extended prophylaxis has been shown to be beneficial include:
  - Abdominal and pelvic cancer surgery patients for up to 28 days after surgery.
  - Total hip replacement (THR) and hip fracture surgery patients (and possibly total knee replacement (TKR)) for 28–35 days after surgery.
  - Because the peak incidence of VTE occurs earlier in TKR, fewer events occur after discharge or 7–10 days; so, extended prophylaxis is less beneficial compared to THR where the risk extends for many weeks after surgery.
- Recommended options for extended prophylaxis are listed in Table 5.3.

5.6 Conclusions

- Most surgical patients are at risk for developing VTE postoperatively. It is important that all patients be screened for VTE risk upon admission to the hospital and given appropriate prophylaxis as per the ACCP guidelines. By doing so, the medical team can minimize the risk of postoperative VTE and improve patient outcomes.

References

1. The Surgeon General's call to action to prevent deep vein thrombosis and pulmonary embolism 2008. US Department of Health and Human Services, Washington DC. Available at: http://www.surgeongeneral.gov/topics/deepvein/http://accpstorage.org/chest08/bestOF/SurgeonGeneralsReport.pdf. Accessed October 22, 2010.
2. Geerts WH, Bergqvist D, Pineo GF, et al. American college of chest physicians. Prevention of venous thromboembolism: American college of chest physicians evidence-based clinical practice guidelines (8th edition). *Chest.* 2008;133(6 suppl):381S-453S. PubMed PMID: 18574271. http://chestjournal.chestpubs.org/content/133/6_suppl/381S.full.pdf+html
3. American Academy of Orthopaedic Surgeons Clinical Guideline on Prevention of Pulmonary Embolism in Patients Undergoing Total Hip or Knee Arthroplasty 2007. http://www.aaos.org/research/guidelines/PE_guideline.pdf. Accessed October 22, 2010.
4. Horlocker TT, Wedel DJ, Rowlingson JC, et al. Regional anesthesia in the patient receiving antithrombotic or thrombolytic therapy: American society of regional anesthesia and pain medicine evidence-based guidelines (third edition). Reg Anesth Pain Med. 2010; 35(1):64–101. PubMed PMID: 20052816. http://journals.lww.com/rapm/Fulltext/2010/01000/Regional_Anesthesia_in_the_Patient_Receiving.13.aspx. Accessed October 22, 2010.

Prevention of Infective Endocarditis (Bacterial Endocarditis Prophylaxis)

6

Steven L. Cohn

6.1 Introduction

- Infective endocarditis (IE) is a serious illness that continues to be associated with significant morbidity and mortality.
- It is thought to result from formation of nonbacterial thrombotic endocarditis (platelets and fibrin) on the surface of a valve or endothelial surface from mechanical disruption or inflammation, bacteremia, bacterial adherence to the fibrin–platelet matrix, and proliferation of the bacteria within the vegetation.
- The incidence of IE ranges from 3 to 10 episodes/100,000 person-years with a ≥2:1 male predominance which is poorly understood.
- Since 1955, the American Heart Association (AHA) has issued evolving recommendations for prevention of IE with antimicrobial prophylaxis before specific procedures such as dental, gastrointestinal (GI), and genitourinary (GU) procedures in patients considered to be at risk for its development.
- The underlying principles were that:
  - IE is uncommon but life threatening, and prevention is preferable to treatment.
  - Certain underlying cardiac conditions predispose to IE.
  - Bacteremia known to cause IE occurs in association with specific procedures.
  - Antimicrobial prophylaxis prevented experimental IE in animals.
  - Antimicrobial prophylaxis was thought to be effective in preventing IE in humans.
- However, various studies, authorities, and societies have questioned the validity of these "guidelines," particularly the efficacy of antimicrobial prophylaxis in humans

S.L. Cohn
Internal Medicine-Medical Consultation Service,
SUNY Downstate - Kings County Hospital Center,
450 Clarkson Ave, Box 68, Brooklyn, NY 11203, USA
e-mail: steven.cohn@downstate.edu

S.L. Cohn (ed.), *Perioperative Medicine*,
DOI: 10.1007/978-0-85729-498-2_6,

since the incidence and mortality of IE have not decreased in the past 30 years despite prophylaxis. Furthermore, these guidelines are actually based on consensus or expert opinion rather than evidence as the incidence of IE is low and there are no randomized controlled trials (RCT).

  - An updated Cochrane systematic review[1] concluded that there remained no evidence about whether penicillin prophylaxis is effective or ineffective against IE in people at risk undergoing an invasive dental procedure. The authors also noted a lack of evidence to support previous guidelines, and they questioned whether the potential harms and costs of prophylactic antibiotics outweighed any potential benefit.

- This chapter will review and summarize the changes in the 2007 AHA guidelines[2] and comment on some of the recommendations from other societies, specifically the European Society of Cardiology (ESC),[3] British Society for Antimicrobial Chemotherapy (BSAC),[4] and the National Institute for Health and Clinical Excellence (NICE)[5] [http://www.nice.org.uk/CG064].

6.2 Rationale for or Against Antimicrobial Prophylaxis (Reasons for Updating the Guidelines)

- The rationale for IE prophylaxis, as noted above, relates to a theoretical link between procedures, bacteremia, and subsequent IE.
- However, the questions to be answered are whether or not:
  - Certain cardiac conditions predispose patients to developing IE
  - Specific procedures induce bacteremia *and* cause IE
  - Antimicrobial prophylaxis can prevent IE
- There are no RCTs and it is unlikely that there will be any, given the huge number of patients required and the ethical issue of using a placebo.
- Acknowledging that it is impossible to determine the relative risk of specific certain cardiac conditions, the various guideline committees tried to identify conditions associated with an IE risk greater than that of the general population over a person's lifetime as well as those conditions associated with the highest risk of adverse outcome should IE occur.
- While certain procedures may be associated with bacteremia, IE is much more likely to result from frequent exposure to random bacteremias associated with daily activities.
- The efficacy of IE prophylaxis is controversial. Although prophylaxis may prevent an extremely small number of cases of IE, the risk of antibiotic-associated adverse events probably exceeds the benefit (if any) from prophylaxis.
- The guidelines had become overly complicated making it difficult for physicians and patients to remember or interpret resulting in both overuse and underuse of prophylaxis.

6.3 Patient-Related Risk Factors/Cardiac Conditions

- Previous AHA guidelines were based on underlying cardiac conditions that over a lifetime were associated with the highest predisposition to acquisition of IE.
  - Conditions with a higher lifetime risk compared to individuals with no known underlying cardiac condition included prosthetic cardiac valves, rheumatic heart disease (RHD), previous IE, congenital heart disease (CHD), and mitral valve prolapse (MVP) with mitral regurgitation.
- Instead, the most recent AHA guidelines recommended that if prophylaxis is effective, it should be restricted to those patients with the highest risk of adverse outcome from IE who would derive the greatest benefit from its prevention.
  - These cardiac conditions included individuals with a prosthetic heart valve, previous IE, CHD, and cardiac transplant recipients who develop valvulopathy.
- Guidelines from other societies differ somewhat in their recommendations and definitions of at-risk patients and cardiac conditions (see Table 6.1).

6.4 Procedure-Related Risk Factors

- Previous AHA guidelines were based on procedures most likely to induce bacteremia and therefore theoretically increase the risk of causing IE in susceptible patients.
  - These included dental procedures, respiratory tract procedures, and GI and GU procedures.
- Because published data proving a cause-and-effect link between these procedures (and potential bacteremia) and subsequent development of IE (with those organisms) is lacking and so few cases occur, the current AHA guidelines modified their recommendations regarding these procedures.
  - The latest AHA recommendations only recommend prophylaxis for dental procedures (only those involving manipulation of gingival tissue or the periapical region of teeth or perforation of the oral mucosa) and for procedures on the respiratory tract or infected skin, skin structures, or musculoskeletal tissue, and only in patients with the highest risk of adverse outcome from IE. For procedures on infected tissue, it is reasonable that the antibiotic regimen include an agent active against *Staphylococci* and beta-hemolytic streptococci.
  - Although endocarditis prophylaxis is not recommended for GI or GU procedures solely to prevent IE, for patients with an established GI or GU tract infection or for those who would receive antibiotic therapy to prevent a wound infection, it may be reasonable for the antibiotic regimen to include a drug active against enterococci.

Table 6.1 Cardiac conditions associated with the highest risk of adverse outcome from endocarditis for which prophylaxis with procedures in Table 6.2 is recommended

Cardiac condition	AHA[2]	BSAC[4]	ESC[3]	(NICE[a])[5]
Prosthetic cardiac valve	Yes	Yes	Yes	No
Previous IE	Yes	Yes	Yes	No
Congenital heart disease (CHD) • Unrepaired cyanotic CHD, including palliative shunts and conduits • Completely repaired congenital heart defect with prosthetic material or device during the first 6 months after the procedure • Repaired CHD with residual defects at the site or adjacent to a prosthetic patch or prosthetic device	Yes	Yes	Yes	No
Cardiac transplant recipients who develop valvulopathy	Yes		No	
Acquired valvulopathy (stenosis or regurgitation)	No	Yes[b]	No	No
Hypertrophic cardiomyopathy	No	Yes[b]	No	No

IE infective endocarditis, *GI* gastrointestinal, *GU* genitourinary, *AHA* American Heart Association, *BSAC* British Society for Antimicrobial Chemotherapy, *ESC* European Society of Cardiology, *NICE* National Institute for Health and Clinical Excellence

[a]Only for GI or GU procedures at "infected" or "potentially infected" sites in patients at risk (essentially all conditions listed)

[b]Only for nondental procedures

- Guidelines from other societies differ in their recommendations and definitions of high-risk procedures (see Table 6.2). For example, the BSAC did not eliminate the recommendation for prophylaxis for GI and GU procedures.

6.5 Antimicrobial Therapy

- If IE prophylaxis is recommended, it should be administered as a single dose 30–60 min before the procedure.
- Antibiotic regimens for IE prophylaxis in patients with cardiac conditions who are undergoing procedures warranting prophylaxis are listed in Table 6.3.
- These antibiotic regimens are based on the most likely causative organisms:
  - *Streptococcus viridans* for dental procedures
  - Enterococci for GI and GU procedures
  - Various microorganisms for respiratory tract procedures – if infected, consider *S. viridans*
  - *Staphylococcus aureus* for cardiac surgery

Table 6.2 Procedures for which endocarditis prophylaxis is recommended (for patients in Table 6.1)

Procedure	AHA[2]	BSAC[4]	ESC[3]	NICE[5]
Dental[a]	Yes	Yes	Yes	No
Respiratory[b]	Yes	Yes	No	No
GI/GU[c]	No	Yes	No	No

GI gastrointestinal, *GU* genitourinary, *AHA* American Heart Association, *BSAC* British Society for Antimicrobial Chemotherapy, *ESC* European Society of Cardiology, *NICE* National Institute for Health and Clinical Excellence

[a]*Recommended* for: dental procedures that involve manipulation of either gingival tissue or the periapical region of the teeth or perforation of the oral mucosa (Not recommended for: routine anesthetic injections through noninfected tissue, dental X-rays, placement/removal/adjustment of prosthodontic or orthodontic appliances/brackets, shedding of deciduous teeth, bleeding from trauma to the lips or oral mucosa)

[b]*Recommended* for invasive respiratory tract procedures involving incision or biopsy of the respiratory mucosa (e.g., tonsillectomy/adenoidectomy)

[c]Sclerotherapy/dilatation of esophageal varices, esophageal laser therapy, ERCP, hepatic/biliary operations, gall stone lithotripsy, surgery involving intestinal mucosa, cystoscopy, urethral dilatation, TURP, transrectal prostate biopsy, vaginal hysterectomy, caesarian section (BSAC list)

Table 6.3 Antibiotic prophylaxis regimens (for patients and procedures at risk)[2]

Situation	Antibiotic	Single dose 30–60 min before procedure
No allergy to penicillin or ampicillin	• Amoxicillin	2 g PO[a]
	Unable to take oral medication	
	• Ampicillin	2 g IM or IV
	or	
	• Cefazolin or ceftriaxone	1 g IM or IV
Allergic to penicillin or ampicillin	• Cephalexin	2 g PO
	or	
	• Clindamycin	600 mg PO
	or	
	• Azithromycin or clarithromycin	500 mg PO
	Unable to take oral medication	
	• Cefazolin or ceftriaxone[b]	1 g IM or IV
	or	
	• Clindamycin	600 mg IM or IV

IM intramuscular, *IV* intravenous

[a]British Society for Antimicrobial Chemotherapy (BSAC) recommends a dose of 3 g or clindamycin 300 mg IV (over at least 10 min); BSAC also recommends prophylaxis for GI and GU procedures with ampicillin or amoxicillin 1 g (if allergic, teicoplanin 400 mg IV) + gentamicin 1.5 mg/kg IV

[b]Do not use a cephalosporin in a patient with a history of anaphylaxis, angioedema, or urticaria with penicillin or ampicillin

- If a patient will be receiving antibiotic prophylaxis to prevent wound infection after specific procedures, it is reasonable that the regimen include an agent that is active against the most likely pathogen for that setting.

- If a patient is already receiving long-term antibiotics with a drug also recommended for IE prophylaxis and the patient has a cardiac condition warranting prophylaxis, it is prudent to change the antibiotic to a different class for the procedure.
  - For example, in a patient who has been receiving penicillin prophylaxis for rheumatic fever who is scheduled for an invasive dental procedure, clindamycin or azithromycin should be given for IE prophylaxis.
- Maintenance of optimal oral health and hygiene may reduce the incidence of bacteremia from daily activities and is more important than prophylactic antibiotics to reduce IE risk for a dental procedure.

6.6 Summary

- Multiple revised guidelines now recommend IE prophylaxis for significantly fewer patients than in the past. This is driven by the lack of scientific evidence-linking procedures and bacteremia to subsequent endocarditis and the lack of efficacy for prophylaxis.
- The effects of these changes need to be monitored, and ideally, RCTs and additional prospective case–control studies are needed to evaluate current regimens and to provide evidence for future recommendations.

References

1. Oliver R, Roberts GJ, Hooper L, Worthington HV. Antibiotics for the prophylaxis of bacterial endocarditis in dentistry. *Cochrane Database Syst Rev.* 2008; (4):CD003813.
2. Wilson W, Taubert KA, Gewitz M, et al. Prevention of infective endocarditis: guidelines from the American Heart Association: a guideline from the American Heart Association Rheumatic Fever, Endocarditis, and Kawasaki Disease Committee, Council on Cardiovascular Disease in the Young, and the Council on Clinical Cardiology, Council on Cardiovascular Surgery and Anesthesia, and the Quality of Care and Outcomes Research Interdisciplinary Working Group. *Circulation*. 2007;116(15):1736-1754.
3. Habib G, Hoen B, Tornos P, et al. Guidelines on the prevention, diagnosis, and treatment of infective endocarditis (new version 2009): the task force on the prevention, diagnosis, and treatment of infective endocarditis of the European Society of Cardiology (ESC). *Eur Heart J.* 2009;30(19):2369-2413.
4. Gould FK, Elliott TS, Foweraker J, et al. Guidelines for the prevention of endocarditis: report of the Working Party of the British Society for Antimicrobial Chemotherapy. *J Antimicrob Chemother*. 2006;57(6):1035-1042.
5. Richey R, Wray D, Stokes T. Prophylaxis against infective endocarditis: summary of NICE guidance. *BMJ.* 2008;336(7647):770-771.

7 Surgical Site Infection Prophylaxis

Amish Ajit Dangodara

7.1 Introduction

- Surgical site infection (SSI) is one of the most common hospital-acquired infections, occurring in up to 5% of clean extra-abdominal surgeries and in up to 20% of intra-abdominal surgeries.[1] It is defined as an infection at the site of surgery that occurs within 30 days after surgery or within 1 year if a foreign body was implanted during surgery.
- Although there are a number of patient-specific risk factors, the type of surgery is the primary risk factor and determines the need for prophylactic antibiotics.
- This chapter reviews the risk factors and recommendations for antibiotic prophylaxis to reduce SSI. Other prophylactic measures to prevent endocarditis, pneumonia, and aspiration are covered elsewhere.

7.2 Patient-Specific Risk Factors

- Medical co-morbidities such as older age, smoking, malnutrition, morbid obesity, poorly controlled diabetes, HIV or AIDS, hypogammaglobulinemia, asplenism, immunocompromised states, active infection, high ASA Class or APACHE score, and prolonged length of stay can all contribute to increased risk of postoperative infection and impaired wound healing. Skin colonization is also a risk factor for SSI.
- Table 7.1 lists patient characteristics associated with surgical site infection. Although most are not modifiable, the risk of SSI may be reduced by:

A.A. Dangodara
UCI Medical Center, UCI Hospitalist Program, University of California,
Irvine, College of Medicine, 101 The City Drive South, Building 26,
Room 1006, Orange, CA 92868, USA
e-mail: aadangod@uci.edu

S.L. Cohn (ed.), *Perioperative Medicine*,
DOI: 10.1007/978-0-85729-498-2_7,

Table 7.1 Characteristics affecting risk for surgical site infection

Patient	Surgical
• Older age • Diabetes mellitus • Cigarette smoking • Immunosuppressive therapy (steroids, DMARDS, immune drugs for transplants, chemotherapy, radiation therapy) • Immunocompromised states (HIV, malignancy) • Malnutrition/cachexia • Obesity • Prolonged preoperative length of hospital stay • Preoperative bacterial colonization (Staphylococcus aureus in nares) • Co-existent active or recent infection at another site • Preoperative transfusion	*Preoperative* • Antiseptic showering • Hair removal (shaving) • Skin prep in or • Handwashing • Infected/colonized or personnel • Antibiotic prophylaxis (inappropriate timing) *Intraoperative* • Or environment (ventilation, environmental surfaces) • Instrument sterilization • Surgical attire • Asepsis and surgical technique *Postoperative* • Incision care • Wound hematoma/contamination • Discharge planning

  - Smoking cessation for >1 month
  - Intensive preoperative nutrition in a patient with moderate to severe malnutrition (enteral is usually preferred and surgery need not be postponed for this purpose)
  - Modest weight reduction (however, very low calorie diets to achieve this goal should not be prescribed just before surgery)
  - Improved glucose control in poorly controlled diabetics
  - Consulting specialist physicians treating the patient to modify immunosuppressant medications as necessary

- Recent or active co-existent infections may seed or infect joint prostheses or endovascular grafts and should be treated prior to surgery.
- Skin colonization with *Staphylococcus*, and increasingly, community-acquired methicillin-resistant *Staphylococcus aureus* (MRSA), can be minimized with proper patient skin preparation.
  - Cleansing of the skin twice with chlorhexidine gluconate-based solutions is more effective at reducing pathologic colonization than alcohol or iodine-based solutions.
  - Minimize colonization by avoiding shaving with razors near the surgical site before surgery. If hair removal is necessary, use clippers or depilatory agents.

7.3 Surgery-Specific Risk Factors

- Surgical site infections are specific to the type of surgery. Surgical risk factors are listed in Table 7.1.
- Surgical wound types[2] can be classified as clean, clean-contaminated, contaminated, or infected (see Table 7.2).
- Aseptic technique requires proper hand and nail hygiene to minimize SSI. Scrub brushes may actually increase the risk of infection as a result of skin damage. Soap and water should be used for the first scrub of the day, followed by a nail pick to clean under the nails, and then an alcohol gel which can be repeated between cases.[3]
  - Soiled hands should be washed with soap and water for minimum of 15 s.
  - Alcohol-based rubs containing ethanol, isopropanol, or *n*-propanol are more effective than either chlorhexidine gluconate or iodine-based scrubs for reducing bacterial colony-forming units on the hands of surgeons and should be used for 3 min.
  - Nail length should be less than 6 mm without chipped or peeling nail polish, or artificial nails.
  - Sterile powder-free gloves are more effective at reducing SSI compared to others.

Table 7.2 Surgical wound classification

Class I: clean	An uninfected operative wound in which no inflammation is encountered and the respiratory, alimentary, genital, or uninfected urinary tract is not entered. In addition, clean wounds are primarily closed and, if necessary, drained with closed drainage. Operative incisional wounds that follow nonpenetrating (blunt) trauma should be included in this category if they meet the criteria
Class II: clean-contaminated	An operative wound in which the respiratory, alimentary, genital, or urinary tracts are entered under controlled conditions and without unusual contamination. Specifically, operations involving the biliary tract, appendix, vagina, and oropharynx are included in this category, provided no evidence of infection or major break in technique is encountered
Class III: contaminated	Open, fresh, accidental wounds. In addition, operations with major breaks in sterile technique (e.g., open cardiac massage) or gross spillage from the gastrointestinal tract, and incisions in which acute, nonpurulent inflammation is encountered are included in this category
Class IV: dirty-infected	Old traumatic wounds with retained devitalized tissue and those that involve existing clinical infection or perforated viscera. This definition suggests that the organisms causing postoperative infection were present in the operative field before the operation

Source: From Mangram et al.[2]

- Intraoperative care should also maintain optimal blood pressure, temperature, oxygenation, and glucose control.
- Minimize blood transfusions (trigger should be 7–8 g/dL assuming adequate cardiopulmonary function).
- Postoperatively, wound contamination may require extended prophylactic antibiotics, avoidance of wound closure, irrigation of the wound, or frequent excisional debridement to reduce the risk of SSI. Wound hematomas or oozing from the wound can become secondarily infected with *Staphylococcus aureus* and extended antibiotic therapy may become warranted.
- Keeping the surgical dressing dry and intact for the first 24–48 h minimizes the risk of SSI.

7.4 Prophylactic Antibiotics: Choice, Timing, and Number of Doses

- The Surgical Infection Prevention (SIP) and Surgical Care Improvement Project (SCIP)[4,,5] are national initiatives to improve outcome for patients having surgery. In conjunction with various specialty societies, these projects have issued guidelines for antibiotic prophylaxis based on the surgical procedure. Institutional data regarding the appropriateness of antibiotic, administration within the proper time interval before surgery, and discontinuation within 24 h is publicly reportable and available on the web.
- Appropriate use of prophylactic antibiotics can significantly reduce the incidence of SSIs.[6] Tables 7.3 and 7.4 list the surgery-specific recommendations for antibiotic prophylaxis from CMS and SCIP.[1,4,5,7]
- The *choice of antibiotic* should be based on the most likely infecting organisms.
  - For most procedures, a first-generation cephalosporin (e.g., cefazolin) which is active against staphylococci and streptococci is usually effective.
  - For intra-abdominal procedures (gastrointestinal and gynecologic) where exposure to bowel anaerobes is possible, a second-generation cephalosporin (e.g., cefoxitin) or a cephalosporin plus metronidazole are preferred. For colorectal surgery and hysterectomy, ampicillin–sulbactam was recently added as an acceptable antibiotic.
  - Where MRSA is a frequent pathogen, vancomycin can be used. Screening for MRSA and decolonization with intranasal mupirocin is controversial but recommended by the Society of Thoracic Surgeons.[8]
- The *timing of administration* of prophylaxis is crucial.[9] The goal is to have therapeutic serum and tissue levels at the time of the skin incision.
  - Most prophylactic antibiotics should be administered within 30–60 min before the initial skin incision.
  - If vancomycin or quinolones infusions are being used, they should be given within 2 h before skin incision.

Table 7.3 CMS/SCIP requirements for inpatients

Surgical procedure	Approved antibiotics	If b-lactam allergy
CABG, other cardiac or vascular	Cefazolin, cefuroxime or Vancomycin**	Vancomycin** or clindamycin
Hip/knee arthroplasty	Cefazolin, cefuroxime or Vancomycin**	Vancomycin** or clindamycin
Colon	Cefotetan, cefoxitin, Ampicillin/sulbactam, or Ertapenem or Cefazolin or Cefuroxime + metronidazole	Clindamycin + aminoglycoside or Clindamycin + quinolone** or Clindamycin + aztreonam or Metronidazole + aminoglycoside or Metronidazole + quinolone**
Hysterectomy	Cefotetan, cefazolin, cefoxitin, cefuroxime or Ampicillin/sulbactam	Clindamycin + aminoglycoside or Clindamycin + quinolone** or Clindamycin + aztreonam or Metronidazole + aminoglycoside or Metronidazole + quinolone**

Source: Adapted from Bratzler and Houck[4]
Dose of antibiotics should be adjusted for patient weight and renal clearance
Preoperative prophylactic antibiotic to be administered within 1 h prior to incision.
**Two hours for Vancomycin or Fluoroquinolones
Administration of antibiotics for more than 24 h after the incision is closed offers no additional benefit to the surgical patient. DOCUMENTATION REQUIRED FOR THERAPEUTIC ANTIBIOTICS

  - In general, for procedures lasting <4 h, a *single preoperative dose* of antibiotic should be sufficient. One or two postoperative doses may be given for prolonged procedures or for specific surgeries; however, antibiotic prophylaxis should be *discontinued no later than 24 h after the surgery*. Note that the Society for Thoracic Surgeons guidelines[8] permit antibiotic prophylaxis to be acceptable for up to 48 h after surgery.

- Discharge Care
  - Educate patients, family members, and care givers about post-discharge care of the surgical site.
  - Stress handwashing and use of protective gloves.
  - Provide adequate supplies for postoperative wound care.

Table 7.4 CMS – SCIP requirements for outpatients

Surgical procedure	Approved antibiotics	If β-lactam allergy
Cardiac (Pacemakers or AICDs) or vascular	Cefazolin, cefuroxime or Vancomycin**	Vancomycin** or Clindamycin**
Orthopedic/Podiatry	Cefazolin, cefuroxime or Vancomycin**	Vancomycin** or Clindamycin
Gastric/Biliary PEG placement, PEG revision	Cefazolin or cefuroxime, cefoxitin or cefotetan or Ampicillin/sulbactam or (Cefazolin or cefuroxime)+ metronidazole	Clindamycin + aminoglycoside or Clindamycin + quinolone** or Vancomycin + aminoglycoside** or Vancomycin + quinolone**
Genitourinary Transrectal prostate biopsy	Quinolone** or Second-generation cephalosporin or Third-generation cephalosporin or Aminoglycoside + metronidazole or Aminoglycoside + clindamycin or Aztreonam + metronidazole or Aztreonam + clindamycin	
Genitourinary Penile prosthesis insertion, removal, revision	Ampicillin/sulbactam or ticarcillin/clavulanate or Pipercillin/tazobactam or Aminoglycoside + first-generation cephalosporin or Aminoglycoside + second-generation cephalosporin or Aminoglycoside + vancomycin** or Aminoglycoside + clindamycin or Aztreonam + first-generation cephalosporin or Aztreonam + second-generation cephalosporin or Aztreonam + vancomycin** or Aztreonam + clindamycin	

Table 7.4 (continued)

Surgical procedure	Approved antibiotics	If β-lactam allergy
Gynecological Pubovaginal sling	First-generation cephalosporin or Second-generation cephalosporin or Ampicillin/sulbactam or Quinolone**	Aminoglycoside + clindamycin or Aminoglycoside + metronidazole or Aztreonam + clindamycin or Aztreonam + metronidazole
Gynecological Laparoscopically assisted hysterectomy, vaginal hysterectomy	Cefazolin or cefuroxime, cefoxitin or cefotetan or ampicillin/sulbactam	Metronidazole + aminoglycoside or Metronidazole + quinolone** or Clindamycin + aminoglycoside or Clindamycin + aztreonam or Clindamycin + quinolone**
Head and neck	Cefazolin or cefuroxime	Clindamycin + aminoglycoside
Neurological	Nafcillin or oxacillin, cefazolin or cefuroxime	Vancomycin** or Clindamycin

Source: Adapted from Bratzler and Houck[4]
Dose of antibiotics should be adjusted for patient weight and renal clearance. Preoperative prophylactic antibiotic to be administered within 1 h prior to incision.
**Two hours for Vancomycin or Fluoroquinolones
Administration of prophylactic antibiotics for more than 24 h after the incision is closed offers no additional benefit to the surgical patient. DOCUMENTATION REQUIRED FOR THERAPEUTIC ANTIBIOTICS

References

1. Bratzler DW, Hunt DR. The surgical infection prevention and surgical care improvement projects: national initiatives to improve outcomes for patients having surgery. *Clin Infect Dis*. 2006;43(3):322-330; Epub 2006 Jun 16. PMID: 16804848.
2. Mangram AJ, Horan TC, Pearson ML, et al. Guideline for prevention of surgical site infection, 1999. Centers for Disease Control and Prevention (CDC) Hospital Infection Control Practices Advisory Committee. *Am J Infect Control*. 1999;27(2):97-132; quiz 133-134; discussion 96. PMID: 10196487.
3. Tanner J, Swarbrook S, Stuart J. Surgical hand antisepsis to reduce surgical site infection. *Cochrane Database Syst Rev*. 2008;(1):CD004288.

4. Bratzler DW, Houck PM. Surgical infection prevention guidelines writers workgroup. Antimicrobial prophylaxis for surgery: an advisory statement from the national surgical infection prevention project. *Clin Infect Dis*. 2004;38(12):1706-1715; Epub 2004 May 26. PMID: 15227616.
5. The Surgical Care Improvement Project (SCIP). MedQIC Website. https://www.qualitynet.org/dcs/ContentServer?c=MQParents&pagename=Medqic%2FContent%2FParentShellTemplate&cid=1228694349383&parentName=Category. Accessed September 21, 2010.
6. Bratzler DW, Ma A, Nsa W. Surgical care improvement project adherence and postoperative infections. *JAMA*. 2010;304(15):1670; author reply 1671-1672. PMID: 20959574.
7. Antimicrobial prophylaxis for surgery. *Treat Guidel Med Lett*. 2009;7(82):47-52.
8. Engelman R, Shahian D, Shemin R, et al. The Society of Thoracic Surgeons practice guideline series: antibiotic prophylaxis in cardiac surgery, part II: antibiotic choice. *Ann Thorac Surg*. 2007;83(4):1569-1576.
9. Weber WP, Marti WR, Zwahlen M, et al. The timing of surgical antimicrobial prophylaxis. *Ann Surg*. 2008;247(6):918-926. PMID: 18520217.

Anesthesiology for the Nonanesthesiologist

8

Vivek K. Moitra and Rebecca S. Twersky

8.1 Definition of Anesthesia

- The practice of modern anesthesiology provides the "5 As" of anesthesia (analgesia, anxiolysis, autonomic stability, amnesia, and areflexia – decreased motor responsiveness) to patients through a pharmacologically induced and reversible state.
- Anesthesiologists administer intravenous and inhalational agents to render patients unconscious and decrease the stress response to surgery.
- Patients who experience anesthesia during surgery will have their vital signs monitored and protected, their acute and chronic pain managed, and their critical care issues treated.

8.2 American Society of Anesthesiologists – Physical Status Classification (ASA-PS)

- The ASA-PS classification, a subjective scale (1–6), considers a patient's comorbidities to estimate risk, including death (Table 8.1).
- Patient's with the following conditions should be medically evaluated and optimized before the day of surgery:
  - ASA-PS classification ≥3
  - Noncompliant with medications
  - Poorly controlled hypertension
  - Poorly controlled seizures
  - Symptomatic asthma, chronic obstructive lung disease, active pulmonary conditions
  - Morbid obesity (Body mass index >35 kg/m^2)
  - Obstructive sleep apnea

V.K. Moitra (✉)
Department of Anesthesiology, Division of Critical Care, College of Physicians and Surgeons of Columbia University, 630 West 168th St, New York, NY 10032, USA
e-mail: vm2161@columbia.edu

S.L. Cohn (ed.), *Perioperative Medicine*,
DOI: 10.1007/978-0-85729-498-2_8, © Springer-Verlag London Limited 2011

Table 8.1 ASA classification system

ASA class	Description	Examples
I	Normal, healthy patient	Healthy patient with good exercise tolerance
II	A patient with one or two mild systemic diseases that are well controlled	Controlled HTN, obesity, controlled DM, asthma, extremes in age, alcohol use, seizure disorder, cancer
III	A patient with multiple systemic diseases that affect activity but is not incapacitating	Poorly controlled HTN, morbid obesity with cardiac or pulmonary involvement, stroke, metastatic carcinoma with end organ damage, DM with end organ disease, ESRD
IV	Severe systemic disease, incapacitating that is a constant threat to life	Unstable angina, CHF, advanced pulmonary, hepatic or renal dysfunction
V	Moribund patient not expected to live 24 h with or without the procedure	Ruptured abdominal aortic aneurysm
E	Modifier added to any of the above classes to signify a procedure that is being performed as an emergency, and may be associated with a suboptimal opportunity for risk assessment	

  - History of myocardial infarction or angina
  - History of stroke
  - Diabetes requiring insulin or HbA1c >8
  - Active alcohol and/or drug abuse
  - End organ dysfunction

8.3 The Role of the Anesthesiologist and Other Health Care Providers

- Throughout the perioperative period, the anesthesiologist evaluates and manages the patient and stratifies organ risks including major adverse cardiac events (MACE), pulmonary complications such as aspiration, and postoperative renal injury.
- Intraoperatively, the anesthesiologist ensures oxygenation and ventilation via airway management; monitors and manages hemodynamic variables such as heart rate, blood pressure, and cardiac output; administers fluids, blood products, and diuretics; evaluates cerebral perfusion; and documents this course in the anesthesia record.
- The anesthesiologist practices in preoperative medicine clinics, the operating room, intensive care units, surgery offices, labor and delivery suites, free standing ambulatory surgical centers, and remote locations such as radiology, endoscopy, and cardiac suites.

- Anesthesia assistants and certified registered nurse anesthetists (CRNAs) administer anesthesia under the direction and supervision of an anesthesiologist.

8.4 Airway Management

- The anesthesiologist evaluates and measures mouth opening, neck circumference, tongue size, range of motion of the cervical spine, the distance between the mandible and the thyroid cartilage, upper airway anatomy, and dentition.
- The modified Mallampati classification describes the visualized portions of the oropharyngeal airway with the patient's mouth open and tongue protruded, and is used to predict difficulty with intubation (Fig. 8.1).[1]
- A dental examination assesses loose teeth, dental prostheses, and infection. Preoperative documentation of missing or chipped teeth prevents erroneous attribution of dental damage to laryngoscopy.
- Difficulty with intubation has been observed in the following conditions:
  - Mallampati classification 3 and 4
  - Limited range of motion of the cervical spine
  - Small mouth opening
  - Congenital facial and airway anatomical abnormalities
  - Poor dentition and prominent incisors
  - Micrognathia
  - Macroglossia

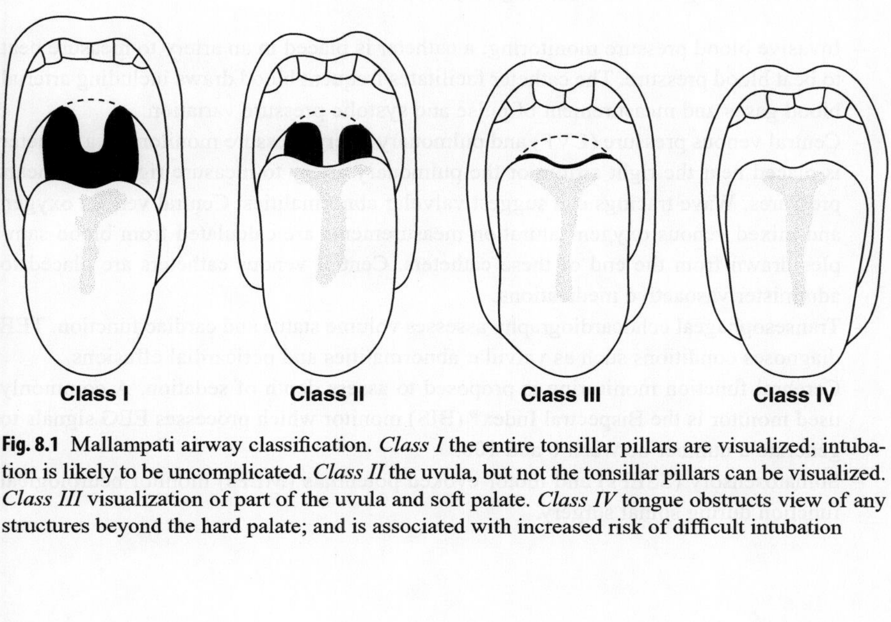

Fig. 8.1 Mallampati airway classification. *Class I* the entire tonsillar pillars are visualized; intubation is likely to be uncomplicated. *Class II* the uvula, but not the tonsillar pillars can be visualized. *Class III* visualization of part of the uvula and soft palate. *Class IV* tongue obstructs view of any structures beyond the hard palate; and is associated with increased risk of difficult intubation

- Short neck
- Obesity
- Patients with a history of head and neck cancer
- Infections such as epiglottitis and Ludwig's angina
- Scleroderma
- Rheumatoid arthritis
- Previous history of difficult intubation

- Endotracheal intubation through the vocal cords is the most predictable method to ensure oxygenation and ventilation, facilitate positive pressure ventilation, and prevent aspiration.
- A laryngeal mask airway (LMA), a supraglottic airway device (it does not pass through the vocal cords) does not prevent aspiration of gastric contents. Patients spontaneously ventilate through an LMA. When intubation is difficult, an LMA can be placed to "rescue" the airway.
- Anesthesiologists manage the airway with devices such as fiberoptic bronchoscopes, fast-track LMAs, video laryngoscopy devices, and Combi-tubes.

8.5 Monitoring

- During administration of anesthesia, ASA standard monitors evaluate oxygenation, ventilation, circulation, and temperature (see Table 8.2).
- Stimulating a peripheral nerve and measuring motor response ("twitch") monitors pharmacologically induced neuromuscular blockade.
- Additional intraoperative monitoring may include:
  - Invasive blood pressure monitoring: a catheter is placed in an artery to measure beat to beat blood pressure. The catheter facilitates frequent blood draws including arterial blood gases and measurement of pulse and systolic pressure variation.
  - Central venous pressure (CVP) and pulmonary artery pressure monitoring: a catheter is placed near the right atrium or the pulmonary artery to measure right-sided heart pressures. Wave tracings can suggest valvular abnormalities. Central venous oxygen and mixed venous oxygen saturation measurements are calculated from blood samples drawn from the end of these catheters. Central venous catheters are placed to administer vasoactive medications.
  - Transesophageal echocardiography assesses volume status and cardiac function. TEE diagnoses conditions such as valvular abnormalities and pericardial effusions.
  - Cerebral function monitoring is proposed to assess depth of sedation. A commonly used monitor is the Bispectral Index® (BIS) monitor which processes EEG signals to generate a number between 0 and 100.
  - Somatosensory (SSEPs) and motor evoked potentials (MEPs) monitor neurological function during spinal surgery.

Table 8.2 ASA standards for basic anesthetic monitoring

Standard	Measurement	Equipment
Oxygenation	• Quantitative measurement of the oxygen concentration in the breathing circuit during general anesthesia • Quantitative assessment of patient's oxygenation	• Oxygen analyzer with low concentration limit alarm • Pulse oximetry
Ventilation	• Qualitative assessment of adequate ventilation • Verification of the correct positioning of an endotracheal tube or a laryngeal mask	• Exhaled CO2 monitoring during monitored anesthesia care (MAC), regional and general anesthesia • Continuous observation of qualitative clinical signs during all sedation/anesthesia. • Clinical assessment at time of insertion or capnography or capnometry
Circulation	• Electrocardiogram • Blood pressure • One other assessment of circulatory function	• ECG monitor (with automated ST segment analysis optional) • BP cuff, usually automated • Pulse oximetry
Body temperature	Continuous monitoring when clinically significant changes in body temperature are intended, anticipated, or suspected	• Temperature probe

8.6 Guidelines Commonly Used by Anesthesiologists

- Fasting guidelines:
  - Preoperative fasting guidelines (national and center specific) are followed to decrease the risk of preoperative aspiration.[2]
  - For elective procedures, adults should not eat fried or fatty food for 8 h before surgery, eat light food (toast) for 6 h before surgery, or drink clear liquids (nonparticulate: water, apple juice, tea, black coffee) for at least 2 h before surgery.
- Anesthesiologists follow guidelines and advisories for conditions such as preoperative evaluation of the cardiac patient for noncardiac surgery, perioperative OSA management, anticoagulation in regional anesthesia, drug eluting stents and antiplatelet therapy, and transfusions.[3-6]

8.7 Types of Anesthesia

- Anesthesiologists provide a pharmacologically induced continuum of sedation, which ranges from minimal sedation to general anesthesia.
- *Minimal sedation/analgesia:* Patients are responsive to verbal stimuli. Respiratory and cardiovascular function is unaffected.
- *Moderate sedation/analgesia:* Often classified as conscious sedation, patients respond to verbal and tactile stimuli. Spontaneous ventilation is usually adequate and cardiovascular function is maintained.
- *Deep sedation/analgesia:* The consciousness of patients is depressed, but patients can purposefully respond to painful stimulation. The anesthesiologist may support the patient's airway to ensure adequate ventilation. Cardiovascular function is usually unaffected.
- *General anesthesia:* Patients are unarousable to painful stimuli. Respiratory, airway, and cardiovascular function may be impaired and require the management of an anesthesiologist.
- *Monitored anesthesia care (MAC):* MAC does not reflect a continuum of sedation per se, rather MAC is a unique anesthetic service distinct from moderate sedation. An anesthesiologist assesses and manages a patient's physiologic or medical problems during a diagnostic or therapeutic procedure. While MAC includes administration of sedatives and/or analgesics, the provider is prepared and qualified to provide general anesthesia when necessary.
- *Regional anesthesia*: Local anesthetics are injected near a nerve to block the transmission of pain signals. Commonly injected sites include the epidural space, intrathecal space (spinal), brachial plexus, and the femoral nerve.

8.8 Pharmacological Agents

8.8.1 Inhalational Anesthetics

- Inhalation anesthetics (isoflurane, sevoflurane, and desflurane) render a patient immobile and amnestic. An advantage of these hypnotic agents administered via the lung is their quick onset, offset, and ease of titration.[7]
- Inhalational anesthesia is associated with a stable hemodynamic profile with little variation; however, vasodilatation, arrhythmias, inhibition of hypoxic pulmonary vasoconstriction, depression of cerebral metabolic rate with an increase in cerebral blood flow (CBF), and cardiac depression can occur.
- The term MAC (minimal alveolar concentration – to be distinguished from monitored anesthesia care) is the end-tidal concentration associated with a particular behavior such as immobility. MAC values differ for each inhaled anesthetic agents and reflect the potency of an anesthetic.

- Inhalation (volatile) anesthetics are bronchodilators and are prescribed as therapeutic agents for the treatment of bronchospasm and status asthmaticus.
- Nitrous oxide is a sedative and analgesic inhalational agent, which commonly is administered in the operating room and dental suites. Administration of nitrous oxide contributes to postoperative nausea and vomiting.

8.8.2 Propofol/Fospropofol

- Propofol is a potent sedative hypnotic, which produces moderate and deep sedation and general anesthesia and has no reversal agent. It causes respiratory depression and apnea.
- Propofol is not an analgesic and should not be prescribed to treat pain.
- The injection of propofol causes venous irritation.
- Because propofol is highly lipid soluble, it is suspended in a 20% fat emulsion that predisposes to infection (the drug must be handled aseptically), hypertriglyceridemia, and pancreatitis. Rarely, administration of high doses of propofol to a patient with shock causes intractable lactic acidosis and myocardial depression, the so-called propofol infusion syndrome (PRIS).
- Fospropofol is a sedative hypnotic pro-drug which is metabolized by the liver into propofol and induces general anesthesia. Compared to propofol, fospropofol's onset time and clinical effect is longer.

8.8.3 Barbiturates

- Barbiturates such as thiopental are short-acting hypnotic agents that induce anesthesia.
- Barbiturates decrease cerebral metabolic rate and cerebral blood flow and manage intracranial hypertension and seizure activity.
- Barbiturates are contraindicated for patients with inducible porphyrias.

8.8.4 Opioids

- Opioids bind mu receptors to decrease the sympathetic response to noxious stimuli such as surgery, drain insertion, and airway management.
- Failure to treat pain exacerbates endogenous catecholamine activity, which predisposes patients to myocardial ischemia, hypercoagulability, hypermetabolic states, sleep deprivation, and delirium.
- Bradycardia, hypotension, respiratory depression, nausea, and skeletal muscle rigidity are potential adverse effects of opioids.
- Opioids have different potencies (Table 8.3).
- Morphine and meperidine should not be prescribed to patients with chronic renal insufficiency because these drugs have active metabolites, which are renally eliminated. Since codeine is converted in vivo to morphine, it should not be administered to patients that have allergies to morphine.

Table 8.3 Opioids

Type	Opioid	Example	Parenteral	Oral
Naturally occurring	Morphine		10 mg	30 mg
	Hydromorphone	Dilaudid	1.5 mg	7.5 mg
Semisynthetic	Oxycodone	Oxycontin	–	30 mg
	Hydrocodone	Vicodin	–	30 mg
Synthetic	Meperidine	Demerol	100 mg	300 mg
	Fentanyl		0.1 μg	~0.4 μg (lozenge on a stick)
	Sufentanil		0.01–0.02 μg	
	Alfentanil		0.5–1 μg	–
	Remifentanil		0.1 μg	–

- Meperidine is administered in the PACU to decrease postoperative shivering. Excessive dosing of meperidine causes seizures.
- Avoidance of meperidine in patients who are taking monoamine-oxidase-inhibitors (MAOIs) prevents neuroleptic malignant syndrome.

8.8.5 Benzodiazepines

- Midazolam, an intravenous benzodiazepine, decreases anxiety and produces amnesia.
- Benzodiazepines decrease ventilatory drive and can cause respiratory insufficiency. This effect is potentiated during co-administration of opioids.
- Although amnesia is essential during general anesthesia in the operating room, the potent anterograde amnesia induced by benzodiazepines – even at sub-hypnotic doses – may predispose patients toward postoperative delirium with confusion and disorientation.
- Flumazenil (Romazicon) reverses benzodiazepine-induced sedation, but the duration of action of flumazenil is brief, and patients should be monitored for resedation.

8.8.6 Dexmedetomidine

- Dexmedetomidine, a highly selective agonist of the α_2-adrenoreceptor, sedates patients in the intensive care unit and the operating room. In contrast to gamma-amino-butyric acid (GABA) agonists, dexmedetomidine sedates without changes in respiratory rate, oxygen saturation, or arterial carbon dioxide tension. Unlike benzodiazepines, clinical doses of dexmedetomidine are not associated with anterograde amnesia. Patients are easily arousable from light levels of sedation and emerge without confusion or disorientation. When left undisturbed, they go back to their previous level of sedation.

Dexmedetomidine *produces* interactive or cooperative sedation and facilitates neurological examination.

- Dexmedetomidine suppresses shivering in patients during therapeutic hypothermia.

8.8.7
Ketamine

- Ketamine binds N-methyl-D-aspartate (NMDA) and sigma opioid receptors to produce intense analgesia.
- Ketamine's popularity has waned because of an undesirable side effect profile: hallucinations, delirium, lacrimation, tachycardia, and potential for an increase in intracranial pressure (ICP) and coronary ischemia.
- Under ketamine anesthesia, patients may appear dissociated from the environment, that is, they keep their eyes open and maintain their reflexes. Blood pressure is maintained and spontaneous breathing and laryngeal reflexes are preserved.
- Recent research suggests that lower doses of ketamine are not associated with untoward effects and may improve outcomes. Ketamine prevents opioid-induced hyperalgesia, decreases inflammation, and reduces bronchoconstriction.

8.8.8
Etomidate

- Etomidate is an induction agent, which has minimal effect on the cardiovascular system.
- Etomidate inhibits adrenocortical synthesis and there are concerns about using etomidate in patients who have relative adrenal insufficiency, i.e., septic patients.
- Among the undesired side effects are burning pain at the injection site, thrombophlebitis, myoclonus, and nausea/vomiting.

8.8.9
Neuromuscular Blocking Agents (Muscle Relaxants)

- Neuromuscular blocking agents do not provide sedation or analgesia.
- The effect of these agents is monitored with a peripheral nerve stimulator.
- Succinylcholine causes rapid muscle relaxation. It is metabolized by plasma cholinesterase (pseudocholinesterase) and has a short half-life.
- Patients who have a genetic variation or decreased activity of pseudocholinesterase experience prolonged apnea from neuromuscular blockade after administration of succinylcholine.
- Patients may experience myalgias after administration of succinylcholine.
- Cisatracurium, vecuronium, and rocuronium are intermediate-acting muscle relaxants with a duration of action of approximately 30 min.

8.8.10
Local Anesthetics and Regional Anesthesia

- Local anesthetics can be injected around nerves to prevent and relieve pain (regional anesthesia).
- The choice of local anesthesia is largely dependent on the medication's duration of action. For example, the effect of a bupivacaine injection can last for 8 h versus a chloroprocaine injection, which has duration of action of 45 min.
- Amino-esters include cocaine, procaine, 2-chloroprocaine, benzocaine, and tetracaine and account for more than 99% of allergic reactions to local anesthetic. Amide anesthetics include bupivacaine, ropivacaine, mepivacaine, and are generally not allergenic.
- Tetracaine and benzocaine can cause methemoglobinemia, even when administered topically.
- Ultrasound technology identifies anatomical landmarks and facilitates regional block placement.

8.9
Effects of Anesthesia on Organ Function and Inflammation

- The inflammatory response to surgery can range from mild hyperglycemia of no clinical consequence to the altered neuroendocrine responses to chronic critical illness. A cascade of stress responses is elicited, mediated by the release of various cytokines and stress hormones.[8]
- Leukocytosis without evidence of infection is common after surgery.
- When inflammation is severe, a systemic inflammatory response syndrome (SIRS) is observed.
- The metabolic consequences of surgery, characterized by elevations in circulating catecholamines, growth hormone, glucagon, and cortisol levels with a concomitant depression in insulin levels, promote hepatic glycogenolysis and gluconeogenesis. Hyperglycemia and insulin resistance marks this metabolic profile.

8.10
Organ Response to Surgery and Anesthesia

- Cardiac, respiratory, renal, hepatic, and cerebral functions are affected to a variable degree in all patients undergoing surgery. Organ dysfunction is often the final common pathway of a confluence of factors such as pre-existing organ dysfunction, low blood flow states, hypovolemia, atheromatous embolism, inflammation, ischemia reperfusion, genetic predisposition, and surgery specific techniques.

8.10.1 Cardiovascular Response

- Catecholamine levels rise with surgery. Tachycardia and hypertension are common during the perioperative period. An increase in sympathetic mediated activity causes coronary vasoconstriction and can induce plaque rupture via shear stress forces.[9]
- Volatile anesthetics cause hypotension via vasodilation and myocardial depression.
- Several studies of isoflurane, sevoflurane, and desflurane demonstrate that these agents afford cardioprotection through pharmacological "preconditioning."

8.10.2 Respiratory

- Atelectasis is common after general anesthesia. In the anesthetized patient, relaxation of the diaphragm and its cephalad movement increase pleural pressures, which compress adjacent lung tissue. In the delivery of intravenous or inhalational anesthesia to the mechanically ventilated patient, atelectasis can occur within 5 min of induction. The diaphragm is displaced cephalad by the abdominal contents, and gas flow is preferentially distributed to the nondependent regions of the lung.[10]
- Inspiring high concentrations of oxygen during the perioperative period can cause atelectasis. When the alveolar capillary concentration of oxygen gradient increases and the capillaries rapidly absorb oxygen, atelectasis follows.
- Heavy smokers with chronic bronchitis develop metaplasia of ciliated columnar epithelium to mucin-producing goblet cells. Cilia clearance of mucus and debris is impaired, surfactant production is diminished, and small airways and alveoli tend to collapse. Obesity causes a reduction in FRC and predisposes to atelectasis in the perioperative period. An increase in extravascular lung water, whether due to congestive heart failure or pulmonary edema, increases the tendency for small airways to collapse.
- Pulmonary vascular constriction in hypoxic lung regions is protective and prevents perfusion of unventilated alveoli. This response is inhibited by inhalational anesthetics.
- Patients with severe pulmonary disease are at risk for prolonged mechanical ventilation after high-risk surgeries where the likelihood of significant fluid shifts and hemodynamic compromise is high.

8.10.3 Renal

- Perioperative acute kidney injury (AKI), characterized by postoperative elevation of S_{Cr}, is uncommon. However, it has a predilection for certain surgical procedures, particularly vascular surgery involving aortic manipulation, where the incidence is between 10% and 25%.

- Although the renal medulla receives less than 10% of renal blood flow (RBF), the medullary process of urinary concentration has a high metabolic requirement. Any compromise to renal blood flow (RBF) increases the regional perfusion imbalance and renders the medulla ischemic.

8.10.4 Cerebral

- The anesthesiologist manages cerebral perfusion pressure (CPP) by monitoring mean arterial blood pressure (MAP) and intracranial pressure (ICP) or central venous pressure (CVP). CPP = MAP – ICP or CVP (whichever is higher).
- Because inhalational agents increase cerebral blood flow (CBF), these medications are deleterious in patients with elevated ICP.
- Propofol suppresses electroencephalogram activity and decreases seizure activity at high doses. Like barbiturates, propofol decreases cerebral metabolic rate and cerebral blood flow (CBF) to decrease intracranial pressure. Hypotension, from propofol-induced vasodilation, decreases cerebral perfusion pressure.
- Benzodiazepines are potent anticonvulsants that inhibit seizure activity when seizures are provoked via antagonism of the gamma-amino-butyric acid (GABA receptor. Benzodiazepines minimally affect ICP and CBF.
- Dexmedetomidine does not decrease intracranial pressure or affect seizure threshold.
- With the exception of morphine, opioids do not affect ICP or cerebral blood flow independent of carbon dioxide arterial tension.
- Sedatives and analgesics depress respiratory rate and cause hypercarbia. Hypercarbia increases intracranial pressure via cerebral vasodilation in at-risk patients. The benefits of sedative therapy to manage ICP, cerebral metabolic rate, and seizure threshold cannot be realized without intensive management of ventilation and avoidance of hypercarbia.

8.11 Anesthesia-Specific Issues

8.11.1 Postoperative Shivering

- Volatile anesthetics impair the thermoregulatory center to cause shivering.
- Patients can experience cardiac complications because oxygen consumption can increase by 400%.
- Medications such as meperidine and dexmedetomidine and forced warming systems decrease shivering and improve patient comfort.

8.11.2
Postoperative Nausea and Vomiting

- Patient characteristics (history of postoperative nausea and vomiting, female gender, nonsmoker), surgery type (laparoscopic, breast, gynecological, eye), and general anesthesia are risk factors for postoperative nausea and vomiting.[11]
- Patients who experience postoperative nausea and vomiting may have a delayed discharge from the postanesthesia care unit.
- Options for prophylaxis and treatment include: 5-HT3 receptor antagonists (i.e., odansetron), scopolamine, dexamethasone, propofol, and acupressure.

8.11.3
Malignant Hyperthermia (MH)

- Malignant hyperthermia is a rare, life-threatening disease, which follows exposure to triggering anesthetic medications (succinylcholine and volatile inhalational anesthetics) in genetically susceptible individuals.
- Patients with malignant hyperthermia have a significant increase in their intracellular calcium. Hypermetabolism, muscle rigidity, elevated creatine kinase, hypercarbia, tachycardia, arrhythmias, myoglobinuria, and fever are presenting symptoms. Death follows disseminated intravascular coagulation, high output congestive heart failure, and acute hyperkalemia.
- Dantrolene, a muscle relaxant that blocks release of calcium from the sarcoplasmic reticulum, is administered to patients with malignant hyperthermia. Additional treatment includes active cooling and correction of acid base, hematological, and hemodynamic abnormalities. Any facility that administers triggering agents (i.e., succinylcholine, inhalation agents) should have sufficient amounts of dantrolene on site.
- Muscle biopsy and genetic testing are ordered to identify patients at risk for malignant hyperthermia.

8.11.4
Anesthesia Awareness

- Rarely, patients experience anesthesia awareness under general anesthesia when they become conscious during surgery and have recall of intraoperative events.
- Potential risk factors for anesthesia awareness include: previous history of awareness; substance abuse or chronic opioid use; trauma; cardiac, obstetric, and emergency surgery; reduced anesthetic doses in the presence of paralysis; and limited hemodynamic reserve.
- Monitoring depth of anesthesia includes ASA standard monitoring and evaluation of clinical signs. The role of brain function monitoring in preventing awareness is still being researched.

8.11.5
Transfusion Therapy

- The decision to transfuse packed red blood cells, fresh frozen plasma, platelets, and cryoprecipitate is controversial (see Chaps. 23 and 41). The ASA has developed a practice guideline for perioperative transfusions.[5]
- If hemoglobin levels are greater than 10 g/dL, patients are rarely transfused. Most patients are transfused when hemoglobin levels are less than 6 g/dL. Monitoring and assessing oxygen delivery and utilization and organ perfusion guide transfusion practices.
- "Cell saver" (blood collected from the surgical site and given back to the patient), acute normovolemic hemodilution (ANH) (blood withdrawn immediately before surgery and replaced with crystalloid or colloid solutions), and preoperative autologous donation of whole blood can reduce the incidence of allogenic transfusion.

8.11.6
The Do Not Resuscitate (DNR) Patient

- End of life care is complex and must consider cultural, religious, personal, and philosophical beliefs. Documentation of discussions among the patient, their surrogate or health care proxy, the surgeon, the primary care physician, and the anesthesiologist should be placed in the chart.
- Because intraoperative care could be considered "resuscitation," clarification of goals of care should be established preoperatively.
- During the perioperative period, DNR orders can be suspended, and resuscitation such as not performing chest compressions or defibrillation can be limited.

References

1. Practice guidelines for management of the difficult airway. An update report by the American Society of Anesthesiologists Task Force on management of the difficult airway. *Anesthesiology*. 2003;98:1269-1277.
2. Warner MA, Caplan RA, Epstein BS, et al. Practice guidelines for preoperative fasting and the use of pharmacologic agents to reduce the risk of pulmonary aspiration: application to healthy patients undergoing elective procedures-a report by the American Society of Anesthesiologists task force on preoperative fasting. *Anesthesiology*. 1999;90:896-905.
3. Fleisher LA, Beckman JA, Brown KA, et al. ACC/AHA 2007 guidelines on perioperative cardiovascular evaluation and care for noncardiac surgery: executive summary. *Circulation*. 2007;116:1971-1996.
4. Gross J, Bachenberg K, Bellingham WA, et al. Practice guidelines for the perioperative management of patients with obstructive sleep apnea. *Anesthesiology*. 2006;104:1081-1093.
5. American Society of Anesthesiologists Task Force on Blood Component Therapy. Practice guidelines for blood component therapy. *Anesthesiology*. 1996;84:732-747.

6. Horlocker TT, Wedel DJ, Rowlingson JC, et al. Executive summary: regional anesthesia in the patient receiving antithrombotic or thrombolytic therapy. *Reg Anesth Pain Med.* 2010;35:102-105.
7. Campagna JA, Miller KW, Forman SA. Mechanisms of actions of inhaled anesthetics. *N Engl J Med.* 2003;348:2110-2124.
8. Desborough JP. The stress response to trauma and surgery. *Br J Anaesth.* 2000;85:109-117.
9. De Hert SG. Volatile anesthetics and cardiac function. *Semin Cardiothorac Vasc Anesth.* 2006;10:33-42.
10. Duggan M, Kavanagh BP. Pulmonary atelectasis: a pathogenic perioperative entity. *Anesthesiology.* 2005;102:838-854.
11. Gan TJ, Meyer T, Apfel CC, et al. Society for Ambulatory Anesthesia guidelines for the management of postoperative nausea and vomiting. *Anesth Analg.* 2007;105:1615-1628.

Part II

Surgery-Specific Risks

Abdominal Surgery

9

Brian Woods

9.1 Introduction

Abdominal surgeries cover a broad spectrum of operations ranging from relatively low-risk procedures, such as elective herniorrhaphy and cholecystectomy, to major high-risk procedures such as pancreatectomy and emergency laparotomy for bowel obstruction, perforation, or bleeding. Patients undergoing abdominal procedures often have multiple comorbidities that need to be optimized to prevent postoperative complications or ameliorate prolonged recovery.

9.2 Preoperative Considerations

- Intra-abdominal pathology can affect every organ system and complicate the anesthetic, the operation, and the postoperative course. Evaluation for abdominal surgery should be initiated with consideration of the organ in question – for example, in appendicitis, has the patient been vomiting or anorexic acutely? Are there signs of systemic inflammation? In the case of bowel neoplasm, has the patient become anemic, had bowel obstruction, or been taking opiates chronically for pain?
- Various patient-related risk factors and metabolic derangement are associated with surgical abdominal pathology (see Table 9.1).
- Preoperative bowel preparation, nausea, and vomiting can acutely or chronically alter volume status, acid-base balance, electrolyte serum levels, and glucose.
- Volume-contracted patients are less able to tolerate anesthesia induction, positive pressure ventilation, and the fluid shifts that result from inflammation and surgical trauma. Correct fluid and electrolyte abnormalities preoperatively if time permits.

B. Woods
Department of Anesthesia, Columbia University College of Physicians and Surgeons, 630 W 168th St, PH 527B New York, NY 10032, USA
e-mail: bw2284@columbia.edu

S.L. Cohn (ed.), *Perioperative Medicine*,
DOI: 10.1007/978-0-85729-498-2_9, © Springer-Verlag London Limited 2011

Table 9.1 Specific preoperative and intraoperative concerns in the abdominal surgery patient

Cardiac	Arrhythmia with CO_2 insufflation Bradycardia with peritoneal stretch Tachycardia from pain or hypovolemia Vascular injury from trochar insertion
Hematologic	Acute versus chronic anemia Adverse transfusion reactions (TACO, TRIM, TRALI, sepsis, hemolysis) Coagulopathies (intrinsic or iatrogenic)
Metabolic	Hypovolemia Hypokalemia Hypo- or hyperglycemia Acidosis or alkalosis Protein malnourishment Acute or chronic kidney injury
Neurologic	Acute and chronic pain Opiate tolerance
Respiratory	Splinting Hypoventilation Hypoxia and atelectasis Aspiration

- Malnutrition, grossly assessed by exam or by albumin levels, has significant implications for perioperative complications including overall patient reserve, wound healing, pneumonia, and survival. Preoperative total parenteral alimentation may improve some outcomes in patients with protein malnourishment.
- Anemia frequently coexists with abdominal pathology, both acutely and chronically. Consideration of how rapidly the anemia developed and how the patient has compensated for the anemia help the perioperative clinician decide how much further anemia could be tolerated and what threshold the individual patient should have for transfusion. The critical care literature provides evidence that lower (Hgb of 7 g/dL) RBC concentrations are tolerated without apparent complication; however, this trial was not conducted specifically on perioperative patients and excluded those with chronic anemia (see Chap. 41).
  - Red blood cell transfusion is not a benign intervention, and the benefit of an increased hemoglobin concentration with improved oxygen delivery should be weighed against possible acidosis and hyperkalemia, fluid overload (transfusion associated circulatory overload or TACO), transfusion-related immunomodulation (TRIM), and transfusion related acute lung injury (TRALI).

- The incidence of pneumonia is higher in patients receiving blood transfusion. Older blood probably conveys more risk and less benefit to the patient because of RBC breakdown and metabolic alterations that increase within the transfusion unit over time.
- Obesity complicates abdominal surgery on multiple fronts. Certain abdominal surgical diseases are more common in the obese, for example, cholecystitis and gynecologic tumors. Abdominal obesity can obscure the physical exam and degrade or even prevent diagnostic imaging. Diabetes, liver disease, sleep apnea, and cardiopulmonary disease are common in the obese. Depression is associated with obesity and pain tolerance may be altered. Airway management might be more difficult in the obese, and blood vessel catheterization can be challenging. Patient positioning for surgery requires particular care to avoid pressure wounds or peripheral nerve injury. Laparotomy or laparoscopy can be more difficult, and wound healing less optimal. The preoperative approach to the obese patient should focus on optimizing the known comorbidities as well as eliciting and managing the undiagnosed, for example, sleep apnea, glucose intolerance, or cardiovascular disease.

9.3 Surgical Approaches

- Laparotomy is the oldest technique for abdominal surgery. Laparoscopy has become widespread and is, for some procedures, a new gold standard, including cholecystectomy. Both techniques offer advantages and disadvantages (see Table 9.2).

Table 9.2 Common laparoscopic procedures

General surgery	Appendectomy Bowel resection Cholecystectomy Gastroesophagectomy Hepatic resection Hernia repair – inguinal, ventral, umbilical Nissen fundoplication Splenectomy Whipple
Gynecologic	Hysterectomy Oophorectomy-salpingectomy Ovarian cystectomy
Genitourinary	Cystectomy Nephrectomy and kidney harvest Prostatectomy

- Patients who have had abdominal surgery in the area of interest, who are unstable, or who would not tolerate abdominal insufflation (see below) often undergo laparotomy instead. Pregnancy is not a contraindication to laparoscopy per se.
- Because carbon dioxide (CO_2) pneumoperitoneum causes profound physiologic changes, patients with cardiorespiratory disease must be optimized to the extent possible before surgery.
- Typically CO_2 pneumoperitoneum at a pressure of 15 mmHg is introduced, which immediately alters ventilation and can decrease lung function residual capacity (FRC). Peak and mean inspiratory pressures rise and tidal volumes fall. Arterial pCO_2 rises as a result of altered ventilation and CO_2 absorption from the abdomen. This rise decreases arterial pH, with its multiple effects on vascular tone, the myocardium, and other systems.
- Cardiovascular effects include reduced venous return decreasing cardiac output, and increased systemic and pulmonary vascular resistance, probably because of elevated pCO_2. Cardiac arrhythmia can occur, particularly during insufflation; bradycardia from vagal stimulation by peritoneal stretch is not uncommon.
- Renal and hepatic perfusion are altered by the increased intra-abdominal pressure; urine output can fall, particularly if the renal perfusion pressure (MAP – IAP) is low, as in the setting of intra-abdominal hypertension.
- Because intracranial pressure (ICP) can increase from abdominal insufflation, laparoscopy may be contraindicated in some patients with CNS pathology. Patient positioning to extremes of head down or head up are often used during laparoscopy, again having significant cardiorespiratory and ICP effects. Ventriculoperitoneal shunts may require clamping during pneumoperitoneum.
- Insufflation can cause reflux of stomach contents; therefore the airway must be secured.

9.4 Anesthetic Considerations

- Primary concerns for the anesthetist with any surgery are patient safety and comfort. Airway and ventilation control, venous access, and perioperative pain management are all important parts of any anesthetic technique. The needs of the patient and the surgeon must be combined under this rubric.
- Simply because the team anticipates a procedure under monitored anesthesia care (MAC) or regional anesthesia does not obviate possible conversion to general anesthesia; every patient should be approached as if requiring a general anesthetic.
- For abdominal procedures, patients with nausea, vomiting, or obstructive processes, or patients presenting acutely are considered to have a full stomach. Therefore rapidly securing the airway against gastric content aspiration, or maintaining the patient's native protection against this, is paramount. Patients in whom difficulty securing the airway (obesity, sleep apnea, challenging-appearing airway exam, history of difficult intubation, for example) is anticipated may require awake intubation.
- The anesthetic is tailored to the patient, the surgery, and the preferences of all involved. Options include monitored anesthesia care (or sedation with an anesthetist present), regional anesthesia (peripheral nerve block or neuraxial), and general anesthesia.

– Superficial procedures can be performed under MAC with local anesthesia. Examples include inguinal hernias and some abdominal wall procedures, e.g., lipoma excisions. Small, targeted procedures such as laparoscopic fallopian tube surgery have been done under local anesthetic.
– Deeper procedures can be done under regional anesthesia (peripheral nerve blocks, paravertebral blocks, spinals, and epidurals). Regional anesthesia can be complicated by patchy block and hypotension, among other problems. Anticoagulation, either spontaneous or iatrogenic, can contraindicate regional techniques. Intraperitoneal procedures typically are done under general anesthesia in current practice, although lower abdominal procedures can be done by neuraxial blockade, for example, Cesarean section and open appendectomies.

• If significant bleeding is expected, then adequate venous access and blood products are necessary.

9.5 Postoperative Considerations

Primary goals are hemodynamic, respiratory, and neurologic stability along with pain control (see Table 9.3).

• Some anesthetic techniques, including regional anesthetics, can be continued or offered in the postoperative period to decrease pain as well as improve gas exchange and patient mobility. Current practice emphasizes a multimodal approach to pain extending beyond the use of opiates.
  – Opiates themselves are associated with respiratory depression, ileus, and delirium. Alternatives or supplements such as acetaminophen, NSAIDs, ketamine, and regional anesthetic techniques should be considered.
  – Behavioral interventions and early mobilization probably help with patients' coping mechanisms and perception of pain.
  – Patient-controlled anesthesia (PCA) has been shown to decrease pain scores and increase patient satisfaction when compared to PRN nurse-administered parenteral opiates.
  – Dexmedetomidine, an intravenous alpha-2 agonist, provides sedation and a degree of analgesia with minimal suppression of respiratory drive.

• Common postoperative complications include pneumonia, hypoxia, venothromboembolism (VTE), bleeding, nausea/vomiting, and ileus.
  – In general, the closer to the diaphragm the abdominal procedure, the more respiratory compromise is likely to result. Part of this results from postoperative pain; patients will not have as great diaphragmatic excursion and will tend to splint with respiration the closer the incision is to the thorax. Early mobilization and incentive spirometry (started preoperatively) are key interventions to improve oxygenation and probably decrease the incidence of pneumonia. Good pain control furthers these postoperative goals.

Table 9.3 Common postoperative complications and solutions

System	Complication	Solution
Neurologic	Pain, delirium, stroke, peripheral nerve injury	Multimodal analgesia, reorientation, minimize opiates, maintain hemodynamics, careful intraoperative positioning
Respiratory	Hypoxia, atelectasis, aspiration, pneumonia	Head of bed up, early mobilization, regional anesthesia, incentive spirometry, smoking cessation
Cardiovascular	Hypo- or hypertension, arrhythmia, MI	Frequent reassessment of volume status, blood pressure control, heart rate control, pain control
GI	Nausea, vomiting, ileus	Antiemetics, fluid balance, avoid opiates; methylnaltrexone
Hepatic	Hyperbilirubinemia, transaminitis	Maintain hemodynamics
Renal	Oliguria, renal injury	Maintain fluid balance and hemodynamics, avoid nephrotoxic drugs
Endocrine	Hypo- or hyperglycemia, adrenal crisis	Follow blood glucose closely, stress dose steroid if indicated
Hematologic	Acute anemia, coagulopathy	Correct as indicated
Immunologic	Immunosuppression, wound infection, resistant pathogen colonization, C. difficile colitis	Limit perioperative antibiotics, limit blood transfusion, high intraoperative FiO_2 might aid wound healing for lower abdominal procedures
Skin	Pressure ulcers	Careful intraoperative positioning

  – Sleep apnea should be guarded against, particularly in the obese. CPAP or BiPAP can treat OSA but may be contraindicated after some abdominal surgeries, particularly those involving the upper GI tract, due to stretch at the anastomosis or altered anatomy and physiology.
  – Vomiting with positive pressure ventilation can precipitate aspiration.

- VTE prevention also benefits from early mobilization, neuraxial anesthesia, as well as standard preventive measures such as intermittent leg compression and anticoagulation.
- Bleeding can result after any surgery, but intra-abdominal bleeding is difficult to diagnose by exam, and signs such as tachycardia and hypotension mimic other common postoperative causes such as pain and hypovolemia.
- Nausea and vomiting are particularly troublesome because they are difficult to treat once started; the focus should be on prevention with less emetogenic anesthetic techniques (regional or total intravenous anesthesia, for example) and intraoperative antiemetics

(e.g., ondansetron or dexamethasone). Postoperative management is largely pharmacologic along with judicious fluid management and gastric decompression if necessary. Nausea and vomiting can be a sign of continued or new postoperative pathology.

- Ileus is frequent after abdominal surgery and increases both length of stay as well as incidence of hospital readmission. Early ambulation and nasogastric decompression have not been shown to help. On the other hand, epidural analgesia, avoidance of bowel preparation, metoclopramide, gum-chewing, early feeding, and opiate antagonists such as methylnaltrexone have evidential support.

9.6 Summary

Patients requiring abdominal surgery frequently have fluid balance, metabolic, and blood count disturbances in addition to the typical comorbidities such as cardiovascular and respiratory disease. Comorbidities should be optimized to the extent possible preoperatively. Obesity is increasingly common, increases certain perioperative complications, and presents several anesthetic and surgical challenges.

- Laparoscopic approaches to abdominal surgery are becoming more frequent, and while laparoscopy conveys certain advantages over laparotomy, it has significant physiologic effects related to insufflation, CO_2 absorption, and patient positioning (see Table 9.4).
- Multiple anesthetic approaches are possible for the patient undergoing abdominal surgery. General anesthesia should be considered as possibly necessary even if not the initial choice. Regional anesthesia may provide certain respiratory, cardiovascular, neurologic, and gastrointestinal benefits but has its own set of risks and is not always appropriate.
- Postoperative complications of abdominal procedures can be anticipated and ameliorated with preoperative preparation, intraoperative management, and postoperative vigilance.

Table 9.4 Laparoscopy versus laparotomy

Laparoscopy	Laparotomy
Advantages	
• Faster recovery • Less pain or pulmonary compromise postoperatively	• Rapid • Simpler equipment requirements • Better surgical exposure
Disadvantages	
• Different surgical skill set and equipment • Limited exposure – multiple small incisions • May need to convert to open procedure • Limited control of bleeding	• Larger wound • More pain • Slower healing • Wound infection • More pulmonary dysfunction

Suggested Reading

Candiotti K, Sharma S, Shankar R. Obesity, obstructive sleep apnoea, and diabetes mellitus: anaesthetic implications. *Br J Anaesth*. 2009;103(Suppl 1):i23-i30.

Gerges FJ, Kanazi GE, Jabbour-Khoury SI. Anesthesia for laparoscopy: a review. *J Clin Anesth*. 2006;18(1):67-78.

Grass JA. Patient-controlled analgesia. *Anesth Analg*. 2005;101(5 Suppl):S44-S61.

Hebert PC, Wells G, Blajchman MA, et al. A multicenter, randomized, controlled clinical trial of transfusion requirements in critical care. Transfusion requirements in critical care investigators, Canadian Critical Care Trials Group. *N Engl J Med*. 1999;340(6):409-417.

Horlocker TT, Wedel DJ, Rowlingson JC, et al. Regional anesthesia in the patient receiving antithrombotic or thrombolytic therapy: American Society of Regional Anesthesia and Pain Medicine Evidence-Based Guidelines (third edition). *Reg Anesth Pain Med*. 2010;35(1):64-101.

Koch CG, Li L, Sessler DI, et al. Duration of red-cell storage and complications after cardiac surgery. *N Engl J Med*. 2008;358(12):1229-1239.

Kuczkowski KM. Laparoscopic procedures during pregnancy and the risks of anesthesia: what does an obstetrician need to know? *Arch Gynecol Obstet*. 2007;276(3):201-209.

Lawrence VA, Cornell JE, Smetana GW. Strategies to reduce postoperative pulmonary complications after noncardiothoracic surgery: systematic review for the American College of Physicians. *Ann Intern Med*. 2006;144(8):596-608.

Story SK, Chamberlain RS. A comprehensive review of evidence-based strategies to prevent and treat postoperative ileus. *Dig Surg*. 2009;26(4):265-275.

Thoracic Surgery

10

Vivek K. Moitra

10.1 Introduction

- Patients who present for thoracic surgery are at increased risk for perioperative cardiovascular and pulmonary morbidity and mortality.
- Given the probable co-morbidities of this patient population (chronic obstructive pulmonary disease (COPD), congestive heart failure (CHF), coronary artery disease, and lung cancer) understanding perioperative risk facilitates an informed consent and directs the preoperative testing process.

10.2 Preoperative Evaluation and Management

- Preoperative evaluation may uncover a history of adequately or inadequately treated CHF, CAD, or COPD.[1-4]
  - Inquire about symptoms of orthopnea, positional dyspnea, smoking, cough, and sputum production.
  - Assessment of functional exercise capacity can be used to anticipate the patient's stress response to anesthesia and surgery.
  - Evaluation of the patient with pulmonary disease and risk reduction strategies is discussed in Chap. 21.

- Order imaging studies such as computed tomography (CT), magnetic resonance imaging (MRI), and tracheal tomography to assess tracheal deviation, pulmonary infiltrates and abscess location, involvement of adjacent structures, and caliber of stenotic airways.

V.K. Moitra
Department of Anesthesiology, Division of Critical Care, Columbia University College of Physicians and Surgeons, 630 West 168th St, New York, NY 10032, USA
e-mail: vm2161@columbia.edu

S.L. Cohn (ed.), *Perioperative Medicine*,
DOI: 10.1007/978-0-85729-498-2_10, © Springer-Verlag London Limited 2011

- Request a pulmonary consult for patients scheduled for lung transplantation, lung volume reduction, or pneumonectomy.
- Consider preoperative steroids in patients with a history of steroid use and risk for relative adrenal insufficiency (See Chap. 22).
- Thoracic surgery patients with COPD or malignancy are at increased risk of venous thromboembolism and warrant prophylaxis (See Chap. 5).

10.3 Pulmonary Function Testing and Thoracic Surgery

- When an adequate history and physical is performed, pulmonary function testing in the setting of non-thoracic surgery rarely changes perioperative management (See Chap. 21).
- Pulmonary function testing, however, is recommended by the ACCP guidelines prior to lung resection surgery because it may guide the extent of surgical resection in patients with lung cancer and regional differences in pulmonary function due to local tissue destruction or COPD.[5] See Fig. 10.1 for an overview of preoperative physiologic assessment of perioperative risk.
- Various guidelines suggest tests such as the forced expiratory volume in 1 s (FEV_1), DLCO (diffusing capacity), the maximum oxygen uptake ($V'O_{2max}$) calculated from cardiopulmonary exercise tests (CPET), or the shuttle walk test to guide surgical intervention, i.e., wedge resection versus lobectomy.
  - No further testing is necessary if the preoperative FEV_1 is >2 L or >80% predicted for pneumonectomy and >1.5 L for lobectomy.
  - Consider measuring DLCO if the patient experiences undue exertional dyspnea or has interstitial lung disease.
  - If the preoperative FEV_1 and DLCO is <80%, determine the amount of functioning lung that would be lost with resection by calculating the percentage of predicted postoperative pulmonary function (PPO).
  - PPO is estimated via ventilation scans, perfusion scans, quantitative CT scans, and anatomic estimation:

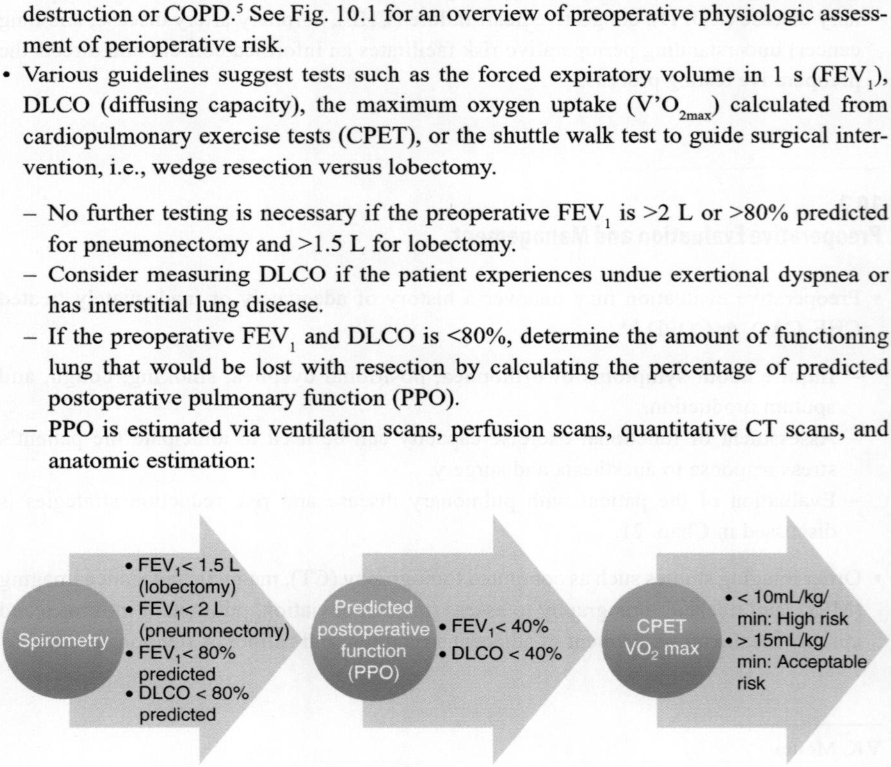

Fig. 10.1 Overview of preoperative physiologic assessment of patients scheduled for lung resection (Adapted from the American College of Chest Physicians Practice Guidelines)

PPO FEV_1 postpneumonectomy = preoperative $FEV_1 \times$ (1 − fraction of total perfusion for the resected lung).
PPO FEV_1 postlobectomy = preoperative $FEV_1 \times$ (1 − [number of functional segments to be removed/total number of functional segments]).

– Patients with PPO FEV_1 or DLCO < 40% predicted should undergo cardiopulmonary exercise testing (CPET) to determine $V'O_{2max}$ values to stratify surgical risk. Consider nonoperative management if the predicted postoperative FEV_1 < 30%.
– Consider nonsurgical options if patients have $V'O_{2max}$ values <10 or <15 mL/kg/min and both PPO FEV_1 and DLCO < 40% predicted.
– Stair climbing and shuttle walk tests (surrogates for CPET) are simpler but less standardized ways of estimating candidacy for lung resection. Patients who cannot climb more than one flight of stairs or walk <25 shuttles on two shuttle walks are at increased risk of perioperative complications.
– Arterial blood gases have not been found to be predictive (e.g., pCO_2 > 45 or O_2 saturation <90%) of postoperative pulmonary complications.

10.4 Surgery-Specific Considerations

10.4.1 Mediastinal Procedures

10.4.1.1 Mediastinoscopy

- Mediastinoscopy is performed to diagnose mediastinal lesions or to determine whether malignancy has spread to mediastinal lymph nodes. If there is nodal involvement, a planned lung resection may be aborted.
- A small incision is made above the sternal notch to introduce the scope for nodal sampling. The pleural space is not entered and complications such as pneumothorax, rupture of the great vessels, and airway damage are rare.

10.4.1.2 Mediastinal Mass Resection

- Mediastinal masses include neurogenic tumors, cysts, teratodermoids, lymphomas, thymomas, parathyroid tumors, and retrosternal thyroids.
- Patients with anterior mediastinal masses may have compression of the tracheobronchial tree, heart, or great vessels such as the superior vena cava or pulmonary artery.

- After induction of anesthesia or changes in patient position, dynamic changes in the patient's anatomy can compress airway structures.
- Occasionally, preparations are made to institute cardiopulmonary bypass if oxygenation or hemodynamic status becomes significantly impaired.

10.4.2 Video Assisted Thoracoscopic Surgery (VATS)

- VATS is a minimally invasive surgery yet this procedure still carries the risks of any intrathoracic procedure. Small incisions are made in the patient's chest wall to facilitate entry of a thoracoscope and surgical instruments.
- Diagnostic and therapeutic procedures (i.e., decortication, pleurodesis, pulmonary resections, pericardial stripping, vagotomy, and sympathetcomy) are performed with VATS.
- Potential benefits of VATS compared to an open thoracotomy include decreased length of stay, improved pulmonary function, decreased postoperative pain, and cosmesis.[6]

10.4.3 Pulmonary Resections

- Pulmonary resections include segmentectomy, wedge or extended wedge resection, and complete anatomical resection by lobectomy or pneumonectomy with removal of involved lymph nodes.
- Resection of pulmonary bulla is performed in patients with bullous compression of normal lung.
- Lung volume reduction surgery is performed in patients with severe upper lobe emphysema and poor exercise capacity.
- A pneumonectomy is frequently performed for bronchogenic carcinoma involving the hilum. Pneumonectomies also are performed in patients with trauma, massive hemoptysis, inflammatory lung disease, and congenital lung disease.[7]
- Tracheal resection and reconstruction is performed in patients with tracheal stenosis. A contingency plan to preserve airway patency in the event of an emergency is necessary. Early yet cautious extubation can preserve tracheal anastomotic suture integrity via a reduction in transtracheal pressure. Postoperatively, the patient's chin may be sutured to the patient's chest to decrease suture line tension.
- Pulmonary resections for cancer and abscesses often require lung isolation for surgical exposure and are performed via a thoracotomy incision.

10.4.3.1 One-Lung Ventilation

- A double lumen endotracheal tube is placed to facilitate one-lung ventilation and enhance surgical exposure.

- During one-lung ventilation, a large alveolar-arterial oxygen tension difference develops from perfusion to the non-ventilated lung.
- Complications of one-lung ventilation and double lumen tubes include hypoxemia, airway trauma (laryngeal, tracheal, bronchial), and difficulty with managing secretions.
- Other airway devices such as a bronchial blocker facilitate differential pulmonary ventilation.

10.4.4 Lung Transplantation

- Candidates for lung transplantation have poor functional capacity. Indications for transplantation include: COPD, alpha-1-antitrypsin deficiency, cystic fibrosis, bronchiectasis, idiopathic pulmonary fibrosis, primary pulmonary hypertension, and Eisenmenger's syndrome.
- Prior to surgery, echocardiography is performed to assess right and left ventricular function.
- Operations include single and double lung, and combined heart–lung transplantation.
- Single lung transplantation is performed via a thoracotomy incision. Double lung transplantation is performed via a "clamshell" transverse sternotomy incision.
- Cardiopulmonary bypass is used if the patient's respiratory and cardiovascular status becomes unstable.
- Neural innervation, lymphatic drainage, and bronchial circulation are disrupted.
- Loss of lymphatic drainage predisposes patients to postoperative pulmonary edema.

10.5 General Postoperative Management

10.5.1 Pulmonary

- Pulmonary complications after thoracic surgery include atelectasis, pleural effusions, respiratory failure from aspiration pneumonia or pneumonitis, pulmonary embolism, pneumothorax, re-expansion pulmonary edema, and acute respiratory distress syndrome (ARDS).
- Atelectasis/pleural effusions: Atelectasis is common and may be exacerbated by narcotics as well as inadequate pain control. Use incentive spirometry and encourage deep breathing preoperatively and postoperatively to improve FRC and decrease atelectasis. Pleural effusions are also frequently encountered and are typically transudates that resolve spontaneously.
- Respiratory failure: Patients with severe pulmonary disease are at risk for prolonged mechanical ventilation if there are significant fluid shifts and hemodynamic compromise during high-risk surgery. Suspect injury to the phrenic nerve when there is an elevation of the hemidiaphragm and weaning from mechanical ventilation is difficult. Paradoxical movement of the diaphragm is observed with fluoroscopy.

- Pneumonia: Risk factors for nosocomial pneumonia include COPD, prior antibiotic use, chronic illnesses, mechanical ventilation, and immobilization. Early extubation decreases the risk of ventilator associated pneumonia[8] and disruption of bronchial suture line integrity. Elevate the patient's head of the bed greater than 30° to prevent aspiration.
- Pulmonary edema: Initiate a conservative fluid management strategy after pneumonectomy or lung transplantation to decrease the risk of acute lung injury or pulmonary edema (postpneumonectomy pulmonary edema). Non-cardiogenic pulmonary edema usually develops within 2–3 days after surgery and is more common after right-sided pneumonectomy. It may also be caused by upper airway obstruction, re-expansion pulmonary edema, and ARDS. Bronchospasm is also common and may be caused by exacerbation of underlying lung disease (COPD), allergic response, histamine release related to medications, and aspiration.

10.5.2 Cardiac

- Cardiac complications include arrhythmias (especially atrial fibrillation), myocardial ischemia/infarction and pericardial tamponade. Risk factors for postoperative atrial fibrillation include age > 60, left ventricular dysfunction, and pneumonectomy or superior lobectomy.[8,9] Treatment considerations in patients with new onset stable atrial fibrillation include adequate analgesia, beta-blockade, and amiodarone.
- Hypoxia, acidosis from an inadequate respiratory effort, and removal of pulmonary vasculature can increase pulmonary vascular resistance (right ventricular afterload) and may lead to right heart failure.

10.5.3 Analgesia

- Inadequate analgesia causes splinting and respiratory compromise and may lead to the need for mechanical ventilation. Use opioid analgesics cautiously in patients whose lungs are not mechanically ventilated. Thoracic epidural analgesia with a continuous infusion of local anesthesia in the epidural space effectively prevents pulmonary splinting and can reduce postoperative pulmonary complications.
- Repeated intercostal nerve blockade anesthetizes the nerves of the chest wall without sedation. Disadvantages of this technique include the need for repeat injections and the risk of local anesthetic toxicity from intravascular uptake of medications.

10.5.4 Chest Tube Management

- Chest tubes in the pleural cavity promote lung expansion and monitor for air leaks.
- Chest tubes are usually placed under water seal and 20 cm H_2O suction.

- Water suction applied to the chest tube of a pneumonectomy patient can cause mediastinal shift, decreased venous return, and cardiovascular collapse.
- Most air leaks stop after a few days. A persistent air leak suggests inadequate closure of the bronchial stump; the development of a bronchopleural fistula; or necrosis of the suture line from ischemia or infection.
- Consider postoperative hemorrhage when there is a large chest tube output (>200 mL/h of fluid), tachycardia, and hypotension. A clot or kink in the chest tube with low output masks major intrathoracic bleeding.

References

1. Jaklitsch M, Billmeier S. Preoperative evaluation and risk assessment for elderly thoracic surgery patients. *Thorac Surg Clin.* 2009;19:301-312.
2. Spiro SG, Gould MK, Colice GL. Initial evaluation of the patient with lung cancer: symptoms, signs, laboratory tests, and paraneoplastic syndromes: ACCP evidenced-based clinical practice guidelines (2nd edition). *Chest.* 2007;132(3 Suppl):149S-160S.
3. Bernstein WK, Deshpande S. Preoperative evaluation for thoracic surgery. *Semin Cardiothorac Vasc Anesth.* 2008;12:109-121.
4. Beckles MA, Spiro SG, Colice GL, Rudd RM. The physiologic evaluation of patients with lung cancer being considered for resectional surgery. *Chest.* 2003;123(1 Suppl):105S-114S.
5. Colice GL, Shafazand S, Griffin JP, Keenan R, Bolliger CT. Physiologic evaluation of the patient with lung cancer being considered for resectional surgery: ACCP evidenced-based clinical practice guidelines (2nd edition). *Chest.* 2007;132(3 Suppl):161S-177S.
6. Fischer GW, Cohen E. An update on anesthesia for thoracoscopic surgery. *Curr Opin Anaesthesiol.* 2010;23:7-11.
7. Slinger P. Update on anesthetic management for pneumonectomy. *Curr Opin Anaesthesiol.* 2009;22:31-37.
8. Vaporciyan AA, Correa AM, Rice DC, et al. Risk factors associated with atrial fibrillation after noncardiac thoracic surgery: analysis of 2588 patients. *J Thorac Cardiovasc Surg.* 2004;127:779-786.
9. Amar D. Postthoracotomy atrial fibrillation. *Curr Opin Anaesthesiol.* 2007;20:43-47.

Vascular Surgery 11

Visala S. Muluk

11.1 Introduction

- Vascular surgery patients are a high-risk group of patients associated with increased incidence of perioperative cardiac complications. Peripheral arterial disease (PAD) is associated with increased risk for vascular disease elsewhere, and these patients typically have a high prevalence of cardiovascular, cerebrovascular, and renal disease.
- The physiologic stress associated with vascular surgical procedures may range from low-stress procedures like amputations to high-stress procedures like repair of a ruptured abdominal aneurysm. However, even low-stress procedures may be associated with high mortality due to patient-specific risks like diabetes, hypertension, and smoking.
- The choice of certain types of procedures requires consideration of the patient's risk factors and life expectancy.
  - Endovascular repair of abdominal aneurysm compared to open repair is associated with lesser morbidity and mortality in the short-term, but no significant difference in the long-term.
  - Carotid endarterectomy versus carotid stenting (CREST trial) showed no significant difference in terms of the combined endpoint of periprocedural stroke, MI or death, and no significant difference in 4-year incidence of ipsilateral stroke. However, there was an increased risk of periprocedural stroke with stenting and MI with endarterectomy. Younger patients had better outcomes with stenting, and older patients had better outcomes with endarterectomy.

V.S. Muluk
VAPHCS, University of Pittsburgh, Pittsburgh, PA, USA
e-mail: visala.muluk@va.gov

S.L. Cohn (ed.), *Perioperative Medicine*,
DOI: 10.1007/978-0-85729-498-2_11, © Springer-Verlag London Limited 2011

11.2 Preoperative Considerations

11.2.1 Patient Related Risk Assessment

- Cardiac risk assessment
  - Coronary artery disease (CAD) is the leading cause of death after vascular surgery. A significant proportion of patients being considered for vascular surgery will have some degree of coronary artery disease because risk factors are the same for CAD and PAD.
  - Decline in functional capacity associated with PAD makes it more difficult to identify patients with potentially significant but asymptomatic CAD.
  - Patient evaluation should include a comprehensive history, focused physical examination, and baseline electrocardiogram (EKG).

    The history should focus on coronary risk factors (particularly those in the RCRI), functional capacity of the patient (inability to achieve 4 METS increases risk of complications), and history of prior cardiac testing and intervention.

    The physical examination should focus on the cardiovascular exam (signs of heart failure, valvular disease, neurologic deficit).

    A resting EKG is recommended even with one clinical risk factor when undergoing vascular surgery (class I).

    Q waves and ST-T wave changes are predictors of postoperative cardiac complications.

  - Based on the ACC guidelines, noninvasive testing before high-risk vascular surgery is:

    Probably recommended (class IIa) with three or more risk predictors (RCRI) and poor (<4 METS) or unknown functional capacity, and may be considered (class IIb) with one to two risk predictors and poor (<4 METS) or unknown functional capacity if it will change management.

    Patients with one to two risk predictors and poor (<4 METS) or unknown functional capacity and undergoing high-risk vascular surgery can usually proceed to surgery with heart rate control.

- Pulmonary disease
  - Cigarette smoking is a risk factor for both PAD and chronic obstructive pulmonary disease (COPD).
  - COPD is associated with a twofold increase in postoperative pulmonary complications.
  - Encourage smoking cessation preoperatively.
  - Screen for obstructive sleep apnea (OSA). Undiagnosed obstructive sleep apnea has a high prevalence in surgical patients (>24%) and is an independent risk predictor of HTN, cardiovascular morbidity and mortality, and sudden death.

- Diabetes Mellitus
  - Hyperglycemia (glucose >180 mg/dL) and autonomic neuropathy may increase risk of postoperative complications.
- Chronic kidney disease
  - Chronic kidney disease (CKD) with a GFR <60 mL/min (Stages III–V) or creatinine >2 mg/dL may be associated with increased perioperative morbidity and mortality.
  - Preexisting renal disease is also an important predictor of postoperative renal failure.
  - Vascular surgery patients who need diagnostic procedures requiring contrast are at an increased risk of developing acute on chronic renal insufficiency.
- Cerebrovascular disease
  - Prior stroke is associated with an increased risk of postoperative stroke but does not warrant further testing preoperatively.
- Anemia
  - A decreased preoperative hematocrit may be associated with increased incidence of perioperative ischemia and postoperative cardiac complications in patients undergoing vascular surgery and prostate surgery, but there are no data to support a specific threshold value.

11.2.2 Surgery Related Risk Assessment

- Surgical decision making process including the type of surgery should take into consideration the following factors: patient-specific risk assessment (including existing co-morbidities) and the life expectancy of the patient.
- For example, patients with multiple co-morbidities may tolerate endovascular repair of abdominal aneurysm better than open procedure.
- Age and risk factors for stroke and myocardial ischemia might play a role in deciding between carotid stenting and carotid endarterectomy.
- The benefits of elective surgical procedures (elective abdominal aneurysm repair and carotid endarterectomy) should be considered carefully especially in patients with decreased life expectancy.

11.3 Perioperative Risk Reduction Strategies

- Preoperative cardiac intervention (see Chap. 20)
  - Preoperative revascularization is rarely necessary just to get a patient through surgery and should be reserved for high-risk patients where it is indicated regardless of surgery.

Angina recalcitrant to maximal medical therapy, evidence of significant left main (LM) disease or severe two or three vessel disease including LAD disease, easily provoked ischemia during exercise stress test or multiple areas of ischemia on imaging test, symptomatic left ventricular dysfunction

- Among patients with known stable coronary arterial disease undergoing major vascular surgery, revascularization did not improve short- or long-term outcomes in the CARP trial. However, patients with LM disease (>50%), EF <20%, and severe aortic stenosis were excluded from the trial.
- Type of revascularization should be decided based on urgency of surgery and consideration of risk of interrupting antiplatelet agents.

• Perioperative medication management

- Consider prophylactic beta-blockers for patients undergoing high-risk vascular surgery based on the ACC/AHA guidelines, assuming time permits dose titration for heart rate control

Beta-blockers are recommended in patients who have evidence of ischemia on preoperative testing and are suggested in patients with evidence of CAD or have multiple risk factors for CAD.
Alpha-2 agonists (clonidine) may have some benefit in vascular surgery patients and can be considered in patients unable to tolerate beta-blockers.

• Perioperative chronic disease management

- Pulmonary disease (see Chap. 21)

Preoperative measures to improve postoperative outcomes include:

Smoking cessation 6–8 weeks prior to surgery, maximizing bronchodilator therapy, and antibiotics or steroid therapy as indicated.

Postoperative measures include:

Incentive spirometry and early mobilization, CPAP and PACU monitoring with continuous pulse oximetry in patients with OSA, and adequate pain control.

- Renal Disease

Measures to prevent postoperative renal failure:

Identification of at risk patients and optimization of renal function with adequate replacement perioperatively to maintain adequate perfusion.
In cases of contrast induced injury, give the kidneys adequate time to recover prior to surgery.

MRA may be associated with lesser renal dysfunction compared to angiography.

Modifications in surgical technique.

EVAR is associated with lesser renal injury compared to open repair of AAA due to less aortic manipulation and renal ischemia.

Currently there are no renoprotective drugs approved by FDA.

Fenoldopam, a newer selective dopaminergic-1 receptor agonist, may have some beneficial effect.

– Diabetes Mellitus

The American College of Endocrinology recommended a preprandial glucose level <110 mg/dL with the maximum level not exceeding 180 mg/dL for hospitalized patients. Several studies have shown that very tight control (<110–140) is potentially harmful.

Continuous intravenous insulin infusion may have better glycemic control than intermittent insulin therapy and may benefit patients undergoing CABG, but it is cumbersome to use outside the ICU setting.

11.4 Surgery-specific Risks and Postoperative Complications

Thrombosis, bleeding, and infection are commonly encountered complications after vascular surgery (Table 11.1).

- Thrombosis
  - Continue aspirin perioperatively to minimize cardiovascular risk as well as peripheral graft thrombosis risk. Clopidogrel and prasugrel are often stopped 5–7 days before surgery to minimize bleeding risk (see Chap. 5).
  - Adding oral anticoagulants to ASA had no added benefit in preventing complications but increased bleeding risk.
  - Heparin, preferably LMWH, can be used for prevention of venous thrombosis.
- Bleeding
  - Vascular surgery patients pose a hemostatic challenge due to tissue injury, use of heparin with or without protamine reversal, and preoperative use of antiplatelet and antithrombotic agents.
  - Postoperative bleeding is usually from the surgical site or GI tract.

    Surgical site bleeding needs immediate attention and may need repeated operation or hematoma evacuation.

    GI prophylaxis with proton pump inhibitors is always recommended.
- Infection
  - Graft infection, early or late, can ultimately lead to limb loss or death.

    To prevent infections, administer prophylactic antibiotics preoperatively and recognize and treat postoperative infections in a timely manner.

Table 11.1 Vascular surgery: complications and surgery-specific issues

Surgery	Postoperative complications	Surgery-specific issues
Open TAAA repair	• Postoperative hemorrhage • Respiratory failure • Renal failure • Spinal cord ischemia	• Associated with highest morbidity and mortality • Coagulopathy with major hemorrhage is associated with 25% mortality rate • The risk of spinal cord ischemia is proportional to the cross clamping time
Open AAA repair	• Leg thromboembolism with ischemia • Respiratory failure • Renal failure • Descending colon ischemia • Ileus • Retrograde ejaculation • Aortoenteric fistula • Ventral hernia	• High perioperative morbidity but long-term mortality similar to EVAR • Longer hospital stay • Aortic manipulation can lead to increased incidence of renal failure due to atheroembolism and renal ischemia
Endovascular infrarenal AAA repair	• Lymphocele • Groin hematoma • IV contrast allergy or renal insufficiency • Endovascular leak • Endotension • Graft migration	• Good alternative for high surgical risk patients • EVR is associated with lower short-term complications and shorter hospital stay • Late reinterventions are common and there is no difference in the long-term mortality benefit • Endoleaks are classified as: Type I leaks are treated with secondary endovascular procedure or an open procedure Type II leaks are usually benign and can be observed Type III leaks are repaired endovascularly Type IV leaks are transient and resolve on their own
Infrainguinal bypass surgery	• Graft thrombosis • Surgical site infection or dehiscence • Leg edema	• Leg edema should be managed by leg elevation • Compression stockings should be used cautiously in the early postoperative period as they can decrease distal arterial flow
Carotid endarterectomy	• Neck hematoma which may lead to airway compromise • Stroke • Cranial nerve injury	• Mortality ranges from 0.5% to 3% and is greater when the hospital and/or surgeon has less experience • Neck hematoma should be explored immediately to prevent airway compression • Higher incidence of MI compared to stenting
Carotid stenting	• Stent thrombosis • Stroke • Groin hematoma • Pseudoaneurysm	• Higher incidence of stroke compared to endarterectomy • Younger patients seem to have better outcomes with stenting

Table 11.1 (continued)

Surgery	Postoperative complications	Surgery-specific issues
A-V fistulas	• High output CHF • Hand ischemia • Arm edema • Later complications include infection, graft thrombosis and false aneurysm	• Native AV fistulas: Higher initial failure rate Lesser incidence of infection and thrombosis • AV synthetic grafts: Higher initial patency rates Higher late failure rates due to thrombosis, infection • Permanent indwelling catheters Can be used immediately High rates of infection and central vein stenosis
Limb amputations	• Poor wound healing due to infection and poor perfusion • DVT • Phantom pain • Emotional problems • Later complications include excessive exposure of transected bone due to muscle retraction	• When infection is suspected cultures should be obtained before starting antibiotics • MRSA infection is highly prevalent and gram negative and anaerobic infections more common in diabetic patients • Wound dehiscence is suggestive of tissue necrosis due to deep seated infection and/or ischemia

Modified from McKean and Muluk[1] with permission. Copyright © 2006, The McGraw Hill Companies, Inc.

Reference

1. McKean SCW, Muluk V. Vascular surgery. In: Cohn SL, Smetana GW, Weed HG, eds. *Perioperative Medicine – Just the Facts*. New York: McGraw-Hill; 2006.

Suggested Reading

Abir F, Kakisis I, Sumpio B. Do vascular surgery patients need a cardiology work-up? A review of pre-operative cardiac clearance guidelines in vascular surgery. *Eur J Vasc Endovasc Surg.* 2003;25:110.

Baker B. Anesthesia and endovascular surgery. *Best Pract Res Clin Anaesthesiol.* 2003;16:95.

McFalls EO, Ward H, Moritz T, et al. Coronary-artery revascularization before elective major vascular surgery. *N Engl J Med.* 2004;351:2795.

Metzler H. Lowering cardiac risk by preoperative interventions. *Minerva Anestesiol.* 2003;69:412.

Prinssen M, Verhoeven EL, Buth J, et al. A randomized trial comparing conventional and endovascular repair of abdominal aortic aneurysms. *N Engl J Med.* 2004;351:1607.

Wennberg DE, Lucas FL, Birkmeyer JD, et al. Variation in carotid endarterectomy mortality in the Medicare population. *JAMA.* 1998;279:1278.

Orthopedic Surgery 12

Ronald MacKenzie and Edwin P. Su

12.1 Introduction

Arthritis is the leading cause of disability in the nation. More than 21% of US adults currently report physician-diagnosed arthritis, a prevalence expected to increase in the future (67 million affected adults by 2030). In 2007, it was estimated that 270,000 primary total hip replacements and 507,000 primary total knee replacements were performed in the US, with projections for the future estimated to increase to over 500,000 hip and 3 million knee replacements by 2030. As many of these patients are elderly and have other chronic medical conditions, orthopedic surgery will remain an important challenge in perioperative medicine.[1-4]

12.2 Preoperative Considerations (Table 12.1)

The preoperative evaluation is the primary focal point of communication between all members of the medical team.[1] Orthopedic surgery has increasingly been performed in the ambulatory setting, and an important benefit resulting from this change is that it moves the preoperative medical evaluation to the outpatient arena thereby enhancing the opportunity for timely communication and collaboration between consulting physicians.

- Arthroscopy, joint replacement, and spine surgery are the most common elective procedures. Indications for surgical intervention include pain and functional limitation (disability) unrelieved by conservative treatment, and severe radiculopathy, nerve dysfunction (e.g., acute foot drop), or myelopathy (in spine surgery).

R. MacKenzie (✉)
Weill Cornell Medical College, Department of Rheumatology,
Hospital for Special Surgery,
New York, NY, USA
e-mail: mackenzier@hss.edu

S.L. Cohn (ed.), *Perioperative Medicine*,
DOI: 10.1007/978-0-85729-498-2_12, © Springer-Verlag London Limited 2011

Table 12.1 Risk factors and complications associated with orthopedic surgery

Preoperative risk factors	Postoperative complications
Patient-related	• Delirium
• Advanced age	• VTE
• Associated comorbidities: cardiac, pulmonary, malnutrition	• Fever/infection – Wound, UTI, pneumonia
• Functional limitations	• Anemia
Procedure-related	• Falls
• Emergency surgery (fracture, cord compression, trauma)	• Peripheral nerve injury
• VTE (highest risk – TKR, THR, HFS)	• Falls
• General anesthesia/intubation (RA, AS)	• Fat embolism

VTE venous thromboembolism, *TKR* total knee replacement, *THR* total hip replacement, *HFS* hip fracture surgery, *RA* rheumatoid arthritis, *AS* ankylosing spondylitis, *UTI* urinary tract infection

- Emergent orthopedic surgery may arise in the setting of hip fracture, acute myelopathy, or septic arthritis (native or prosthetic joint).
- With the aging of the population, orthopedic surgery is increasingly offered to patients with extensive burdens of comorbidity and age-related surgical-anesthesiological vulnerability.
- Exercise intolerance, although often attributed to underlying joint disease, makes cardiac risk assessment somewhat more challenging.
- Orthopedic surgery patients are also at risk for venous thromboembolism, falls, and postoperative delirium.
- Connective tissue diseases are relatively prevalent in orthopedic populations and present specific challenges to perioperative care (Chap. 28).
- General anesthesia with endotracheal intubation may present a particular danger in patients with rheumatoid arthritis or ankylosing spondylitis. Two forms of cervical spine disease are encountered: the unstable spine of the patient with rheumatoid arthritis and the rigid spine of the patient with ankylosing spondylitis.
- For RA, cervical spine instability should be ruled out prior to surgery with flexion/extension films as there may or may not be symptoms (such as neck pain, neck crepitus on range of motion testing, radicular symptoms, arm and/or leg weakness, or bladder and bowel dysfunction). Affected patients should wear a soft cervical collar to the operating room, and when possible, epidural or spinal anesthesia should be employed.
- For ankylosing spondylitis, the patient's rigid cervical spine may also present technical challenges for the anesthesiologist during intubation, and fiberoptic methods are often employed in this clinical setting.
- Advantages of regional anesthesia include a reduction in blood loss, venous thromboembolism, postoperative respiratory events, and in death.

12.3 Postoperative Considerations (Table 12.1)

12.3.1 Venous Thromboembolism (VTE)

- A complex balance exists between a possible life-threatening pulmonary embolus and the potential for postoperative bleeding.
- Total knee replacement, hip replacement, and hip fracture surgery are associated with the highest risk for VTE.[2] Strategies to reduce this risk include combined pharmacologic and mechanical prophylaxis, short intraoperative time, and epidural anesthesia.
- The mainstay of prevention is prophylactic anticoagulation which should begin immediately following (day of) surgery. ACCP recommended regimens include warfarin, low molecular weight heparin, or fondaparinux, often used in combination (multi-modal) with various mechanical compression devices. Although not recommended by the ACCP, aspirin is an alternative in the AAOS guidelines. Mechanical approaches to DVT prophylaxis include graded compression stockings and various pneumatic devices, foot flexion/extension exercises, and early ambulation (see Chap. 5 VTE Prophylaxis).

12.3.2 Postoperative Infection

- Postoperative fever (>38.0°C) is commonly seen in the first 24–48 h postoperatively after major orthopedic surgery. This phenomenon, which is associated with transient rises in the ESR and CRP, arises as a consequence of inflammatory mediator release after surgery. Other causes account for late onset fever (>48 h) and include atelectasis, drug fever, pneumonia, and surgical site/wound infection.
- Efforts to prevent and detect any infectious processes perioperatively are of utmost importance.
- The skin and urinary tract are sites of specific concern and infection can be ruled out by a careful history and physical examination. Routine urinalysis and culture are of questionable value but are often performed routinely before total joint replacement.
- Dental consultation may be appropriate in patients with poor oral hygiene and dentition.
- Prophylactic antibiotic therapy for total joint arthroplasty patients should begin <2 h before surgery and continue for at most 24 h.
  - A common protocol involves cefazolin (Ancef) 1 g q8h (total of three doses) or, in penicillin allergic patients, vancomycin 1 g q12h (total of two doses). (See Chap. 7-Surgical Site Infection Prophylaxis).
- Indwelling urinary catheters should be removed as soon as possible (24–48 h).

12.3.3
Peripheral Nerve Injuries

- Peripheral nerve injuries arise more often after upper and lower extremity surgery. Mechanisms include excessive traction on the nerve, compression resulting from prolonged positioning of the extremity during surgery, or from a cast.
- Patients with chronic neurological disease or conditions such as neuropathies in the setting of diabetes or spinal stenosis are at increased risk of nerve injury from surgery.
- Early detection and intervention is critical to the outcome in these circumstances.

12.3.4
Fat Embolism Syndrome

- Fat embolization may also occur after procedures involving instrumentation of the femoral medullary canal.
- One to three percent of patients undergoing joint replacement surgery (particularly simultaneous bilateral procedures) develop fat embolism syndrome (FES).
- Signs and symptoms involve the respiratory, neurological, hematological systems, as well as the skin. Time of onset is variable with hemodynamic instability developing almost immediately in some or insidiously over the first 2–3 postoperative days. In the latter, patients gradually become hypoxemic, may be hypotensive and are often confused. Transient thrombocytopenia is common.
- The majority of patients develop mild to moderate hypoxemia or radiographic changes (mainly bilateral alveolar infiltrates), but only a minority will develop life-threatening adult respiratory distress syndrome.
- Neurological manifestations range from mild drowsiness to acute confusional states or to severe obtundation and coma, all consequences of the hypoxemia and the direct effect of the embolization of fat on the brain.
- The skin eruption, which is rare in the total joint arthroplasty patient, takes the form of a petechial rash involving the conjunctiva and oral mucosa and may be distributed over the folds of the neck and axillae. Retinal edema and hemorrhage is also commonly seen.
- Treatment is supportive and includes the administration of oxygen and the prevention of pulmonary hypertension (by fluid restriction and the use of diuretics and vasodilators). Corticosteroids are not effective.
- In the majority, the condition resolves within 3–7 days although in severe cases the mortality rate has remained in the 5–15% range even with modern aggressive therapy.

12.3.5
Heterotopic Ossification

- Heterotopic ossification (HO) may complicate both total hip and knee replacement. Risk factors include hypertrophic OA, Ankylosing Spondylitis, and the performance of trochanteric osteotomy. It occurs more often in men.
- Effective approaches to the prevention of this condition include the use of NSAIDs in the postoperative period or irradiation.

12.3.6
Anemia

- A degree of postoperative anemia usually occurs after major joint arthroplasty.
- Preoperative autologous donation of blood and the use of erythropoietin (EP) have been employed to reduce the transfusion requirement of patients undergoing major orthopedic surgery. The use of postoperative iron is usually ineffective and often contributes to postoperative constipation.

12.3.7
Postoperative Confusion

- Acute confusional states (delirium) after orthopedic surgery are a common problem. Usually multifactorial in etiology, such states are particularly common in the elderly with hip fracture patients at especially high risk (60%).
- Confusional states are known to increase length of stay, risk for complications, mortality, and they interfere with rehabilitation resulting often in a need for long term institutionalization.
- Modifiable risk factors include the correction of hypoxia, electrolyte and metabolic disorders, the elimination of psychoactive medications (those with sedative, hypnotic, and anti-cholinergic properties). The prompt recognition of various conditions that may be associated with postoperative cognitive decline is vital. Such conditions include myocardial infarction, stroke, drug and alcohol withdrawal, adverse reactions to medication and fat embolism.
- Environmental considerations and supportive measures often prove "orienting" and may reduce the incidence and severity of postoperative confusion and delirium.

12.3.8
Nutritional Considerations

- Malnutrition is associated with increased surgical morbidity and mortality and is particularly common in the elderly hip fracture patient (20%).
- Oral protein supplementation is believed to improve postoperative complications. In the severely depleted patient, enteral tube feeding may be required.

12.4
Common Orthopedic Procedures

Surgical treatment of joint disease is focused on the relief of pain with secondary objectives such as improved joint range of motion, a reduction in joint swelling, and return to function. Due to the limitations and complications of surgical intervention, the decision to move forward is one that must be individualized for each patient. Factors such as disease severity, the patient's desired activity level, as well as the patient's anticipated life span are all relevant to decision-making. Typically patients who are candidates for the surgical treatment of joint diseases have failed conservative measures (NSAIDS, physical therapy, intra-articular injections) and have daily pain that hinders their quality of life.

12.4.1 Osteotomy

- In circumstances where a structural abnormality around a joint has lead to mechanical overload, an osteotomy may be an option to correct alignment problems.
- The most common sites for osteotomy are hip (for acetabular dysplasia) and the tibia (for knee realignment).
- Osteotomy is generally performed in younger patients (<40 years); beyond this age, the loss of cartilage is such that more beneficial results are attained with total joint arthroplasty.

12.4.2 Arthroscopy

- Arthroscopic surgery is performed by inserting a camera and specialized instruments into a joint via small, puncture-type incisions.
- Arthroscopic surgery is effective in the treatment of intra-articular pathology such as meniscal tears of the knee, labral tears of the hip, cartilage flaps, small chondral defects and loose bodies.
- Arthroscopic reshaping of the bones of the femur and acetabulum is becoming a popular procedure (for femoro-acetabular impingement).

12.4.3 Synovectomy

- Synovectomy refers to removal of the synovial lining of the joint, either via an open or arthroscopic approach. In conditions such as rheumatoid arthritis, where the disease process involves an actively inflamed synovium, debulking the pathologic tissue may reduce symptoms and slow the destruction of cartilage.
- Synovectomy can be effective at relieving pain as long as there is remaining cartilage.
- The most common joints that benefit from synovectomy are the knee and elbow.

12.4.4 Arthrodesis

- Arthrodesis achieves the goal of pain relief by creating a non-mobile joint. This surgical fusion of the articulating bones creates a construct that can bear weight and is stable.
- Gait mechanics after fusion are altered requiring more energy for ambulation.

12.4.5
Total Joint Replacement

- Joint arthroplasty refers to the re-creation of congruent joint surfaces, typically with artificial parts. Once the articular cartilage is completely worn or destroyed on both sides of the joint, arthroplasty, in which the articular surfaces are replaced by shaped materials designed to recreate the joint kinematics, is the most predictable option to relieve pain.[5]
- The most common procedures are that of total hip and knee replacement but numerous other joints can be replaced (small joints of the hand, wrist, elbow, shoulder, ankle).
- Recovery from total knee is more difficult than for total hip replacement due to greater postoperative pain and the emphasis on regaining motion.
- Current studies demonstrate implant survival to be 90–95% at 15 years, depending upon patient factors such as weight and activity.

12.4.6
Surgical Innovations in Total Joint Replacement

- There has been a movement toward "minimally invasive surgery" across all surgical subspecialties. Non-surgical advances have also resulted in improved outcome. These include the use of peripheral nerve blocks and preemptive analgesia and a more expeditious approach to rehabilitation. Improvements in implant technology have focused on more wear-resistant prostheses.
- Hip resurfacing is growing as an alternative treatment to total hip replacement in the younger, active patient. Rather than removing the femoral head and portion of the femoral neck as in THR, the bone is sculpted to accept a metal resurfacing cap (like a tooth), preserving an additional 4–5 cm of bone.
- Computer navigation is a tool used to aid in the reproducible positioning of implants.

12.4.7
Hip Fracture

- Hundreds of thousands of hip fractures, most commonly due to falls, occur annually resulting in major costs to society.
- Within the first year of fracture, 20% of such patients die and of the survivors many require assistive devices or help from others in order to complete activities of daily living.
- Femoral neck and intertrochanteric fractures occur with equal frequency. Severely displaced femoral neck fractures may require total joint replacement due to the higher incidence of vascular damage and subsequent avascular necrosis. Subtrochanteric fractures are more difficult to treat. Healing is impaired due to the abundance of cortical bone and decreased vascularity. Intramedullary nail fixation is the preferred treatment.

- As this is usually an elderly population, providing the perioperative medical care for this patient population can be challenging. The optimal timing of surgery is significantly influenced by existing medical comorbidities but current practice is to operate early (24–48 h) as the outcomes associated with delayed surgery, appear worse.
- Postoperative medical comanagement may positively influence outcome. Early surgical intervention is strongly encouraged in order to mitigate against postoperative complications and to allow for timely institution of rehabilitation.

12.4.8
Spine Surgery

- The sequelae of spinal arthritis is spinal stenosis which may require decompressive surgery. Newer surgical treatments such as lumbar disc replacement may be used in certain cases to treat spinal disorders. Whereas the gold standard, vertebral fusion, eliminates painful motion at degenerative disc levels, disc replacement attempts to preserve motion of the spinal unit. Acute herniated discs, if accompanied by neurological deficits (i.e., foot drop) respond well the microdiscectomy, a relatively benign procedure associated with a brief length of stay (i.e., <24 h).

References

1. MacKenzie CR, Paget SA. Perioperative care of the rheumatic disease patient. In: Hochberg MC, Silman AJ, Smolen JS, Weinblatt ME, Weisman MH, eds. Rheumatology, 5th ed. Philadelphia: Elsevier, 2010. *This book chapter is a comprehensive review or perioperative medicine as it pertains to the patient with rheumatic disease.*
2. Memtsoudis SG, Della Valle AG, Mazumdar M, et al. Perioperative outcomes after unilateral and bilateral total knee arthroplasty. *Anesthesiology*. 2009;111:1206-1216. *This study examines the trends in joint replacement in the United States.*
3. Kurtz S, Ong K, Lau E, et al. Projections of primary and revision hip and knee arthroplasty in the United States from 2005 to 2030. *J Bone Joint Surg Am*. 2007;89:780-785. *This study examines the trends in joint replacement in the United States.*
4. Graves SE, Davidson D, Ingerson L, et al. The Australian Orthopaedic Association National Joint Replacement Registry. *Med J Aust*. 2004;180(5 suppl):S31-S34. *This document provides information from a National Registry regarding the survival rates of commonly performed joint replacement procedures.*
5. Kirkley A, Birmingham TB, Litchfield RB, Giffin R, et al. A randomized trial of arthroscopic surgery for osteoarthritis of the knee. *N Engl J Med*. 2008;359:1097-1107. *This study is one of only a few randomized controlled clinical trials of an important orthopedic surgical procedure.*

Neurosurgery 13

Victor Duval

13.1 Introduction

- The perioperative management of neurosurgical patients requires special considerations – an adequate history may be difficult to obtain, the procedure may be technically challenging, and bleeding may be catastrophic.
- The preoperative assessment must address the patient's primary pathology, as well as cardiopulmonary comorbidities. It should always include, when possible, a thorough and focused history and physical exam. Laboratory and other studies should be ordered based on the patient's specific risk factors for perioperative complications.
- Neurologic deficits are common. These will influence the choice of airway management technique, the precautions taken during intraoperative positioning, and the hemodynamic parameters that will be adhered to in the intraoperative and postoperative period.
- The central nervous system is well vascularized. Achieving hemostasis can be particularly challenging due to the ischemic potential of common techniques used for other nonneurosurgical procedures. These, along with other factors, significantly increase the risks for massive perioperative hemorrhage.
- Routine prophylactic measures should be taken to minimize the risk of postoperative infection, and deep vein thrombosis in all patients (see Chaps. 5 and 7). Prophylaxis against gastric ulcers and seizures can be limited to selected patients.
- Neurosurgical patients are prone to unique postoperative complications. Patients often require close monitoring in an intensive care setting.

V. Duval
David Geffen School of Medicine at UCLA, Department of Anesthesiology,
Ronald Reagan UCLA Medical Center, 757 Westwood Plaza,
Los Angeles, CA 90095, USA
e-mail: vduval@mednet.ucla.edu

S.L. Cohn (ed.), *Perioperative Medicine*,
DOI: 10.1007/978-0-85729-498-2_13,

13.2
Preoperative Considerations

13.2.1
Assessment

- It is important to carefully evaluate the patient's baseline neurologic status, as well as assess for signs of elevated intracranial pressure, risk for hemorrhage, and vasospasm based on the size and location of the lesion.
- The preoperative assessment must also take into account the patient's co-morbidities.
  - Patients with intracranial pathology often present with seizures.
  - Vascular lesions are often associated with hypertension.
  - Patients presenting with a subarachnoid hemorrhage (SAH) are at risk for stunned myocardium and neurogenic edema.
  - Hyperglycemia may exacerbate the extent of neurologic injury and should be tightly controlled.
  - Obesity is associated with a higher incidence of postoperative respiratory complications, including airway compromise.
- Consider the patient's current medication history.
  - Continue beta blockers perioperatively.
  - Calcium channel blockers may exaggerate the hemodynamic response to volatile anesthetic agents.
  - Monitor glucose levels closely, especially with concomitant use of glucocorticosteroids, and adjust antihyperglycemic medications appropriately to avoid significant hypo- or hyperglycemia.

13.2.2
Special Preparation

- Preoperative laboratory tests should be based on the presence and the extent of co-morbidities uncovered from the history and physical examination.
  - Obtain a baseline hemoglobin concentration and platelet count have a type and screen available in the blood bank should the need for a transfusion arise.
- The neurosurgical patient often presents with neurologic deficits that lead to deconditioning precluding the ability to assess exercise tolerance.
  - Cardiopulmonary studies should be obtained based on the history and physical examination as recommended by current guidelines (see Chaps. 20 and 21).
- Prescribe antibiotic prophylaxis for all neurosurgical cases, with therapy directed against gram positive organisms. Administer cefazolin, clindamycin, or vancomycin within 60 min of surgical incision (see Chap. 7).

- For prevention of deep vein thrombosis in neurosurgical patients, compression devices in the lower extremities are the most appropriate since anticoagulants can potentially interfere with hemostasis.
- Patients who receive perioperative steroid treatment and patients undergoing intracranial procedures are at increased risk for developing peptic ulcers. H_2 histamine antagonists, such as famotidine, are the most commonly prescribed agents. Proton pump inhibitors are also effective (see Chap. 27).
- Maintain therapeutic levels of antiepileptic agents for patients who undergo manipulation of cortical structures, as is almost always the case for supratentorial surgery, and those who have a preexisting seizure disorder. Phenytoin and levetiracetam are commonly used agents that can be administered intravenously (see Chap. 29).

13.3 Postoperative Considerations

13.3.1 General Considerations

- All patients undergoing neurosurgical procedures are at risk of developing airway compromise, especially in the initial 30 min after general anesthesia. Risk factors include duration of surgery, airway manipulation during anterior cervical procedures, lower cranial nerve injury following brain stem procedures, and altered level of consciousness secondary to surgical factors or narcotic requirement. Monitor patients in a setting where airway complications can be diagnosed and corrected quickly.
- Assess neurologic function frequently, typically hourly, for the first 24 h postoperatively in an appropriate setting, such as an ICU or a neuro-observation unit, for most neurosurgical patients.
- Monitor patients undergoing intracranial neurosurgical procedures for signs of intracranial hypertension, such as altered level of consciousness, changes in pupil reactivity, or any new focal neurologic findings.
- Maintain hemodynamic parameters within 20% of baseline in the acute postoperative phase. This commonly requires the use of antihypertensive agents, such as beta blockers and calcium channel blockers. In patients with subarachnoid hemorrhage, vasoactive agents, such as norepinephrine, may be necessary to decrease the risk of vasospasm. A central venous catheter and invasive blood pressure monitoring can be very useful.

13.3.2 Complications

- Neurosurgical hemorrhage can have devastating consequences. It is therefore important to achieve optimal hemostasis both surgically and medically. When bleeding develops, rule out coagulopathy and promptly manage surgically as necessary.

- Infections can have devastating consequences in the neurosurgical patient but are very rare. Prescribe appropriate prophylactic antibiotics and recognize and treat postoperative infections promptly.
- The risk and nature of neurologic deficits depends on the size and location of the lesion. These can include generalized seizures after supratentorial surgery, aphasia after surgery on the dominant frontal, temporal, or parietal lobe, visual changes in occipital lobe and suprasellar surgery, altered level of consciousness after brain stem procedures, sensory deficits after posterior spine surgery and motor deficits after anterior spine surgery. Previously untreated and large arteriovenous malformations present the greatest risk for malignant brain swelling.
- As many as 70% of patients will develop vasospasm after a subarachnoid hemorrhage, which can lead to permanent neurologic deficits and death. Initial size of the hemorrhage and neurologic status are known to correlate with the risk developing vasospasm. Monitor patients with daily transcranial doppler imaging.
- Patients undergoing pituitary surgery or spine surgery requiring durotomy are at an increased risk of developing a CSF leak. These patients usually complain of a positional headache and frequently require surgical repair.
- Pneumocephalus is another potential complication of craniotomy, transsphenoidal surgery, and after spine surgery requiring durotomy. Clinically significant pneumocephalus can impair consciousness but rarely requires surgical intervention.
- Visual loss can occur after any surgical procedure in the prone position. Conjunctival edema is a relatively common complication leading to a transient decrease in visual acuity and discomfort. Bilateral visual loss is most often the result of ischemic optic neuropathy and is more common after prolonged procedures, associated with large amounts of intraoperative blood loss, and intraoperative hypotension. Unilateral visual loss is usually the result of direct pressure on the eye leading to central retinal artery occlusion. The intraoperative use of a horseshoe and certain protective goggles has been reported to increase the risk of this complication.

13.4 Surgical Procedures

13.4.1 Spine Surgery

- Indications include osteoarthritis, rheumatoid arthritis, spinal stenosis, scoliosis (see Chap. 12), tumor, syringomyelia, tethered chord, and trauma.
- Associated preoperative factors include advanced age, tobacco use, and decreased exercise tolerance. Patients with rheumatoid arthritis are at additional risk for atlanto-occipital joint subluxation, and may require administration of stress dose of steroids in the perioperative period (see Chap. 28).
- Patients with cervical and high thoracic spine lesions are also at risk of autonomic dysfunction. This can range from relatively benign conditions, such as orthostatic hypotension, to

more serious phenomena such as autonomic hyperreflexia associated with quadriplegia or spinal shock in acute spinal trauma.

- Patients undergoing cervical spine surgery are at higher risk of intraoperative airway complications. Patients undergoing combined anterior–posterior cervical procedures are also at risk of developing airway edema in the postoperative period, which should be carefully considered when extubating the patient.
- Postoperatively, patients may benefit from the use of muscle relaxants such as methocarbamol as an adjunct to narcotics for pain control. Patients may require frequent neurologic assessment in an intensive care setting.
- An epidural hematoma can lead to permanent neurologic deficits if not recognized and surgically evacuated promptly. Order a STAT MRI whenever progressive lower extremity weakness or sensory deficit develops.

13.4.2 Intracranial Surgery

- The most common indications include tumor, abscess, hematoma, subarachnoid hemorrhage, arteriovenous malformation, hemangioma, aneurysm, trauma, and intractable epilepsy.
- Preoperative considerations center around the mass effect created by the lesion. The goal is to preserve cerebral perfusion pressure and to avoid bleeding of vascular lesions. Many patients have decreased intracranial compliance. They may have been started on a steroid therapy, most commonly dexamethasone, and may need stress dose steroids in the perioperative period (see Chap. 22). Seizure prophylaxis is controversial. The American Heart Association and American College of Cardiologists consider intracranial surgery an intermediate risk procedure.
- Postoperatively, patients are usually monitored in the ICU setting overnight for possible complications. These include intracranial bleeding, pneumocephalus, increased intracranial pressure, seizures, stroke, and hyponatremia, the latter possibly due to the syndrome of inappropriate antidiuretic hormone (SIADH) or cerebral salt wasting (CSW) (see Chap. 39).
- Hypertension is very common and responds well to labetalol.
- Brain stem surgery may also compromise the cranial nerves responsible for the gag and swallow reflex. Take aspiration precautions with these patients to minimize the risk of airway complications.
- Patients recovering from aneurysm clipping are at an increased risk of vasospasm. Keep mean arterial pressure elevated, assure adequate hydration, and maintain their hematocrit around 30%. Recent evidence suggests that calcium channel blockers, such nicardipine administered as a drip, may be effective in preventing vasospasm in patients who are at risk.
- The mortality rate for patients suffering from subarachnoid hemorrhage (SAH) approaches 40%. The risk peaks at the age of 55. Other factors include hypertension, family history of SAH, and peripheral vascular disease. Despite treatment, the rate of cognitive dysfunction is almost 25%. The goal of therapy is to decrease systolic blood

pressure and heart rate while maintaining cerebral perfusion and reducing the risk of vasospasm, which peaks between 5 and 7 days. Beta blockers are effective in achieving the former, whereas calcium channel blockers (nimodipine) and alpha agonists can be used to attain the latter. Nonspecific ST elevations are present in up to 8% of patients, but are more frequently reflective of the underlying increase in sympathetic tone leading to stunned myocardium (a reversible condition) rather than ischemia. Nonetheless, cardiac enzymes should be obtained and the patient should be closely monitored for life-threatening arrhythmias.

- Transphenoidal surgery is performed for the resection of pituitary masses. The most common indications include prolactin secreting microadenomas and nonsecreting macroadenomas. Secondary amenorrhea is a common finding in the former while headache, visual field defects, and hypopituitarism are more typical of the latter. Nonsecreting suprasellar masses can in addition cause SIADH and hydrocephalus. Growth hormone secreting tumors leading to acromegaly, adrenocorticotropic hormone secreting tumors causing Cushing's disease, and thyroid stimulating hormone secreting tumors resulting in hyperthyroidism are rarer. The workup for patients suspected of having a pituitary lesion should include endocrine studies and an MRI. Hypocortisolism should be treated with steroids while monitoring, and correcting glucose and sodium levels preoperatively. Hypothyroidism should also be corrected as it can exaggerate the cardiovascular suppressant effects of anesthetic agents. Postoperative complications can include adrenal crisis, which should be treated with glucocorticoids and central diabetes insipidus, which responds to desmopressin. In addition, a CSF leak, characterized by a positional headache may develop requiring aggressive hydration, supine positioning, and eventual surgical repair. The risk of meningitis is significant when this complication develops.
- Other late complications may include infection (from meningitis or a shunt) and pressure ulcers (from immobility and steroid use).

Suggested Reading

Gerlach R, Krause M, Seifert V, Goerlinger K. Hemostatic and hemorrhagic problems in neurosurgical patients. *Acta Neurochir*. 2009;151:873-900.

Pasternak JJ, Lanier WL. Neuroanesthesiology review–2007. *J Neurosurg Anesthesiol*. 2008;20(2):78-104.

Warner DS. Anesthesia for craniotomy. *Can J Anesth*. 2002;49(6):R1-R8.

Gynecologic Surgery 14

Bruce E. Johnson

14.1 Introduction

Preoperative medical consultations are less common for gynecologic surgery than in some other surgical specialties. The main reason for this is that with the exception of gynecologic oncology and perhaps some urogynecology, much of gynecologic surgery occurs in younger women who are less likely to have co-morbid conditions that would warrant preoperative consultation.[1] Also, the use of prophylactic antibiotics has decreased postoperative infection which was another reason medical consultation was requested. Special considerations in patients undergoing gynecologic surgery to be addressed include the widespread performance of laparoscopic procedures, specifics related to vaginal and vulvar procedures, and the use of estrogen-based products.

14.2 Preoperative Considerations

14.2.1 Cardiovascular Risk Factors

- The increase in obesity[2] means more women are at risk for the metabolic syndrome. Since menstrual irregularities and infertility are common in the metabolic syndrome, more women may be having diagnostic and therapeutic procedures due to these complaints. Common consequences of the syndrome include glucose intolerance, hypertension, lipid abnormalities, and increased risk for coronary artery disease (CAD). Obese women are more likely to be deconditioned, making it difficult to assess exercise tolerance, an important consideration when evaluating cardiopulmonary function.

B.E. Johnson
Virginia Tech Carilion School of Medicine, Roanoke, VA, USA
e-mail: bejohnson@carilionclinic.org

S.L. Cohn (ed.), *Perioperative Medicine*,
DOI: 10.1007/978-0-85729-498-2_14, © Springer-Verlag London Limited 2011

- CAD in women may present with different symptoms than in men. Instead of crushing, substernal chest pain, women with angina may only have symptoms of fatigue, perspiration, neck or jaw achiness, or shoulder/arm discomfort.

14.2.2 Pulmonary Risk Factors

- Lower abdominal and pelvic procedures can reduce pulmonary function by approximately 25%. This change combined with the use of general anesthesia and the presence of obesity[2] may increase the gynecologic surgery patient's risk of postoperative pulmonary complications and warrant use of lung expansion maneuvers and other risk reduction strategies (see Chap. 21).

14.2.3 Anesthesia

- Most laparoscopic, open abdominal and extensive vaginal/vulvar procedures are done under general anesthesia which tends to carry more risk than regional or local anesthesia.

14.2.4 Thromboembolic Disease

- Oral contraceptive pills (OCP) and postmenopausal hormone therapy (HT) contain supraphysiologic doses of estrogen, a well-recognized risk for venous thromboembolism (VTE). Similarly, selective estrogen receptor modulators (SERM) such as tamoxifen carry risk of thromboembolism. In relatively non-elective surgery, there is little advantage to discontinue these agents. However, in truly elective cases, one must weigh the risk of VTE if the drug is continued versus the risk of pregnancy or postmenopausal symptoms (hot flashes) if temporarily stopped before surgery.
  - To decrease risk of VTE, OCPs should be discontinued at least 6 weeks before surgery to allow all the stimulated coagulation factors to return to baseline. This is a relatively long time for a woman who had been taking OCPs for contraception to utilize other, perhaps less reliable, measures. If the risk of pregnancy is greater than the perceived risk of postoperative thromboembolism, the surgeon and consultant may decide simply to continue the medication (which is usually the case).
  - For the same reason, HT should be discontinued at least 6 weeks before surgery. However, a woman taking HT for hot flashes is likely to experience a resurgence of that symptom.
  - If the woman is taking a SERM for treatment of breast cancer, the oncologist should be contacted to discuss whether temporary discontinuation is feasible. If she is taking a SERM as prophylaxis, there is little risk in stopping it.

14.2.5 Infection

- Antibiotic prophylaxis is indicated for most vulvar and vaginal procedures. Even abdominal procedures that involve entering the vagina, the most common example being hysterectomy, are preceded by prophylactic antibiotics.[3] Such treatment has dramatically reduced previously common infections such as cuff cellulitis, pelvic cellulitis or abscess. A common practice is to give a second generation cephalosporin 30–60 min before surgery with some gynecologists following this with a second dose postoperatively. Metronidazole or clindamycin can be used in penicillin-allergic patients (see Chap. 7).

14.3 Postoperative Considerations

Complications encountered after gynecologic surgery include bleeding, infection, VTE, urinary tract injury, neuropathy, bowel dysfunction, and cardiopulmonary complications.[4]

- *Bleeding*: Blood loss is greater after myomectomy than hysterectomy and also greater after more extensive surgical procedures. If postoperative hemorrhage is suspected, repeat the hemoglobin/hematocrit every few hours, transfuse as necessary, and plan for re-exploration.
- *Infection*: Besides Staphylococcus and Streptococcus organisms often responsible for surgical site infections, a number of other pathogens are commonly isolated from postoperative pelvic infections. These include aerobic gram-negative bacilli, anaerobes, and Mycoplasma. Types of infection include pelvic cellulitis, cuff cellulitis, pelvic abscesses, and later osteomyelitis pubis.
  - Autoimmune and inflammatory conditions are more common in younger women. These diseases are often treated with corticosteroids as well as chemotherapeutic or immune-modulating agents which may predispose to poor tissue healing and increased risk of infection. Prophylactic antibiotics should be given and the surgeon (and consultant) should maintain a higher index of suspicion for postoperative infection in these settings.
- *VTE*: Risk factors germane to gynecologic surgery include malignancy (both ovarian and endometrial carcinoma),[5] prior radiation therapy, chemotherapy, use of estrogen or estrogen-like hormones, obesity, and pelvic surgery itself. Pulmonary embolism remains a significant cause of postoperative morbidity and mortality.
  - While early ambulation and use of pneumatic compression devices may suffice in some circumstances (short procedures, benign disease), women undergoing major pelvic operations (oncologic, infections) should receive pharmacologic prophylaxis with or without mechanical devices (see Chap. 4).
  - Pelvic thrombophlebitis may be sterile and attributed to the same risk factors noted above, or it can be complicated by infection. Such complications are difficult to

detect and diagnose. Complaints of pain specific to phlebitis are difficult to separate from usual postoperative pain and fever may be low-grade or non-existent. Imaging studies, including magnetic resonance angiography, have a disappointingly low sensitivity. Often, clinical suspicion is most relevant. Treatment with both anticoagulation (heparin) and antibiotics should be started.

While embolism from infected ovarian veins rarely causes clinically evident pulmonary embolism, septic complications in the lungs may ensue so heparin is used to reduce likelihood of embolization. Antibiotics use should be directed by cultures obtained at the time of operation; if not available, then empiric treatment for gram-negative and anaerobic organisms is indicated.

- *Urinary tract injury*: Every gynecologist-in-training is taught that there are two crucial complications to avoid during pelvic surgery–injuries to the bladder and inadvertent suturing of the ureter.
  - Injuries noted during the procedure can be directly repaired, usually with satisfactory results.[6] Bladder injury can usually be repaired primarily. Ureteral complications can require stenting with urological follow-up.
  - Postoperative hematuria is more likely to be associated with bladder than ureter complications. However, both may lead to flank/pelvic pain, infection, fluid collection, and even fistula. Obstruction of a ureter may lead to acute hydronephrosis; if a leak also happened, collection of urine in the abdomen may result in either ascites-type accumulation or a more localized fluid collection (urinoma).
  - The medicine consultant is typically called to help manage renal dysfunction resulting from ureter damage or infectious complications.
- *Neuropathies*: Many gynecologic procedures are done in the lithotomy position. Gynecologists and anesthesiologists are well aware of the possible neurological complications that can occur from inadvertent compression injuries during surgery. Examples of such complications include:
  - Injury to the femoral nerve: occurring because of retractor injury, the patient may experience pain and/or numbness of the anterior thigh and instability of the knee especially on standing. Findings would include absent patellar reflex and quadriceps weakness.
  - Injury to the sciatic/peroneal nerve: occurring because of stretch/pressure due to the lithotomy position, the patient may experience lower limb and foot numbness. Findings would include decreased sensation in the lower leg and weakness with foot eversion.
  - Injury to the obturator nerve: occurring because of inadvertent transaction, the patient would experience pain and numbness of the medial thigh. Findings include weakness of hip adduction.
- *Bowel dysfunction*: Routine use of a nasogastric (NG) tube should be avoided as it increases risk of aspiration.[7] It should only be used for refractory nausea and vomiting or significant abdominal distention. Postoperative ileus can be managed with a nasogastric (NG) tube if necessary, bowel rest, electrolyte repletion, and hydration. It needs to be differentiated from small bowel obstruction which usually presents later.

- *Cardiopulmonary complications*: Risk of cardiovascular death after gynecologic surgery is relatively low; however, risk has to be individualized. Postoperative atelectasis is common, and risk of pneumonia is related to the type of surgery and specific patient risk factors (e.g., chronic obstructive pulmonary disease (COPD), smoking, obesity). This can be minimized by incentive spirometry and other strategies as noted previously (see Chap. 21).
- *Adrenal suppression:* Repeated or prolonged treatment with corticosteroids may result in adrenal suppression and hypoadrenalism when confronted with the stress of surgery. Women who otherwise appear to be functional may have poor appetite, undue fatigue, delayed ambulation, altered electrolytes, and even hypotension or cardiovascular collapse while trying to recover from surgery. Stress dose steroids may be warranted (see Chap. 22).

14.4 Common Procedures

- Many gynecologic procedures are laparoscopic, done in younger, healthier women, and performed in ambulatory surgicenter locations (Table 14.1). The women are rarely seen for preoperative evaluation and postoperative medical complications are infrequent, but there are several considerations for the consultant.

Table 14.1 Gynecologic surgery-specific considerations

Type of surgery	Preoperative considerations	Postoperative considerations
Laparoscopic	Few specific issues	Air embolism rare. Hypercapnea and postop pulmonary dysfunction due to Trendelenburg position, pressure of abdominal organs on diaphragm, or obesity.
Hysterectomy	Prophylactic antibiotics. If on hormones (OCP or HT) consider discontinue if time permits.	Bladder or ureter injuries may occur. VTE risk high; consider routine prophylaxis.
Vulvar/vaginal	If cancer, usually older woman with attendant risks. Prophylactic antibiotics, especially for vaginal.	Surgical exenteration with high complication rate, including infection, bowel ileus, bedrest, and VTE.
Malignancies	Often older women, with attendant cardiovascular (CV)/pulm risks. Prophylactic anticoagulation common. Preop chemo- or radiotherapy may leave patient anemic or infection-prone.	Ovarian cancer-induced ascites may be associated with fluid shifts. Postop bowel ileus common.

Adapted from Porter and Johnson[7]

- Both thrombophlebitis and urologic complications may occur. Prophylactic anticoagulation may not be used and estrogen-based treatments are not usually stopped. Ureteral injury is less common during laparoscopic surgery than during open procedures though injuries to the bladder still happen.
- Insufflation of the abdomen with air uncommonly results in problems, but pneumothorax and pneumomediastinum can occur from air passing through congenital defects in the diaphragm. Unless truly large, with functional pulmonary compromise, these generally resolve quickly and do not require chest tube insertion.
- Many laparoscopic procedures are done in the Trendelenburg position, deliberately allowing abdominal organs to drift out of the pelvis. This plus obesity plus insufflation may combine to compromise diaphragmatic function, occasionally leading to hypoventilation. Preexisting poorly controlled asthma or other lung disease can exacerbate the problem.

- Gynecologic oncology cases often occur in older women, with a greater likelihood of co-morbid medical conditions and debility.[8] Procedures are often lengthy and can involve bowel resection. Postoperatively, these women are likely to have ileus, nasogastric tubes, and prolonged bedrest. Vulvar and vaginal cancer cases carry a relatively high risk of infection. Ovarian cancer is often associated with ascites, which may not be fully controlled following a debulking operation; rapid reaccumulation of ascites can result in fluid shifts with resultant alteration in renal function and even blood pressure control.
- Urogynecology procedures carry risks of bladder or urethral damage. Short term concerns include prolonged catheter placement; longer term issues include both incontinence (often the very reason for the procedure) and urinary retention.
- Operations for infertility range from laparoscopic repair of altered tubes or ovaries to harvesting of eggs following stimulation (frequently with clomiphene). Each procedure, no matter how many times previously performed, carries equal risk.
- Therapeutic (induced) abortion remains a common surgical procedure in obstetrics/gynecology with upward of 1.3 million procedures performed in the USA each year. It is quite safe with mortality of less than 1 in 100,000. Complications of the procedure are also low, depending on the time in pregnancy the abortion is performed and the procedure chosen.

  - Therapeutic (induced) abortion is safest when done at less than 12 weeks gestation using the vacuum extraction technique. For pregnancies of greater than 12 weeks (second trimester), the more common procedure is the dilation and extraction (D&E). D&E procedures have more risk of bleeding, infection, and uterine perforation.
  - Induction of uterine contractions (labor) can be stimulated by prostaglandin products; there is a small but present risk of uterine rupture in women who previously had cesarean section.
  - Most therapeutic (induced) abortions are done under some form of anesthesia. Early terminations may be done with local, cervical blocks. Most other operative procedures are typically done under general anesthesia.

References

1. Johnson BE, Porter J. Preoperative evaluation of the gynecologic patient: considerations for improved outcomes. *Obstet Gynecol*. 2008;111:1183-1194.
2. Pandey S, Bhattacharya S. Impact of obesity on gynecology. *Womens Health*. 2010;6:107-117.
3. ACOG Committee on Practice Bulletins. ACOG Practice Bulletin No. 74. Antibiotic prophylaxis for gynecologic procedures. *Obstet Gynecol*. 2006;108:225. American College of Obstetricians and Gynecologists.
4. Katz VL, Lentz GM, Lobo RA, Gershenson DM, eds. *Comprehensive Gynecology*. 5th ed. Philadelphia: Mosby Elsevier; 2007.
5. Gerestein CG, Damhuis RA, de Vries M, et al. Causes of postoperative mortality after surgery for ovarian cancer. *Eur J Cancer*. 2009;45:2799-2803.
6. Cholkeri-Singh A, Narapalem N, Miller CE. Laparoscopic ureteral injury and repair: case reviews and clinical update. *J Minim Invasive Gynecol*. 2007;14:356-361.
7. Porter J, Johnson BE. Gynecologic surgery. In: Cohn SL, Smetana GW, Weed HG, eds. *Perioperative Medicine: Just the Facts*. New York: McGraw-Hill; 2006:74-81.
8. Mains LM, Magnus M, Finan M. Perioperative morbidity and mortality from major gynecologic surgery in the elderly woman. *J Reprod Med*. 2007;52:677-684.

Urologic Surgery

15

Bruce E. Johnson

15.1 Introduction

Urologic surgery encompasses a wide variety of surgical techniques including laparoscopic, cystoscopic/resectoscopic, open abdominal, open flank/thoracic, vascular, and extracorporeal shock-wave lithotripsy. Patients undergoing urologic procedures span a broad spectrum of ages and comorbidities. Perioperative consultation in urologic surgery requires both attention to these comorbid conditions and a working knowledge of operative-specific complications.[1]

15.2 Preoperative Considerations

- Many urologic patients are older. It was estimated that as much as 50% of men over age 70 would undergo some form of prostate surgery, with upward of 70% of these surgical candidates having at least one medical diagnosis that conferred surgical risk. A thorough evaluation seeking any modifiable risk is essential.
- Assess older patients for cardiopulmonary disease, anemia, renal dysfunction, and other common age-related conditions.
  - Mild chronic kidney disease (stage 1 or 2) can become worse if the patient is dehydrated or hypervolemic, anemic, or hyperkalemic.[2] Advanced stages of chronic kidney disease (CKD) are associated with cardiorespiratory disease, dysfunctional hemostasis, and anemia.
  - As many older urologic patients have anemia, determine if the surgery is likely to result in significant blood loss (e.g., retropubic prostatectomy, cystectomy, nephrectomy); if so consider the use of erythropoietin, iron, or preoperative transfusion.

B.E. Johnson
Virginia Tech Carilion School of Medicine, Roanoke, VA, USA
e-mail: bejohnson@carilionclinic.org

S.L. Cohn (ed.), *Perioperative Medicine*,
DOI: 10.1007/978-0-85729-498-2_15, © Springer-Verlag London Limited 2011

- Obtain a screening urinalysis and treat bacteriuria as it may be associated with the development of bacteremia after instrumentation of the genitourinary tract. Prescribe preoperative prophylactic antibiotics based on the type of procedure and likelihood of bacteremia and postoperative infection (see Chap. 7).[3]
- Consider venous thromboembolism (VTE) prophylaxis for open urologic procedures. Transurethral and minor procedures do not usually mandate prophylaxis in the absence of other risk factors (see Chap. 5).

15.3 Postoperative Considerations

- Bleeding, in several different manifestations, can present postoperative complications; most of these are commonly known to urologists and routinely managed.
  - Bleeding that requires catheter placement, and even flushing, is common following certain bladder and prostate procedures and lithotripsy.
  - Bleeding following prostate procedures is common as the prostate releases plasmin and thromboplastin which are anticoagulants, and the urologist has only indirect access to the bleeding site via the cystoscope during transurethral procedures. Blood clots may form and result in urinary tract obstruction.
  - Lithotripsy results in "gravel" that, in addition to causing pain, may injure the kidney pelvis and/or ureters causing bleeding, or result in obstruction.
  - Both the bladder and the kidney are vascular organs, making blood loss during even routine cystectomy and/or nephrectomy common. Persistent bleeding following procedures that might involve the ureter could be an indication of incomplete repair or inadvertent injury.
- Electrolyte abnormalities are common, especially after trans-urethral resection of the prostate (TURP). Many patients undergoing urological procedures have some renal function compromise. Stress of surgery, along with occasional large volume fluid replacement, may affect electrolytes, especially sodium and potassium. Marginal renal function limits the ability to self-correct. Hyponatremia can develop quickly and may present immediately after surgery as confusion, altered mental status, or seizures.
  - Patients undergoing TURP operations used to be at considerable risk for postoperative hyponatremia. Large volumes of hypotonic solution were commonly used to flush the operative site, allowing the urologist better visibility. Absorption of this fluid via the bleeding vessel and prostatic plexus could change the serum sodium rapidly. This complication is less commonly seen now with the use of laser resection (rather than cold knife) and with the use of glycine or mannitol osmotic agents in the flushing solution.
  - Urinary diversion surgeries still carry risk of electrolyte abnormalities due to inconsistent absorption of urine by the ileum or colon.

- Postoperative delirium is also seen frequently since many patients undergoing urological procedures are elderly, and surgical stress is often significant.[4]
  - Identify and treat true metabolic or neurologic events.
  - Protect the patient from self-injury while the delirium improves on its own.
- Complications specific to laparoscopy or robotic surgery are rare. These may include gas insufflation embolus and absorption of gas with alterations of acid/base or electrolytes.

15.4 Common Procedures

There are some specific issues that should be considered relative to the proposed urologic operation (Table 15.1).

Table 15.1 Urologic surgery-specific considerations

Type of surgery	Preoperative considerations	Postoperative considerations
Lithotripsy	Urine for culture: treat any bacteriuria. If pacemaker, EP cardiac consultation.	
TURP	Urine for culture: treat any bacteriuria.	Severe hyponatremia in as many as 4% of patients. Volume overload/ hypo-osmolality. Hemolysis.
TURBT	Some recommend treat all with prophylactic antibiotics.	Bladder/catheter clot may cause urinary retention.
Cystectomy (esp. radical)	Some recommend treat all with prophylactic antibiotics. If possible, treat anemia. Preop renal function may allow or reject urinary diversion.	Closely monitor H/H. If diversion, closely monitor electrolytes, creatinine, acid–base. High risk for delirium. High risk for VTE; consider pharmacologic and mechanical prophylaxis.
Nephrectomy (esp. radical)	If possible, treat anemia.	Closely monitor H/H. Awareness of atelectasis. If tumor, awareness of tumor embolism. High risk for VTE; consider pharmacologic and mechanical prophylaxis.
Renovascular	Evaluate for coexistent CV, other vascular disease.	Postop monitor with arterial line for BP management. Atheroembolic injury to kidney, lower extremities.

Adapted from Porter and Pfeifer[1]

CV cardiovascular, *EP* electrophysiologist, *H/H* hemoglobin/hematocrit, *TURBT* transurethral resection of bladder tumor, *TURP* transurethral resection of the prostate, *VTE* venous thromboembolism

- Extracorporeal shock wave lithotripsy used to involve almost full immersion in a tub of water, even while the patient is anesthetized. Although spinal or epidural anesthesia can be used, general anesthesia is preferred. Several postoperative issues are relevant[5]:
  - The "gravel" produced and passed through the ureter and bladder may result in pain and hematuria. While most lithotripsy procedures are relatively short, fluid shifts may occur. Water immersion can cause renal adaptations that result in diuresis (and possibly kaliuresis and natriuresis as well), but this rarely causes problems unless large quantities of intravenous fluids were administered during the procedure.
  - Water immersion in an anesthetized patient reduces functional residual capacity and may lead to postoperative atelectasis. Patients should be instructed in incentive spirometry preoperatively and should continue to use the device once discharged home.

- Urinary diversion operations are complicated procedures usually performed because of urinary tract malignancies or other lower abdominal/pelvic malignancies (e.g., cervical, rectal).[5] These include:
  - Ureterosigmoidostomy in which the ureters are mobilized from the bladder and anastomosed to the sigmoid colon; no external stoma is created.
  - Ureteroileal cutaneous diversion in which an isolated loop of ileum serves as the urinary exit to the outside through a stoma, the ureters having been anastomosed from the bladder to the ileal loop. A bag is continuously worn to collect the urine
  - Continent diversions are a variation of the ureteroileal cutaneous diversion in which the ileum serves as a repository for urine, a "nipple" is created, and intermittent catheterization is possible. A urinary bag is not needed if the procedure is successful.
  - These operations can produce interesting, and sometimes difficult-to-resolve electrolyte abnormalities, due to the inconsistent absorption of urine products by the diverted bowel.

    Hyperchloremic metabolic acidosis is relatively common, and hypokalemia occurs as well.

    Oral potassium supplements and occasionally sodium bicarbonate are usually sufficient to correct these abnormalities.

    Preexisting renal insufficiency may complicate treatment.

- The TURP, and to some degree the TURBT, remains a prototypical urologic operation.[1] As mentioned above, the greatest concern with these surgeries, especially the TURP, is hyponatremia resulting from absorption of hypotonic irrigating solutions, resulting in hyponatremia
  - Greater awareness, the use of solutions with glycine or mannitol, and the use of "hot" laser knives which cause coagulation at the site have decreased the likelihood of this complication.
  - After the operation is over, the patient's normal response to the hyponatremia (once it is recognized) is to hold onto sodium and excrete free water. Treatment involving fluid restriction or normal saline and administration of a loop diuretic can assist this process.

- Vascular repair of the renal artery, whether with an open repair or percutaneous angioplasty, is usually a procedure with low complications.[5]
  - The most common cause of death is a postoperative MI. Other complications include electrolyte abnormalities from hyperaldosteronism, renal failure, and rarely rupture of the renal artery or renal artery thrombosis.
  - With percutaneous angioplasty and/or stenting, small emboli into the kidney parenchyma may occur.

    Hematuria, sometimes pyuria, and even short-term elevations in blood pressure may ensue.

    Cholesterol or blood clots may also embolize to lower extremities.
- Some urological procedures carry a moderate risk for postoperative venous thromboembolism.[6]
  - These generally are procedures performed in the pelvis or retroperitoneum and include retroperitoneal lymph node dissection, radical nephrectomy, open prostatectomy/radical prostatectomy, urinary diversion operations, and cystectomy.
  - Consider VTE prophylaxis even though some procedures (e.g., cystectomy) are bloody (see Chap. 5).
  - While early ambulation is always a goal, use of compression stockings and subcutaneous heparin or low molecular weight heparin should be strongly considered.
- Adrenalectomy can be performed by urologists or general surgeons.[1] Sometimes adrenalectomy is done as part of a radical nephrectomy by an urologist for cancer. On other occasions, adrenalectomy is done for endocrine-related conditions (e.g., Cushings syndrome, Conns syndrome, and others).
  - Unless bilateral adrenalectomy is planned, most patients will not require postoperative steroid supplementation. An important exception is the person with a single adrenal adenoma or carcinoma producing excess corticosteroid. In such cases, the contralateral adrenal gland may be suppressed and postoperative "stress" steroids would be indicated (see Chaps. 3 and 22).
  - Preoperatively check catecholamines and start an alpha-blocker.
  - Intraoperative hypertension and postoperative hypotension may complicate the procedure, regardless of whether a pheochromocytoma has been identified.
  - Monitor the patient postoperatively in an ICU setting.
- Radical nephrectomy, cystectomy, and prostatectomy are complex operations with relatively high morbidity and mortality.[7,8]
  - The operations can be quite bloody, requiring both intraoperative and postoperative transfusion

    Frequent postoperative measurement of hemoglobin/hematocrit is important
  - Because of blood and fluid shifts, intraoperative and postoperative hypotension is not unexpected.
  - Management of postoperative bleeding is further complicated due to likelihood of using prophylactic anticoagulation.

– A complication unique to renal cell carcinoma, a common reason for radical nephrectomy, is tumor emboli. Indeed, tumor may migrate from the kidney parenchyma along the renal vein and even enter the vena cava. Separation of portions of tumor from the tumor bulk leads to pulmonary emboli; the clinical presentation is little different from blood clot (though the longer term consequences certainly are).

References

1. Porter J, Pfeifer K. Urologic surgery. In: Cohn SL, Smetana GW, Weed HG, eds. *Perioperative Medicine: Just the Facts*. New York: McGraw-Hill; 2006:82-88.
2. West SE. Urologic surgery. In: Merli GJ, Weitz HH, eds. *Medical Management of the Surgical Patient*. 2nd ed. Philadelphia: Saunders; 1998:368-373.
3. Yamamoto S, Kanamaru S, Kunishima Y, et al. Perioperative antimicrobial prophylaxis in urology: a multi-center prospective study. *J Chemother*. 2005;17:189-197.
4. Hamann J, Bickel H, Schwaibold H, et al. Postoperative acute confusional state in typical urologic population: incidence, risk factors, and strategies for prevention. *Urology*. 2005;65:449-453.
5. Tanagho EA, McAninch JW, eds. *Smith's General Urology*. 17th ed. New York: McGraw-Hill; 2008.
6. Scarpa RM, Carrieri G, Gussoni G, et al. Clinically overt venous thromboembolism urologic cancer surgery: results from the @RISTOS study. *Eur Urol*. 2007;51:130-135.
7. Prasad SM, Ferreria M, Berry AM, et al. Surgical apgar outcome score: perioperative risk assessment for radical cystectomy. *J Urol*. 2009;181:1046-1052.
8. Wallner LP, Dunn RL, Sarma AV, et al. Risk factors for prolonged length of stay after urologic surgery: the National Surgical Quality Improvement Program. *J Am Coll Surg*. 2008;207:904-913.

Bariatric Surgery

16

Brian Harte

16.1 Introduction

- Bariatric surgery refers to surgical procedures which alter the functioning of the gastrointestinal tract with the purpose of facilitating weight loss.
- Obesity is defined as body mass index (BMI) of 30 or greater; a BMI of 40 or greater is considered "severely" or "morbidly" obese. Morbidly obese individuals are potential candidates for surgery to achieve substantial weight loss.
- Those with BMI between 35 and 40 may also be candidates for surgery if their condition is complicated by severe comorbidities such as obstructive sleep apnea (OSA), obesity-hypoventilation, or difficult-to-control diabetes.
- Bariatric surgery has a low complication rate (operative mortality is less than 1.5%), but patients should demonstrate understanding of lifestyle and dietary changes necessary after surgery. The screening process should be rigorous and include behavioral, psychosocial, and medical evaluations.
- From the perspective of chronic disease management and obesity-related morbidity and mortality, bariatric surgery can be associated with impressive outcomes: greater weight loss, better quality of life, and improvements in diabetes, sleep apnea, hypertension, and dyslipidemia.
- Bariatric surgery encompasses numerous specific surgical procedures, which fall into one of three categories:
  - *Restrictive procedures* lower the storage capacity of the stomach. Weight loss tends to be gradual, and modern techniques (such as adjustable gastric banding) tend to be well tolerated.
  - *Malabsorptive procedures* (e.g., jejuno-ileal bypass and biliopancreatic bypass) decrease caloric (and nutrient) absorption by shortening the length of the digestive tract. The weight loss induced by pure bypass procedures may be impressive, but the

B. Harte
Department of Hospital Medicine, Cleveland Clinic,
9500 Euclid Avenue, M2 Annex, Cleveland, OH 44195, USA
e-mail: harteb@ccf.org

S.L. Cohn (ed.), *Perioperative Medicine*,
DOI: 10.1007/978-0-85729-498-2_16, © Springer-Verlag London Limited 2011

complications related to malabsorption may also be severe, including diarrhea, electrolyte abnormalities, and liver failure.

 - *Combination procedures* include both restrictive and malabsorptive components. The Roux-en-Y gastric bypass can be performed laparoscopically and can result in significant weight loss, although nutrient malabsorption can be problematic.

- The best choice of bariatric procedure depends on the available expertise (surgeon and institution), patient preferences, BMI, metabolic variables, comorbidities, and preoperative risk stratification.

16.2 Preoperative Assessment and Management

- Obesity has associations with many chronic diseases. The goal of the preoperative evaluation should be to determine that the patient meets the recommended criteria for bariatric surgery, to identify issues that increase the patient's operative risk and intervene to reduce risk when possible, and to identify and modify factors that may reduce the probability of long-term weight loss and subsequent complications.
- Specific contraindications to bariatric surgery include:
  - Unstable psychiatric conditions or inability to understand lifestyle implications of weight-loss reduction surgery
  - Alcohol or drug dependence
  - Severe pulmonary hypertension or biventricular congestive heart failure
  - Nephrogenic diabetes insipidus (due to potential short- and long-term fluid and electrolyte management issues)

- Factors that may increase risk of perioperative complications include history of venous thromboembolism (VTE), decompensated CAD or heart failure, unrecognized or untreated OSA, smoking, and superobesity (BMI > 50 kg/m^2).
- An Obesity Surgery Mortality Risk Score (OS-MRS) has been validated and includes five equally weighted variables: BMI ≥ 50 kg/m^2, male gender, hypertension, VTE history, and age ≥ 45 years.[1]

Table 16.1 Obesity Surgery Mortality Risk Score (OS-MRS)

Risk factors:
BMI ≥ 50 kg/m^2
Male gender
Hypertension
VTE risk (i.e., prior VTE, right heart failure, pulmonary hypertension, or venous stasis)
Age ≥ 45 years

Table 16.1 (continued)

OS-MRS class	# Risk factors	Mortality (%)
A	0–1	0.2
B	2–3	1.2
C	4–5	2.4

- The definitions of the low, intermediate, and high risk groups and their corresponding mortality rates are seen in Table 16.1.
- The most common causes of death were pulmonary embolism, cardiac causes, and gastrointestinal leak.

16.2.1 Cardiac Evaluation

- Obesity is associated with an increased risk of coronary artery disease as well as a higher prevalence of clinical cardiac risk factors: hypertension, hyperlipidemia, and diabetes. Although laparoscopic techniques are generally associated with low cardiac morbidity and mortality, the rates are still higher than other forms of laparoscopic general surgery.
- A standard risk-assessment of cardiac risk, based on the patient's clinical risk factors and self-reported capacity, is appropriate but limited because physical examination and routine electrocardiogram are insensitive to the presence of heart disease in this patient population. In addition, morbid obesity can be associated with a limited or difficult-to-assess functional capacity.
- "Cardiomyopathy of obesity" results from hemodynamic derangements related to an increased body mass, including an increase in circulating blood volume and increased cardiac output, which in turn may result in ventricular dilation and cardiomyopathy, with or without pulmonary hypertension. Diastolic heart failure is more common, and symptoms of obesity cardiomyopathy are seen most often in patients ≥75% above their ideal body weight or with BMI ≥40 kg/m^2.
- Both coronary artery disease and left-ventricular systolic dysfunction are associated with perioperative morbidity and mortality. However, aside from optimal medical therapy (e.g., chronic beta-blocker administration), specific interventions to attenuate these risks are limited.

16.2.1.1 Assessment (see Chap. 20)

- Patients with no clinical cardiac risk factors and good functional capacity may in general proceed to surgery without further cardiac or pulmonary testing.
- In addition to the Obesity Surgery Mortality Risk Score (Table 16.1), the American Heart Association guidelines for assessing cardiac risk in severely obese patients contain several differences from the standard assessment algorithm, based on expert opinion[1]:

– A routine electrocardiogram (EKG) is appropriate for patients with coronary disease or at least one cardiac risk factor, and chest radiography is recommended for all patients. Findings suggesting coronary disease or pulmonary pathology should be pursued.
– Patients with one or more cardiac risks and a functional capacity equal to or greater than four metabolic equivalents (METS) can generally proceed to surgery after chest radiography and EKG.
– Consider noninvasive stress testing for patients with one or more risk factors and those with poor functional capacity (<4 METS) if a positive finding will change management (although it rarely does). Transesophageal dobutamine stress testing may provide the best images in severely obese patients.
– Cardiopulmonary exercise testing may also help predict a composite complication rate which was significantly increased with peak oxygen consumption<15.8 mL/kg/min, and length of stay was also highest in the group with lowest peak oxygen consumption.
– A finding of new decreased systolic ejection fraction on cardiac testing suggests obesity or other cardiomyopathy, and may warrant further evaluation such as angiography prior to surgery. However, routine preoperative echocardiography is not necessary and is appropriate only if otherwise clinically indicated (e.g., unexplained dyspnea, physical findings suggestive of heart failure or valvular disease).

16.2.1.2 Interventions

- Patients on beta-blockers should continue them through surgery.
- Patients with an indication for beta-blockers should have them started preoperatively provided there is adequate time for dose titration to achieve optimal heart rate control.
- Continue or initiate statin therapy for dyslipidemia.
- Optimize blood pressure control.

16.2.2 Pulmonary Evaluation (see Chap. 21)

- The underlying mechanics of respiration are compromised in obese patients, especially when they are supine. Morbidly obese patients typically have restrictive lung disease physiology:

  – Critical lung volumes are reduced – specifically, expiratory reserve volume, forced vital capacity, forced expiratory volume, and functional residual capacity.
  – In addition, obese patients experience diminished respiratory system compliance, increased intra-abdominal pressure from the increased body mass, and increased work of breathing. These derangements result in ventilation-perfusion mismatch and hypoxemia.

- In general, obesity is not clearly associated with an increased risk of major pulmonary complications after surgery but patients are more likely to develop atelectasis based on altered closing volumes. Obese patients commonly suffer from clinically evident or indolent pulmonary disease, most commonly OSA, pulmonary hypertension, and obesity-hypoventilation, all of which may be associated with specific perioperative risks.

– Obstructive Sleep Apnea

  The prevalence of OSA in the obese population is higher than in the population overall.

  OSA has been associated with an increased risk of poor wound healing after surgery, postoperative reintubation, unplanned transfer to intensive care, length of hospital stay, and cardiac ischemia after orthopedic surgery.

  Clinical screening tools for OSA have limited overall predictive value. However, for patients suspected of having OSA who do not have a history of sleep disorders, the STOP-Bang questionnaire (Table 16.2) has a high sensitivity for moderate and severe OSA (defined as an apnea–hypopnea index ≥15 and 30 respectively), although the specificity is low.

  There is no clear consensus on the utility of routine complete polysomnographic testing prior to bariatric surgery. In patients with STOP-Bang scores suggestive of OSA (i.e., ≥3 answers of "yes") consider formal testing preoperatively, in particular if additional comorbid conditions are present (e.g., CHF, diabetes, and hypertension).[2]

– Pulmonary Hypertension

  A true association between pulmonary hypertension and obesity is unclear, in part because of frequent confounding comorbidities which may result in secondary pulmonary hypertension (e.g., OSA, heart failure, and thromboembolic disease).

  Pulmonary hypertension may predict poor postoperative survival, but rigorous prospective data is lacking.

– Obesity-hypoventilation consists of chronic daytime hypoxemia and hypoventilation in the absence of chronic obstructive lung disease and may clinically suggest OSA or pulmonary hypertension.

Table 16.2 The STOP-Bang questionnaire[2]

Do you **S**nore loudly (louder than talking or loud enough to be heard through closed doors)?
Do you often feel **T**ired, fatigued, or sleeping during daytime?
Has anyone **O**bserved you stop breathing during your sleep?
Do you have or are you being treated for high blood **P**ressure?
BMI ≥ 35 kg/m^2?
Age ≥ 50 years old?
Neck circumference ≥ 40 cm^2?
Gender is male?

An answer of "yes" to three or more questions in patients without a history of sleep disorders has a sensitivity of 84% for OSA (56% specificity), and 93% and 100% for moderate and severe OSA, respectively (specificity 43% and 37%)

16.2.2.1
Assessment

- Airway management is a particular concern in the obese population. A careful assessment of the neck, mouth, jaw, and upper airway should be undertaken by an experienced anesthesiologist.
- For most patients, the AHA recommends preoperative chest radiography (see above).
- As stated above, there is no clear consensus on the usefulness of polysomnography. It may be appropriate in patients with STOP-Bang scores of 3 or greater, especially if additional comorbidities are present.
- Pulse oximetry is reasonable to assess for obesity-hypoventilation syndrome, with follow-up arterial blood gas sampling if abnormal. Other tools to help assess pulmonary function include radiography, echocardiography, and pulmonary function tests. However, as in the general population, these should be used selectively, only when clinical findings warrant further evaluation.

16.2.2.2
Interventions

- Initiate incentive spirometry and lung-expansion exercises preoperatively and continue them in the postoperative setting.
- Consider preoperative polysomnography in patients with suspected OSA and initiate a treatment plan. Continue CPAP postoperatively in patients who were using it at home.
- Avoid or minimize the general use of benzodiazepines and narcotics in this population, and observe patients on these medications in monitored settings.

16.2.3
Venous Thromboembolism (See Chap. 5)

- Obesity is a major risk factor for venous thromboembolism (VTE), and pulmonary embolism is the leading cause of mortality after bariatric surgery (although the overall rate is low, less than 1%).

16.2.3.1
Assessment

- Perform risk assessment for a personal or family history of VTE and other comorbid conditions that may increase VTE risk.

16.2.3.2
Interventions

- Pharmacological VTE prophylaxis, adjusted for patient weight, is indicated.
- In addition, the American Society for Metabolic and Bariatric Surgery recommends early postoperative ambulation and perioperative use of lower extremity sequential compression devices.
- There are no established recommendations regarding the role of inferior vena cava filters as a prophylactic intervention.

16.2.4
Diabetes Mellitus

- Obesity predicts the development of diabetes mellitus. Uncontrolled diabetes may predict postoperative morbidity including infections and poor wound healing.

16.2.4.1
Assessment

- Consider routine screening for diabetes via random or fasting glucose.

16.2.4.2
Intervention

- Glycemic control should be optimized prior to surgery (see Chap. 22).

16.2.5
Thyroid Disease

- Thyroid function testing, looking for hypothyroidism, is often performed in the evaluation of obesity. However, obese patients are not inherently more likely to have abnormal thyroid stimulating hormone tests than normal-weight individuals.

16.2.6
Liver Disease

- Accumulation of fat in the hepatocytes (hepatic steatosis) is common in obese patients, although the pursuit of specific manifestations of liver disease (such as coagulopathy, ascites, and cirrhosis) is only indicated if history or examination suggests underlying pathology.

- Gallstones are associated with obesity and with rapid weight loss. If present, prophylactic cholecystectomy may be performed in conjunction with the bariatric procedure.

16.2.7 Complications

- Anastomotic leaks occur in approximately 2% of cases. Although patients may have fatigue, anorexia, abdominal pain, fever, or tachycardia, clinical identification of this complication can be difficult because the textbook findings of peritonitis may not be present. Surgical re-exploration is the optimal approach to diagnosis.
- Wound dehiscence is rare but should be entertained by the presence of serosanguinous wound drainage.
- Wound infections are less common with laparoscopic surgeries than with open techniques. However, when they occur they can be challenging to treat, and can lead to further complications including incisional hernia.
- Long-term management includes medical, surgical, and psychological support. Although many medical conditions may improve, malabsorption and electrolyte abnormalities may occur. After significant weight loss, the patient may develop sagging skin causing cosmetic and other problems and may require plastic surgery.

References

1. Poirier P, Alpert MA, Fleisher LA, et al. Cardiovascular evaluation and management of severely obese patients undergoing surgery: a science advisory from the American Heart Association. *Circulation*. 2009;120:86-95.
2. Chung F, Yegneswaran B, Liao P, et al. STOP questionnaire: a tool to screen patients for obstructive sleep apnea. *Anesthesiology*. 2008;108:812-821.

Suggested Reading

Buchwald H, Avidor Y, Braunwald E, et al. Bariatric surgery: a systemic review and meta-analysis. *JAMA*. 2004;292:1724-1737.

Collazo-Clavell ML, Clark MM, McAlpine DE, et al. Assessment and preparation of patients for bariatric surgery. *Mayo Clin Proc*. 2006;81(10 suppl):S11-S17.

Colquitt J, Clegg A, Sidhu M, et al. Surgery for morbid obesity. *Cochrane Database Syst Rev*.2004; 4: CD003641.

Flegal KM, Carroll MD, Ogden CL, et al. Prevalence and trends in obesity among US adults, 1999-2000. *JAMA*. 2002;288:1723.

Kaw R, Aboussouan L, Auckley D, et al. Challenges in pulmonary risk assessment and perioperative management in bariatric surgery patients. *Obes Surg*. 2008;18:134-138.

Keating CL, Dixon JB, Moodie ML, et al. Cost-effectiveness of surgically induced weight loss for the management of type 2 diabetes: modeled lifetime analysis. *Diab Care*. 2009;32:567-574.

McGlinch BP, Que FG, Nelson JL, Wrobleski DM, Grant JE, Collazo-Clavell ML. Perioperative care of patients undergoing bariatric surgery. *Mayo Clin Proc*. 2006;81(10 suppl):S25-S33.

Mechanick JI, Kushner RF, Sugerman HJ, et al. American Association of Clinical Endocrinologists, The Obesity Society, and American Society for Metabolic & Bariatric Surgery Medical guidelines for clinical practice for the perioperative nutritional, metabolic, and nonsurgical support of the bariatric surgery patient. *Surg Obes Relat Dis*. 2008;4(5 suppl):S109-S184.

Perugini RA, Mason R, Czerniach DR, et al. Predictors of complication and suboptimal weight loss after laparoscopic Roux-en-Y gastric bypass: a series of 188 patients. *Arch Surg*. 2003;138:541-545.

Sergio H, Scott D, Robert S, et al. Safety and efficacy of postoperative continuous positive airway pressure to prevent pulmonary complications after Roux-en-Y gastric bypass. *J Gastrointest Surg*. 2002;6:354-358.

The Longitudinal Assessment of Bariatric Surgery Consortium. Perioperative safety in the longitudinal assessment of bariatric surgery. *N Engl J Med*. 2009;361:445-454.

Ophthalmic Surgery

17

Deborah C. Richman

17.1 Introduction

- Cataract (and lens) surgery is the most common ambulatory surgery procedure performed in the United States, with over four million of these procedures being done annually. Glaucoma and retinal surgery are the next most common ophthalmic procedures.
- Ophthalmologic surgery is considered low risk surgery (mortality <0.2%) and is generally done on an ambulatory basis with topical or regional local anesthetic.
  - Some major ocular plastic–craniofacial procedures which belong in category of head and neck surgery are intermediate risk.
  - General anesthesia is indicated in those who are unable to cooperate, for the more extensive procedures, and for dacryocystorhinostomy and enucleation.
  - When postoperative complications occur, they are usually related to the patient's underlying medical conditions.

17.2 Preoperative Assessment

- Since the majority of cases are ambulatory, efficient ambulatory centers need to rely on adequate preoperative assessment not only for medical optimization but also for screening out patients that would delay on time starts or affect turnover times. Patients with transport issues, known for "no show" at physician appointments, difficult intravenous (IV) access, and combative patients should be scheduled at a time when, and in a facility where, they would have the least impact on operating room (OR) efficiency.

D.C. Richman
Department of Anesthesiology, Stony Brook University Medical Center,
Stony Brook, NY 11794-8480, USA
e-mail: drichman@notes.cc.sunysb.edu

S.L. Cohn (ed.), *Perioperative Medicine*,
DOI: 10.1007/978-0-85729-498-2_17, © Springer-Verlag London Limited 2011

- The preoperative evaluation requires an assessment of known comorbidities. In the majority of cases, a focused history and physical is all that is needed. A landmark study[1] of almost 20,000 cataract procedures found that preoperative testing made no difference to outcomes. These findings can probably be extrapolated to other low-risk ophthalmic surgeries done under local anesthesia with sedation. However, any new or previously undiagnosed findings on history and physical *do* need evaluation and treatment as indicated, unrelated to upcoming surgery.
- As many eye patients are elderly, there are all the common comorbidities associated with age. The most common diseases are cardiovascular disease, hypertension, and diabetes. Cataracts are more common in diabetics and also in those on steroids. Usually a stress dose of steroids is not indicated for minor eye procedures.

17.3 Specific Diseases

- Cardiovascular disease (coronary artery disease, atrial fibrillation, and mechanical valves) – according to the 2007 AHA guidelines,[2] patients without active cardiac conditions need no further work up for low risk procedures (see Chap. 20).
  - Cardiac medications should be continued on the day of surgery, especially beta blockers and statins. Diuretics are typically withheld in these awake patients under local anesthesia.
  - Aspirin and warfarin can usually be safely continued for cataract surgery.[3] Risk of bleeding is increased with combination anticoagulant and antiplatelet therapies. In most cases it is acceptable to continue clopidogrel and other platelet inhibitors, as the risk of thrombosis on stopping the drug is higher than the risk of hemorrhage. For vitreo-retinal procedures, risk benefit of withdrawing the drug preoperatively for 3–4 days should be reviewed in each case. Oculo-plastic outcomes are dependent on good hemostasis. Warfarin and clopidogrel may need to be stopped to achieve this – again, on a case-by-case basis, in discussion with the prescribing physician.
- Diabetes mellitus – book early in the day with as minimal interruption to their medication and meals as possible. Oral hypoglycemics and short-acting insulin can be withheld on the morning of surgery and given postoperatively if desired once the patient can eat.
- Chronic obstructive airways disease – may need general anesthesia if unable to control cough and movement during the procedure. Optimize bronchodilator therapy preoperatively.
- Deafness – hearing aids should be worn for any procedure under sedation to allow for understanding and cooperation.
- Mild dementia – may be cooperative for loco-regional procedures – tend to do better with propofol (avoid opiates and benzodiazepines). The block should be done under sedation and adequate time allowed for the sedation to wear off, so that the patient is

cooperative for the procedure. Congenital syndromes can have ocular features requiring surgery. Two examples are mentioned below, but further discussion is beyond the scope of this chapter.

- Down's syndrome – cataract and strabismus

  Cardiac anomalies (third of cases).
  Airway and c-spine stability are also important to evaluate, especially when control and positioning of the neck is shared with the surgeon. Atlanto-axial instability is evaluated by lateral flexion and extension cervical spine films. Some patients have had this study in the context of a "sports clearance."

- SturgeWeber – 50% have glaucoma.

  Airway hemangiomas
  Seizures

17.4 Intraoperative Management

- Anesthesia for eye surgery includes (Table 17.1):

  - Topical local anesthesia – most comfortable at the time of administration, lowest risk of hematoma, higher intra-operative pain.
  - Sub-tenon capsule block – blunt needle, small volume.
  - Peri-bulbar block.
  - Retro-bulbar block – largest volume, surgery easier and more comfortable.
  - General anesthesia – airway is usually inaccessible and needs to be secured; endotracheal intubation or laryngeal mask airway (LMA) insertion are both acceptable alternatives.[4]

    Risks of general anesthesia specific to eye surgery: closed claims analysis found 30% were due to inadvertent patient movement with eye injury.[5] Muscle relaxation with nerve stimulator monitoring is recommended, especially with an open eye.

- Contraindication to local anesthesia:

  - Absolute: Allergy to local anesthesia; patient refusal
  - Relative: lack of patient cooperation or communication difficulty (deafness, language difficulties, mental incapacity); inability to lie flat and still (severe GERD, chronic cough, orthopnea, back or joint pain affecting position, severe Parkinson's disease)

Table 17.1 Anesthetic options

Type of anesthesia	Indication	Akinesis	Ocular cardiac reflex	Pain on injection/application	Comments	Complications
Topical	Laser refractive surgeries Cataract Pterygium	No	Present	Mild		• Chemosis • Eye movement
Sub-tenon	Cataract Trabeculectomy Vitreo-retinal (strabismus)	Adequate	Blocked	Mild to moderate	Blunt needle May fail after scleral buckle	• Minor: subconjunctival hemorrhage or swelling
Peri-bulbar	Cataract Trabeculectomy Vitreo-retinal (strabismus)	Good	Blocked	Mild to moderate	Sharp needle	• Globe perforation • Brainstem anesthesia (loss of consciousness/seizures/respiratory arrest/contralateral loss of vision) • Intravascular injection
Retro-bulbar	Cataract Trabeculectomy Vitreo-retinal (strabismus)	Good	Blocked	Mild to moderate	Sharp needle	• Retro-bulbar hemorrhage and IOP increase • Globe perforation • Brainstem anesthesia (loss of consciousness/seizures/respiratory arrest/contralateral loss of vision) • Intravascular injection • Optic nerve damage • Muscle atrophy
General	Local contraindicated Open eye Strabismus Dacryocystorhinostomy	Good	Present	Mild to moderate – IV only		• Postop pain if no block • IOP effects • Postoperative nausea and vomiting (PONV)

17.5 Intraoperative Concerns

- Ocular cardiac reflex (OCR) is a common complication of ocular surgery.
  - Caused by traction on the extraocular muscles, pressure on the globe (often from the anesthesia injection) and pain, it may result in vagal-mediated bradycardia, hypotension, ectopic beats, malignant ventricular arrhythmias, and even asystole.
  - Treatment is to stop the stimulus, deepen anesthesia/treat the pain, intravenous atropine (0.007 mg/kg). Tolerance to the stimulus develops with time.
- Intraocular pressure (IOP): control affects surgical outcome (normal IOP is 12–20 mmHg).
  - Factors affecting IOP include drugs, laryngoscopy and intubation, extraocular muscle tone, mydriasis, changes in choroidal blood volume.
- Hemorrhage: more common in the retro-bulbar block; raises intraocular pressure and surgery may need to be postponed.
- Fire risk: surgical fires are devastating complications and ocular surgery can be a high risk setting. The Silverstein fire risk assessment score is discussed as part of the time out, before the start of surgery.
  - Risk factors contributing to the score (1 point each) are surgery above diaphragm, open oxygen source, heat source; any eye procedure under monitored anesthesia care (MAC) with supplemental oxygen automatically scores 2 points. Adding laser equipment or electrocautery makes this very high risk.
- Intraocular gas – occasionally a gas bubble [poorly absorbed gases like SF_6 (sulfur hexafluoride) and C_3F_8 (octafluoropropane)] is injected in to the eye to hold retinal repair in place. Nitrous oxide, if used, will significantly increase the size of the bubble leading to raised IOP.
- Open-eye injury with full stomach – concern about the use of succinylcholine and its temporary effect on intraocular pressure and extrusion of eye contents. Precurarization prior to succinylcholine has been advocated, as has use of rapid onset longer acting non-depolarizers at high doses.
- Ocularplastic surgery requires the patient to be arousable and cooperative. Dexmedetomidine has been used effectively as a sedative for this purpose. Dexmedetomidine is also used (off label) for retinal surgery with the positive effects of lower blood pressure and lower IOP.

17.6 Postoperative Complications

- Hypertension is a frequent finding and anesthesiologists and medical consultants are often asked to help with management to prevent raised IOP.

- Common causes are postoperative pain and failure to take the patient's usual antihypertensive medications; addressing these causes is usually adequate.
- Elevated intraocular pressure – control by removing the cause, elevating the head of the bed.
- PONV is common in eye surgery, especially after strabismus repair. Administer antiemetics prophylactically intra-operatively, keep the patient well hydrated, and treat PONV early.
- Cough can be minimized by:
  - Optimizing COPD and obstruction preoperatively
  - Treating postnasal drip at the start of the procedure
  - Treating reflux
  - Avoiding endotracheal intubation, which has a higher incidence of cough at the end of the procedure than the use of the LMA or local blocks
- Patients with obstructive sleep apnea may not be able to wear their continuous positive airway pressure (CPAP) masks and are at increased risk of sedative induced apneas. They need appropriate monitoring in the recovery period (ASA guidelines).[6] Oculo-plastic surgery is specifically implicated. Patients at high risk should be advised to get a temporary nasal cushion-type CPAP device, which does not press on the eye or face in any way. The highest risk of apnea- and hypoxic-related events is during rebound REM sleep which occurs 2–5 days after anesthesia or sedation. Emphasize compliance with CPAP.
- Fall risk – poor vision is a risk factor for falls, and often fall prevention is an indication for eye surgery. The risk is highest in the immediate postoperative period, and patients and families need to be aware of this.
- Nitrous oxide is contraindicated in repeat surgery within a month after the use of intraocular gas bubble. This gas bubble can take 3–4 weeks to resorb and the high solubility of nitrous oxide can cause raised IOP and permanent visual loss.

17.7 Conclusion

This brief chapter covers the key perioperative management issues of ophthalmic surgery. Attention to detail in these low-risk procedures facilitates the patients' expectations – a good outcome and improved quality of life.

References

1. Schein OD, Katz J, Bass EB, et al. The value of routine preoperative medical testing before cataract surgery. Study of medical testing for cataract surgery. *N Engl J Med.* 2000;342(3):168-175.
2. Fleisher LA, Beckman JA, Brown KA, et al. ACC/AHA 2007 guidelines on perioperative cardiovascular evaluation and care for noncardiac surgery: a report of the American College of

Cardiology/American Heart Association Task Force on Practice Guidelines (Writing Committee to revise the 2002 guidelines on perioperative cardiovascular evaluation for noncardiac surgery): developed in collaboration with the American Society of Echocardiography, American Society of Nuclear Cardiology, Heart Rhythm Society, Society of Cardiovascular Anesthesiologists, Society for Cardiovascular Angiography and Interventions, Society for Vascular Medicine and Biology, and Society for Vascular Surgery. *Circulation*. 2007;116(17):e418-e499.

3. Katz J, Feldman MA, Bass EB, et al. Risks and benefits of anticoagulant and antiplatelet medication use before cataract surgery. *Ophthalmology*. 2003;110(9):1784-1788.
4. Denny NM, Gadelrab R. Complications following general anaesthesia for cataract surgery: a comparison of the laryngeal mask airway with tracheal intubation. *J R Soc Med*. 1993;86(9):521-522.
5. Gild WM, Posner KL, Caplan RA, Cheney FW. Eye injuries associated with anesthesia. A closed claims analysis. *Anesthesiology*. 1992;76(2):204-208.
6. Gross JB, Bachenberg KL, Benumof JL, et al. Practice guidelines for the perioperative management of patients with obstructive sleep apnea: a report by the American Society of Anesthesiologists Task Force on Perioperative Management of patients with obstructive sleep apnea. *Anesthesiology*. 2006;104(5):1081-1093; quiz 1117-1088.

18 Otolaryngologic Procedures

Paul J. Primeaux

18.1 Introduction

It should be understood that head and neck surgery encompasses a broad range of procedures from brief endoscopic outpatient procedures to complex tumor resections with reconstruction lasting 10–12 h or more. Although the 2007 AHA/ACC Guidelines on Perioperative Cardiovascular Evaluation classify head and neck surgery as "intermediate risk" with an expected cardiac complication rate of 1–5%, the risk of perioperative medical complications in this diverse group of patients cannot be described as uniform. Risk assessment in otolaryngology patients (like all surgical patients) requires an understanding of both the risk posed by existing physiologic derangements (heart disease, renal failure, diabetes, etc.) and the risk inherent in the procedure to be performed.

18.2 Preoperative Considerations

- Patients facing brief uncomplicated head and neck procedures will rarely require medical consultation unless advanced systemic disease makes coordination of care necessary. These patients include:
  - Renal failure patients who must adjust their dialysis schedule
  - Patients on anticoagulants at high risk of complications from thrombosis/embolism if these agents are discontinued
- Patients most likely to experience serious medical complications perioperatively are those undergoing surgery for invasive head and neck cancer. Rates of serious medical complications in these patients are reported to be as high as 28%.

P.J. Primeaux
Tulane University School of Medicine, Tulane Medical Center,
New Orleans, LA, USA
e-mail: pprimeau@tulane.edu

S.L. Cohn (ed.), *Perioperative Medicine*,
DOI: 10.1007/978-0-85729-498-2_18, © Springer-Verlag London Limited 2011

- Cigarette smoking and alcohol abuse place patients at higher risk of developing head and neck cancers and also increase the likelihood of coexisting cardiac, pulmonary, hepatic, and renal disease.
- Medical complications following head and neck surgery include cardiac, pulmonary, neurologic, and infectious complications as well as renal insufficiency, and ETOH withdrawal.
- Risk factors associated with postoperative complications in various studies are listed in Table 18.1.
  - Systematic approach to the preoperative risk assessment and medical optimization:
    1. Understand the particulars of the procedure (site, duration, expected blood loss, airway manipulation, etc.) and determine surgical risk. This may require direct communication with the surgical team.
    2. Cardiac evaluation. Follow the AHA/ACC guidelines for noncardiac surgery (see Chap. 20). Despite the fact that many of these patients are older, males, and smokers, stress testing is usually not necessary and coronary revascularization is rarely needed simply to get a patient through surgery. Remember that delaying a resection for invasive cancer until after coronary revascularization may not be in the best interest of the patient. However, understanding the territory of myocardium at particular risk following noninvasive stress testing or knowing ventricular performance and severity of valvular abnormalities from a preoperative echocardiogram may be immensely valuable to the perioperative monitoring and individualized care of the patient.
    3. Pulmonary evaluation. Otolaryngology patients undergoing major surgery tend to be older, smokers, overweight, poorly nourished, and more likely to have COPD. They may have swallowing difficulties, increasing risk for aspiration, and be more likely to develop mucus plugs. These factors place them at increased

Table 18.1 Risk factors for postoperative complications

Anesthesia time of ≥ 8 h[a]
History of hepatitis[a]
Preoperative gastrostomy tube placement[a]
Large volume intraoperative fluid replacement[b]
Oncologic surgery (especially invasive head and neck)[b]
Comorbidity (ACE-27 grade 2, ASA ≥ 3, APACHE II, POSSUM, Charlson index)
Smoking within 6 weeks of surgery
Intraoperative transfusion
Flap reconstruction
Preoperative radiation therapy

ACE-27 Adult comorbidity evaluation 27 index, ASA American Society of Anesthesiologists
[a]Predicted medical complications
[b]Predicted surgical complications

risk of pulmonary complications. In addition, surgery near the airway and procedures of >3 h duration further increase the risk of pulmonary complications. Consider the following in your preoperative assessment:

(a) ABG to quantify CO_2 retention in COPD.
(b) PFTs to measure response to bronchodilator therapy in patients with wheezing or significant dyspnea. (Any patient with marked improvement after bronchodilator therapy should receive at least 3 days of treatment with bronchodilators prior to surgery.)
(c) Administer oral steroids in severe asthma.
(d) Start antibiotics to treat any active infections.
(e) Instruct patients with obstructive sleep apnea to bring their CPAP/BiPAP devices with them on the day of surgery.
(f) Start incentive spirometry preoperatively, with instruction on proper use.
(g) Delay elective surgery in patients with active pulmonary infections and in those with acute exacerbations of asthma or COPD.

4. Renal evaluation. Renal failure is a possible complication of major otolaryngologic surgery. Laboratory evaluation of preoperative renal function and electrolytes as well as a complete blood count should be reviewed for patients with preexisting renal dysfunction or those with risk factors for renal disease (such as diabetes mellitus or hypertension) who are undergoing complex procedures.

(a) Dialysis patients should have the following documented on the preoperative assessment:

- Dry weight
- Dialysis schedule
- Volume typically removed
- Typical post-dialysis blood pressure
- Whether or not the patient makes urine (and how much in 24 h)
- Sites and type of hemodialysis access (tunneled catheter or AV fistula)
- Electrolytes (following dialysis immediately prior to surgery)

(b) Renal failure patients with anemia or electrolyte abnormalities will need to have these corrected prior to surgery.

5. Hepatic evaluation. Patients with cancer of the head and neck are more likely to have a history of alcohol abuse and are therefore at risk for hepatic dysfunction. Additionally, a history of hepatitis may independently place patients at risk for medical complications following complex head and neck cancer resection.[1] As a result, it may be prudent to evaluate the hepatic function in those at risk for liver disease (history of ETOH abuse or hepatitis). Consider the following:

(a) Check serum Na+. Hyponatremia is common in cirrhotic patients and should be corrected if <130 meq/L or is below normal and decreasing.
(b) Check synthetic function with PT/PTT. It may be necessary to correct coagulopathy prior to surgery. Document preoperative hepatic enzymes.

(c) Measure preoperative albumin. Cachexia is common in cancer patients and made worst in concomitant liver disease. Intense enteral nutritional support may be required if albumin <2.5 g/dL. (Provide enteral support for about a week prior to surgery if scheduling permits.)

(d) Careful screening and counseling is necessary for patients with alcohol dependence. Referral to psychiatry and careful support for preoperative abstinence with prophylaxis for alcohol withdrawal may be necessary.

6. Search for specific electrolyte abnormalities common after preoperative radiation therapy or associated with certain head and neck cancers:

   (a) Hypercalcemia: Parathyroid-like hormone may be secreted by squamous cell tumors of the head and neck. Symptomatic patients ("moans, groans, bones, stones, and psychic overtones" – pneumonic for symptoms of hypercalcemia) should have a serum calcium measured and hypercalcemia treated. Therapy includes fluids and diuretics, bisphosphonates, and calcitonin.

   (b) Hypothyroidism:
   - Primary hypothyroidism may occur within several months following radiation of the neck, and secondary hypothyroidism can occur following radiation of the skull base and subsequent hypopituitarism.
   - Patients with previous neck radiation should have a TSH (+/−free T4) measured and hypothyroidism treated.

   (c) Adrenal Insufficiency: May also occur following skull base radiation. Obtain serum cortisol, ACTH, aldosterone, renin, and potassium or perform an ACTH simulation test.

18.3 Postoperative Concerns

- The list of medical complications following extensive head and neck surgery is quite broad and is listed in Table 18.2.
- The risk of medical complications increases dramatically with increasing duration of surgery and anesthesia (>8 h) and the need for large volume fluid replacement intraoperatively. Admission to the ICU postoperatively in these patients should be considered and is the standard for any patient with a new surgical airway (tracheostomy/cricothyrotomy).
- Cardiac or pulmonary complications are increased following procedures associated with considerable surgical stress. Fluid and electrolyte derangements are common. The 2008 British Consensus Guidelines on IV fluid therapy in Surgical Patients is a valuable tool to guide postop fluid therapy (see Chap. 39).
- In patients with surgical airways, the need for fastidious pulmonary nursing care and frequent suctioning cannot be overemphasized. The reduced ability of head and neck surgery patients to clear airway mucous leads to plugging and potential obstruction of the airway. If obstruction does occur, prepare for and treat post-obstructive pulmonary

Table 18.2 Postoperative medical complications following extensive head and neck surgery

Cardiac	Ischemia Infarction Arrhythmias CHF
Pulmonary	Prolonged ventilation Pneumonia Hypoxia Bronchospasm DVT/PE ARDS
Miscellaneous	Renal insufficiency/failure Hemorrhage Airway loss/obstruction ETOH withdrawal ICU admission
Surgery specific	Hypocalcemia Phrenic nerve injury Recurrent laryngeal nerve injury[a] Facial nerve injury ⇑ HR and ⇑ BP CSF leak/meningitis Vision impairment Thoracic duct injury Vertigo Nausea/vomiting

Modified from Farwell et al.[1]

[a]Recurrent laryngeal nerve injury can result in acute airway compromise. Have airway specialists at the bedside when extubating patients after surgery on/near the neck

edema following the successful removal of the obstruction. Positive end expiratory pressure is typically required to maintain oxygen saturation and reduce edema formation.

18.4 Selected Surgical Procedures

18.4.1 Thyroidectomy

- Indications: Thyroid cancer, thyroid nodule, hyperthyroidism, Grave's disease, goiter.
- Duration: 1–2 h
- Estimated blood loss: Typically <100 mL, however bleeding will likely increase with the size and complexity of the thyroid mass.

- Morbidity and postoperative concerns:
  - Thyroid storm – monitor for tachycardia, fever, cardiovascular collapse, delirium; treat with beta-blocker, thionamides (PTU), iodines, steroids, antipyretic (non-aspirin), and supportive care in a monitored setting.
  - Hematoma – monitor for signs of airway obstruction; may require emergent re-intubation.
  - Hypoparathyroidism – monitor for hypocalcemia
- Check calcium after surgery and q 8 h for 24–48 h
- Check for tetany – Trousseau's or Chvostek's signs, or for prolongation of the QT interval on EKG
- Severe hypocalcemia can cause laryngospasm resulting in loss of airway, seizures, mental status changes, hypotension, circumoral paresthesia, or cardiac arrhythmias
- Treat hypocalcemia with IV calcium gluconate 1–2 g over 10–20 min followed by an infusion of 0.5–1.0 mg/kg/h. (IV calcium will cause tissue necrosis upon extravasation. Ensure properly placed venous access.)
  - Recurrent laryngeal nerve damage (will cause acute airway obstruction if bilateral)

18.4.2 Parathyroidectomy

- Indications: Parathyroid carcinoma, hyperparathyroidism, parathyroid adenoma
- Duration: 1–2 h
- Estimate blood loss: <100 mL
- Morbidity and postoperative concerns: similar to thyroidectomy (except for thyroid storm and hypothyroidism)
  - Hypoparathyroidism with hypocalcemia
  - Hematoma with airway compromise
  - Recurrent laryngeal nerve injury

18.4.3 Mandibulectomy (Marginal or Segmental) with Neck Dissection (Radical or Modified Radical) and Free Flap Reconstruction

- Indications: Invasive squamous cell carcinoma or osteosarcoma
- Duration: 6–8 h for mandibulectomy (+3–6 h for free flap reconstruction, +2–4 h for neck dissection)
- Estimated blood loss: 300–1,000 mL or greater
- Morbidity:
  - Surgical stress is significant in cases of long duration, large volume fluid resuscitations, and those requiring blood transfusions.
  - Serious medical complications may occur in 25–30% of patients and include:

Hemorrhage
DVT/PE
Chyle leak
Nerve injury (facial, recurrent laryngeal, vagus, trigeminal, hypoglossal)
Ischemia/MI
Pneumonia

- Postop Concerns:
  - These patients should be initially placed in the ICU
  - Monitor BP and HR closely. Elevations may be due to carotid sinus denervation and will require aggressive therapy.
  - New tracheostomy: aggressive pulmonary toilet (see airway concerns above)
  - Pneumothorax possible; get postop CXR and check for position of the tracheostomy tube and rule out pneumothorax.
  - Begin tube feeds POD #1
  - Phrenic nerve injury may cause diaphragmatic paralysis with subsequent atelectasis and respiratory difficulty

18.4.4 Laryngectomy (May Also Include Neck Dissection and Flap Reconstruction)

- Indications: Laryngeal cancer or intractable aspiration
- Duration: May vary widely based on the extent of the tumor resection
  - 2–4 h for laryngectomy (4–8 h if pharyngolaryngectomy is required) + 2–4 h for neck dissection + 2–4 h for flap reconstruction
- Estimated Blood Loss:
  - 50–300 mL for laryngectomy (add 200–300 mL of neck dissection and add 100–200 if flap reconstruction required)
- Morbidity and postoperative concerns: see mandibulectomy above

18.4.5 Otologic and Neurotologic Procedures

These procedures include those procedures on the ear and surrounding structures. They include: myringotomy, simple and radical mastoidectomy, tympanomastoidectomy, stapedectomy and cochlear implantation.

- Indications: chronic otitis media, cholesteatoma, temporal bone tumors, hearing loss, otosclerosis, and temporal bone fracture
- Duration: Can vary widely with simple procedures lasting an hour or less and complex tumor resections lasting up to 8 h. Consult with the surgical team to assess the likely duration and extent of surgery.

- Estimated blood loss: Typically minimal
- Morbidity:
  - Vertigo
  - Nausea and vomiting
  - Facial nerve injury
  - Hearing loss
  - CSF leak
- Postoperative concerns
  - Steroids are sometimes administered intraoperatively to reduce swelling and prevent nausea and vomiting. This may induce or worsen DM.
  - Severe nausea and vomiting following middle ear surgery may cause damage to delicate middle ear reconstructions. Potent anti-emetic therapy with 5-HT3 antagonists and/or transdermal scopolamine may be necessary.
  - Screen for facial nerve damage
  - CSF leak may be associated with subsequent meningitis. Lumbar puncture may be required to diagnose and identify the organism responsible. Empiric coverage should begin while awaiting gram stain and culture results.

18.5 Conclusion

Patients undergoing head and neck surgery represent a wide variety of pathology and preexisting medical conditions. Close consultation between the medical and surgical teams preparing patients for surgery and caring for them postoperatively is often necessary to ensure high quality care.

Reference

1. Farwell DG, Reilly DF, Weymuller EA, et al. Predictors of perioperative complications in head and neck patients. *Arch Otolaryngol Head Neck Surg*. 2002;128:505-511.

Suggested Reading

Cooper CB. Assessment of pulmonary function in COPD. *Semin Respir Crit Care Med*. 2005;26:246-252.

Fleisher LA, Beckman JA, et al. ACC/AHA 2007 guidelines on perioperative cardiovascular evaluation and care for non cardiac surgery. *J Am Coll Cardiol*. 2007;50:159-242. doi:doi:10.1016/j.jacc.2007.09.003; [Published online 27 Sept 2007].

Geerts W, Ray JG, Colwell CW, et al. Prevention of venous thromboembolism. *Chest.* 2005;128:3775-3776.

Johnson RG, Arozullah AM, Neumayer L, et al. Multivariable predictors of postoperative respiratory failure after general and vascular surgery: results from the patient safety in surgery study. *J Am Coll Surg.* 2007;204(6):1188-1198.

Kaplan MJ, Damrose E, Nekhendzy V, et al. Otolaryngology – head and neck surgery. In: Jaffe RA, Samuels SI, eds. *Anesthesiologists manual of surgical procedures.* 4th ed. Philadelphia: Lippincott, Williams, and Wilkins; 2009; Section 3.0.

McAlister FA, Khan NA, Straus SE, et al. Accuracy of the preoperative assessment in predicting pulmonary risk after non thoracic surgery. *Am J Respir Crit Care Med.* 2003;167:741-744.

Powell-Tuck J, Gosling P, Lobo DN, Allison SP Carlson GL, Gore M et al. British Consensus Guidelines on Intravenous Fluid Therapy for Adult Surgical Patients GIFTASUP, reducinglength ofstay.org.uk; 2008.

Qaseem A, Snow V, Fitterman N, et al. Risk assessment for and strategies to reduce perioperative pulmonary complications for patients undergoing non cardiothoracic surgery: a guideline from the American College of Physicians. *Ann Intern Med.* 2006;144:575-580.

Electroconvulsive Therapy

19

Howard S. Smith

19.1 Introduction

- Electroconvulsive therapy (ECT) is the practice of inducing seizure activity with an external electrical current while the patient is under general anesthesia.
- The most common indication for ECT is major depressive disorder with or without features of psychosis, severe suicidality, catatonia, or in pregnancy where a rapid response is required. It is often used for patients whose depression has been refractory to antidepressant medications or who do not tolerate adverse effects of antidepressants, as it is considered to be at least as effective and possibly more effective than antidepressant medications.
- According to the American Psychiatric Association (APA), other potential indications for ECT in certain circumstances may include: schizophrenia, bipolar disorder, organic delusional disorder, organic mood disorder, obsessive compulsive disorder, neuroleptic malignant syndrome, neuroleptic-induced Parkinsonism, and tardive dyskinesias.
- The mortality of ECT is estimated to much less than 1% (4/100,000 treatments). Morbidity is limited, but may include cardiovascular effects, central nervous system effects, and other symptoms (e.g., headaches, myalgias).

19.2 Preoperative Management

- The APA does not feel that ECT has any "true" absolute contraindications because of the life-saving potential of ECT and low risk of adverse effects; however, several conditions may significantly increase risk and may be considered relative contraindications (see Table 19.1).
- Ensure resuscitative medications and equipment are available and personnel in the ECT suite and recovery area are trained for cardiopulmonary resuscitation.

H.S. Smith
Department of Anesthesiology, Albany Medical College,
47 New Scotland Avenue, MC-131, Albany, NY 12208, USA
e-mail: smithh@mail.amc.edu

S.L. Cohn (ed.), *Perioperative Medicine*,
DOI: 10.1007/978-0-85729-498-2_19,

Table 19.1 Potential contraindications for ECT/GA

• Unstable or severe cardiovascular disease (including recent MI)
• Space-occupying intracranial lesion with increased intracranial pressure
• Recent cerebral hemorrhage or stroke
• Bleeding or unstable vascular aneurysm
• Severe pulmonary dysfunction
• American Society of Anesthesiologists Class 4 or 5

19.2.1 Patient Risk Factors

19.2.1.1 Cardiac Disease

- Cardiac events related to ECT are relatively uncommon and usually minor. The most frequent complication is transient "benign" arrhythmias which tend to occur more often in older persons and in those with known cardiovascular disease.
- Since ECT is considered to be a low-risk procedure, only patients with "active cardiac conditions," defined by the ACC guidelines as unstable coronary syndromes (recent MI or severe coronary artery disease, decompensated heart failure, severe cardiac valvular disease, and significant arrhythmias), may not be appropriate candidates for ECT (the risks versus benefits need to be carefully weighed).
  - Most patients who experience benign cardiac morbidity are able to complete the series of ECT treatments.
  - Patients with mild to moderate hypertension can generally safely undergo ECT, but because of the risk of post-procedure hypertension, the blood pressure should be reasonably well controlled prior to ECT.
  - In general, patients should continue their usual blood pressure medications.

    Patients with stable ischemic heart disease can safely undergo ECT, continuing anti-anginal medications.

    Postpone ECT for unstable angina or recent myocardial infarction (within the past 4–6 weeks).

- Patients with compensated heart failure can safely undergo ECT and should continue their usual medications.
  - Postpone ECT if the patient has decompensated heart failure.
- Patients with controlled arrhythmias, pacemakers, and defibrillators can safely undergo ECT and should continue their usual anti-arrhythmic medications.
  - Have a magnet available to deactivate pacemakers should there be problems.
  - Proactively deactivate defibrillators via programming immediately prior to ECT and re-activate immediately after treatment.

- Monitor patients with continuous electrocardiography intraoperatively and in the post-anesthesia care unit.

- The QTc interval may be increased significantly in patients on various antidepressant and antipsychotic medications, and may be associated with increased risks of ventricular arrhythmias.[1] The QTc interval may also be prolonged by ECT treatment and general anesthesia, but continuous infusion of landiolol can partially attenuate this prolongation.[2]

19.2.1.2
Anticoagulation

- Patients who are anticoagulated can probably be safely treated with ECT if the INR is less than 3.5.[3]

19.2.1.3
Chronic Obstructive Pulmonary Disease (COPD)

- Although no specific studies address the risk of ECT among patients with COPD, pulmonary function should be optimized with bronchodilators and/or inhaled or systemic steroids prior the procedure.
- Postpone ECT if COPD is uncontrolled.
- Although not frequently used, theophylline may increase the risk of status epilepticus with ECT. If feasible, discontinue theophylline and allow adequate time for its metabolism before ECT.

19.2.1.4
Diabetes Mellitus (DM)

- Patients with DM can usually receive ECT without complication. Although there are no randomized controlled trials, anecdotal data have not found specific problems attributable to mild to moderate hyperglycemia.
  - Attempt to normalize blood glucose prior to ECT although there is no known reason to postpone ECT in asymptomatic patients with mild to moderate hyperglycemia.
  - Avoid hypoglycemia before, during, or after ECT.
  - Adjust diabetes medications appropriately knowing that patients will not be eating before or shortly after ECT.

19.2.1.5
Stroke

- Case reports and retrospective studies demonstrate that ECT has been safely performed after patients have recovered from lacunar infarctions, hemorrhagic infarctions, and in the setting of structural brain changes including cortical atrophy and ventricular enlargement.

- Avoid ECT within 1 month after a stroke.
- Obtain brain MRI or CT to rule-out intracranial mass, vascular malformation, and acute hemorrhage prior to ECT in post-stroke patients.

19.2.1.6 Dementia

- Patients with dementia are at low risk for major complications after ECT. The most common post-ECT minor complications are confusion, somnolence, and memory impairment, but these are usually self-limited.
- Acetylcholinesterase inhibitors, unilateral ECT, and bilateral ECT with the electrode placement in a Left Anterior (frontal)/Right Temporal [LART] location may diminish post-ECT adverse cognitive effects.[4]

19.2.1.7 Seizure Disorders

- Antidepressant medications may lower the seizure threshold, thus ECT may be a better alternative in some patients with epilepsy.
  - Continue the patient's anticonvulsant medications through ECT. Although the ECT-induced seizure threshold will be higher, ECT is generally still effective.
  - Spontaneous epileptic seizures after ECT are rare if patients have maintained therapeutic anticonvulsant levels.

19.2.1.8 Intracranial Space Occupying Lesions

- ECT may not be appropriate for these patients because of the risks of hemorrhage and increased intracranial pressure. However, for severe, refractory depression, ECT is sometimes undertaken with extreme caution.
  - ECT is relatively contraindicated if there is evidence of increased intracranial pressure on clinical examination or on brain imaging.
  - Obtain consultation from colleagues from neurology and/or neurosurgery when ECT is planned for patients with intracranial space occupying lesions.

    Maintain blood pressure and heart rate control throughout ECT (e.g., using esmolol, an ultra-short acting beta blocker).
    Consider using steroids to minimize brain swelling and intracranial pressure.

19.3
Anesthetic Technique and Operative Pathophysiology

- ECT is typically delivered three times per week usually (e.g., M-W-F) for 6–12 treatments; however, more treatments may be needed.
- To induce a seizure that is considered effective (usually lasting 30–60 s) electrodes are placed either unilaterally or bilaterally on the scalp and a pulse or sine wave of current is applied. A significantly shorter seizure duration may also be somewhat beneficial.[5]
- The procedure is performed under general anesthesia with short-acting induction agents, most often propofol or methohexital.
- "Neuromuscular blocking paralytic" agents such as succinylcholine (or atracurium in the case of pseudocholinesterase deficiency) are delivered to prevent musculoskeletal injury during the seizure.
- Airway management usually involves a bite block and mask ventilation.
- The seizure usually has two phases: a tonic phase followed by a clonic phase.
  - The tonic phase causes an initial 15–20 s parasympathetic discharge which can lead to bradyarrhythmias and even asystole.
  - The clonic phase results in a sympathetic discharge results with a catecholamine surge that may cause tachyarrhythmias and hypertension.
  - These hemodynamic changes usually resolve within 15–20 min.
- ECT-induced neurohumeral discharges may lead to increased cerebral blood flow and intracranial pressure, and may increase blood–brain barrier permeability. It has been postulated that medical therapy for ECT may be more effective post-ECT as the levels of antidepressants and other psychiatric medications may increase in the central nervous system.

19.4
Preoperative Preparation Including Prophylaxis

19.4.1
History and Physical

- The history and physical examination should focus on airway assessment and evaluation for cardiac, pulmonary, and neurologic abnormalities. Assess the patient's mental status and perform a fundoscopic examination for evidence of elevated intracranial pressure.

19.4.2
Pre-procedure Laboratory Evaluation

- Pre-procedure laboratory evaluation is discussed in Chap. 2 and should be based on the patient's medical comorbidities and medications.
  - Check a basic metabolic panel for patients taking diuretics, ACE inhibitors or ARBs, or with DM. Obtain a pregnancy test in women of childbearing potential.
  - Check a PT/INR in patients taking warfarin.
  - Obtain a screening pre-procedure EKG in patients who have, or are at risk for, heart disease.
- Correct electrolyte abnormalities and blood glucose prior to ECT.
- Use continuous electrocardiography and other standard American Society of Anesthesiology (ASA) monitoring through ECT for all patients.

19.4.3
Medications

- Continue the patient's usual antihypertensive medications.
- Short-acting IV beta-blockers can be used to treat periprocedural hypertension and tachycardia.
- Pretreatment atropine or glycopyrrolate may be useful for patients at significant risk of bradyarrhythmias or who developed significant bradyarrhythmias or asystole during previous ECT.

19.4.4
Common Postoperative Problems and Solutions

- Monitoring in the post-anesthesia care unit (PACU) should be done per usual PACU standards for patients recovering from general anesthesia.

19.4.5
CNS Effects

- Similar to a post-ictal state, headache, somnolence, short-term memory impairment and confusion are relatively common after ECT and usually resolve within 24 h. Persistent symptoms should trigger further evaluation.
- Transient muscle pains (myalgias) may occur (generally from succinylcholine).
  - Simple headaches and/or muscle pain can be treated with the usual analgesics.

Table 19.2 Approaches to lower seizure threshold and produce adequate ECT seizures

• Hyperventilation
• Theodur 300 mg PO
• Caffeine sodium benzoate 125 mg intravenously on call to OR
• Increase energy of ECT machine
• Discontinue all pre-ECT benzodiazepines, anticonvulsants, etc.
• Use etomidate as the induction agent

19.4.6 Seizure Duration

- If the seizure lasts longer than 3 min, then anticonvulsant agents such as benzodiazepines or barbiturates should be administered in efforts to break the seizure. Initial treatment attempts are generally successful; however, if status epilepticus occurs, it should be aggressively treated until the seizure is terminated which may rarely require the patient being intubated, mechanically ventilated, and "placed in a barbiturate coma."
- If there is no seizure or inadequate seizure activity, an ECT treatment may be attempted again (or at most two more times); generally waiting at least a minute to avoid delivering electricity during the refractory period. If the seizure is much too short or does not occur at all, various approaches may be tried in efforts to produce "adequate seizure" activity (see Table 19.2).

19.4.7 Arrhythmias

- Bradyarrhythmias and asystole may complicate ECT and can be treated with atropine.
- Other arrhythmias can be managed with the appropriate antiarrhythmic medications.

References

1. Tezuka N, Egawa H, Fukagawa D, et al. Assessment of QT interval and QT dispersion during electroconvulsive therapy using computerized measurements. *J ECT*. 2010;26(1):41-46.
2. Matsura M, Fujiwara Y, Ito H, et al. Prolongation of QT interval induced by electroconvulsive therapy is attentuated by landiolol. *J ECT*. 2010;26(1):37-40.
3. Mehta V, Mueler P, Gonzalez-Arriaza H, Pankratz VS, Rummans TA. Safety of electroconvulsive therapy in patients receiving long-term warfarin therapy. *Mayo Clin Proc*. 2004;79(11):1396-1401.
4. Swartz CM, Nelson AI. Rational electroconvulsive therapy electrode placement. *Psychiatry*. 2005;2:37-43.
5. Scott AI. Electroconvulsive therapy, practice and evidence. *Br J Psychiatry*. 2010;196:171-172.

Part III

Preoperative Evaluation and Management of Co-existing Medical Diseases

Cardiac Disease

20

Steven L. Cohn

20.1 Introduction

- Preoperative cardiac risk assessment has evolved over the past 40 years from a simple global assessment of a patient's physical status (the ASA classification[1]) to multivariate risk analyses (Goldman[2], Detsky[3]) to a simplified scoring system (Lee RCRI[4]) to guidelines (ACC/AHA, ACP).
- The latest of these is the ACC/AHA guidelines for perioperative cardiac evaluation and management, originally published in 1996 and updated in 2007[5] to incorporate the RCRI factors.
- Using these guidelines, which emphasize clinical evaluation and selective cardiac testing (pharmacologic stress tests only in situations where it is likely to change management), physicians are now better able to provide a more accurate assessment of perioperative risk, and the focus has turned to risk reduction strategies. These include revascularization (CABG or PCI), medical therapy (beta-blockers, alpha-agonists, statins), and other intraoperative measures (normothermia, anesthetic technique).
- Although surgical and anesthetic techniques have improved and perioperative cardiac events have decreased, operative mortality and cardiac morbidity remain significant, especially among high-risk patients or high-risk procedures.
- This chapter reviews the current state of the art for perioperative risk assessment and risk reduction in patients with cardiac disease.

S.L. Cohn
Internal Medicine-Medical Consultation Service,
SUNY Downstate - Kings County Hospital Center,
450 Clarkson Ave, Box 68, Brooklyn, NY 11203, USA
e-mail: steven.cohn@downstate.edu

S.L. Cohn (ed.), *Perioperative Medicine*,
DOI: 10.1007/978-0-85729-498-2_20,

20.2 Patient-Related Risk Factors

- Prior cardiac disease
  - Coronary artery disease (CAD):

    Previous MI: The time interval between a prior MI and the planned noncardiac surgery influences risk. A recent MI is associated with greater risk than an "older" MI and mandates further investigation prior to elective surgery. The definition of "recent" has changed from <6 months (Goldman and Detsky) to <3 months (Larsen) to <1 month (ACC) . The reason for this change is that previously, time selected out high-risk patients; now most patients with an acute MI either undergo cardiac catheterization or have noninvasive testing done during or shortly after hospitalization and are identified as high risk on that basis or are treated.

    Angina: The severity and stability of angina influence risk. Unstable angina and severe angina (NYHA Class III–IV) are associated with a risk similar to a recent MI. Mild stable angina (Class I–II) is an ACC and RCRI clinical risk predictor but did not predict major postoperative cardiac complications in the older indices of Goldman and Detsky.
  - Congestive heart failure (CHF): Decompensated or symptomatic heart failure (S3, JVD, rales and symptoms) is associated with greater risk of postoperative complications than compensated CHF or a previous history of CHF, and it requires further evaluation and treatment before elective surgery.
  - Arrhythmias: Hemodynamically significant arrhythmias (ventricular tachycardia, SVT, symptomatic bradyarrhythmias, advanced heart block) are major clinical predictors of risk and should be controlled prior to surgery.
  - Valvular heart disease: Severe symptomatic aortic stenosis (AS) is the valvular lesion that carries the greatest risk of postoperative cardiac complications.
  - Prior cardiac intervention: Although having had a revascularization procedure may reduce risk of complications, prophylactic coronary revascularization for the sole purpose of getting the patient through surgery has not been shown to be better than optimal medical therapy. Prior coronary artery bypass grafting (CABG) may be protective for up to 5 years if no new (or worsening) symptoms are present. Prior percutaneous coronary intervention (PCI) with balloon angioplasty or stenting (depending on the timeframe) may also be somewhat protective.

- Risk factors for CAD
  - Age: Age >70 is a risk factor in various risk indices but is no longer a clinical predictor in the ACC guidelines. However, it may improve risk prediction when added to the RCRI. Age represents a marker for decreased cardiac reserve, silent cardiac disease, and increasing comorbidity rather than a risk factor by itself.

- Hypertension (HTN): HTN per se is not a risk factor unless the blood pressure is significantly elevated. Even then, it is unclear at what level it increases perioperative risk.
- DM: Diabetes is a risk factor for CAD and is a risk factor in the RCRI (taking insulin) and the ACC guidelines (any diabetes).
- Dyslipidemia: Although hyperlipidemia is a risk factor for CAD, it has not been found to be an independent risk factor for postoperative cardiac complications.
- Cigarette smoking: While smokers are at higher risk for underlying CAD and pulmonary disease, cigarette use is not an independent risk factor for postoperative cardiac complications.

• Associated comorbid diseases

- PVD and CVA: Peripheral vascular disease and stroke are coronary equivalents that often coexist with CAD.
- CKD: Renal insufficiency (creatinine >2.0 or 2.5 mg/dl) was an independent risk predictor in all of the published cardiac risk indices.
- COPD: Concomitant pulmonary disease may be associated with increased cardiac complications.
- Clinical symptoms

  Chest pain and dyspnea: The presence, severity, and stability of these symptoms as well as related symptoms (orthopnea and paroxysmal nocturnal dyspnea) are related to risk of cardiac complications.

  Functional status/exercise capacity: Functional dependence, the need for assistance with the activities of daily living, and the inability to walk 2–4 blocks or climb 1–2 flights of stairs, regardless of the reason, are associated with increased risk of postoperative complications.

• Prior cardiac evaluation

- Noninvasive tests (NIT): Knowing a patient's ischemic threshold or severity of disease may help predict risk. More extensive test abnormalities (reperfusion defects or wall motion abnormalities) are associated with increased risk. Detailed results of prior cardiac tests are helpful.

  For exercise ECG tests, note the peak heart rate, systolic blood pressure, and rate pressure product (RPP) along with the number of METS achieved, percent of target heart rate attained, symptoms or ECG abnormalities, and the reason the test was stopped.

  For nuclear tests, the presence, number, and severity of reperfusion abnormalities are important. Fixed defects are less predictive of short-term risk.

  For echocardiograms, note the presence and extent of systolic wall motion abnormalities and the LVEF (in addition to any valvular pathology).
- Coronary angiography: Symptomatic left main or three-vessel coronary artery disease are associated with increased risk and should be corrected, if time permits, as they are indications for revascularization independent of the need for noncardiac surgery.

20.3 Surgery-Related Risk Factors

20.3.1 Type of Surgery

Although the 2007 ACC guidelines changed the categories for surgery-related risk in order to have better evidence for noninvasive test recommendations, the following definitions are still valid for predicting postoperative cardiac complications.

- High-risk procedures: usual risk of cardiac complications >5%.
  - *Emergent major operations*: Emergency surgery increases the risk for cardiac complications due to increased emotional and physiological stress and lack of time to optimize the patient's condition.
  - *Major vascular surgery*: Aortic aneurysm repair and infrainguinal arterial bypass surgery are the highest risk procedures for perioperative cardiac events. These procedures are associated with significant hemodynamic changes, and vascular surgery patients frequently have underlying CAD.
  - *Prolonged procedures with significant blood loss or fluid shifts*: Examples of these include major operations, such as Whipple's procedure or debulking of intra-abdominal tumor masses, where blood loss and fluid shifts pose increased risk to patients with CAD or CHF.

- Intermediate risk procedures: complication rate 1–5%
  - *Intraperitoneal or intrathoracic surgery*: Intrathoracic operations alter the normal pressure gradients in the thoracic cavity, while potentially limiting blood oxygenation, both can lead to increased myocardial oxygen demand and ischemia.
  - *Carotid endarterectomy/endovascular AAA (stent/coil)*: Cardiac risk with carotid endarterectomy and endovascular procedures is lower than with other vascular surgeries. Nonetheless, many patients with peripheral arterial disease also have significant CAD.
  - *Major orthopedic procedures*: Patients undergoing these procedures are often elderly and have comorbid illnesses, including known or suspected CAD. Due to their joint disease, it may be difficult to assess their functional status.
  - *Major head and neck surgery*: These procedures, done under general anesthesia, are often prolonged. Additionally, most patients with oral head and neck malignancies have significant smoking histories and may have underlying CAD.

- Low-risk procedures: complication rate <1%
  - *Superficial and minor operations* on the skin, breast, or eyes (e.g., cataract), or endoscopic procedures, usually portend minimal risk.

20.3.2 Type of Anesthesia

- Whether or not neuraxial (spinal or epidural) anesthesia is safer than general anesthesia remains controversial. However, the decision as to the type of anesthesia is still best left to the anesthesiologist.
- Although earlier research suggested no clear morbidity or mortality benefit of either general or neuraxial (spinal or epidural) anesthesia, a meta-analysis by Rodgers[6] and colleagues including 9,559 patients indicated a lower risk for overall mortality (OR 0.7) with neuraxial blockade. Risk of myocardial infarction, renal failure, venous thromboembolism, transfusion requirements, pneumonia, and respiratory depression was also reduced.
  - A practical advantage to neuraxial anesthesia is that the awake patient may be able to alert the anesthesiologist if symptoms of cardiac ischemia occur.
- For minor procedures performed with local anesthesia, the expected risk of coronary ischemia is minimal. Patient anxiety may be a factor but can usually be alleviated with anxiolytics.

20.4 Preoperative Evaluation

- A detailed history and focused physical examination are key in clinical risk assessment. Several basic diagnostic tests may also helpful. Various risk indices have been developed, based mainly on simple clinical evaluation, to help refine preoperative risk stratification.
- Current risk assessment is usually based on the Lee RCRI and the ACC/AHA guidelines[5] which now include the RCRI factors.

20.4.1 Preoperative Risk Indices

- Goldman[2] and colleagues published the original cardiac risk index based on a prospective multivariate analysis of preoperative cardiac risk in 1,001 patients undergoing noncardiac, nonneurologic surgery. They identified nine independent predictors of death or major postoperative cardiac complications and assigned points to them based on their relative importance. Higher point totals were correlated with increased complication rates.
- Detsky[3] and colleagues modified this risk index by expanding the list of risk factors and factoring in the pretest probability of complications based on the risk of the surgery itself.
- Eagle[7] and colleagues identified 5 factors (age, DM, angina, MI, and CHF) associated with perioperative cardiac events and used these to risk stratify patients and decide when further cardiac testing was indicated.

- Lee[4] and colleagues identified and validated 6 factors associated with increased risk of perioperative complications (RCRI). These factors were high-risk surgery, CAD, CHF, cerebrovascular disease (stroke or TIA), DM requiring insulin, and renal insufficiency (creatinine >2.0 mg/dL). Higher complication rates were associated with having more risk factors – 1% with 0–1 factors, 4–7% with 2 factors, and 9–11% with ≥3 risk factors.

20.4.2 ACC/AHA Guidelines

- The ACC developed a stepwise approach to preoperative cardiac risk evaluation using the information obtained from the history, physical examination, and laboratory tests. Their algorithm is based on the patient's clinical risk factors, surgery-specific risk and self-reported exercise capacity, and the underlying theme is to avoid testing if the result will not change management.

20.4.2.1 Clinical Risk Factors

- What the ACC previously defined as "major clinical predictors" are now called "active cardiac conditions". These are unstable coronary syndromes (MI<30 days, unstable or severe angina), decompensated heart failure, hemodynamically significant arrhythmias, or severe (symptomatic) valvular heart disease.
- The group of risk factors previously called "intermediate clinical predictors" is now called "clinical risk factors". This category includes five of the six Lee RCRI factors (MI>30 days or stable mild angina, compensated or history of HF, DM, renal insufficiency, and stroke) – the type of surgery is considered separately.
- The "minor risk predictors" in the 2002 guidelines were dropped (hypertension, dyslipidemia, cigarette smoking) with the exception of cerebrovascular disease which was moved up to the clinical predictor group. Most studies found that these factors were not significant predictors of postoperative cardiac complications.

20.4.2.2 Procedural Risk

- The type of surgery has its own inherent risk which is independent of the patient's clinical risk factors. This pre- and post-test probability concept, used in Detsky's modified cardiac risk index, is factored into the ACC algorithm.
  - For example, a patient undergoing cataract surgery, a low-risk operation, is unlikely to have a complication regardless of the patient's clinical risk. Conversely a patient with no clinical risk factors undergoing high-risk surgery, such as a Whipple's procedure, is more likely to have a postoperative complication than would have been predicted

based on clinical pretest probability alone. Therefore, the risk of the surgery itself may alter management and influence the decision to do further testing.

- The ACC risk stratifies surgical procedures into three categories – vascular, intermediate, and low risk.
  - The previous designation of "high risk" has been changed to "vascular surgery". Patients undergoing these procedures have a greater likelihood of underlying cardiac disease and perioperative complications, and the preponderance of evidence for cardiac testing comes from patients undergoing aortic and major vascular surgery. Hence, the approach to these patients may be somewhat different than for nonvascular surgery.
  - The "intermediate risk" category includes most intrathoracic, intra-abdominal, head and neck, orthopedic, and urologic procedures as well as some lower risk vascular procedures such as carotid endarterectomy and endovascular abdominal aortic aneurysm repair.
  - "Low-risk" surgery includes procedures not invading a body cavity (chest or abdomen) such as endoscopic or superficial procedures, eye surgery, and breast surgery.

20.4.2.3 Functional Capacity

- Goldman and colleagues noted that patients with good functional capacity, even with mild, stable angina, tend to do well. This follows the concept of the ischemic threshold in which a patient developing symptoms or ischemia on a stress test at 8–10 METS is at lower risk than a patient who has ischemia at a lower exercise level and with a lower rate–pressure product. Reilly[8] and colleagues found that a patient's self-reported exercise capacity correlated with the risk of postoperative complications, and the ACC guidelines incorporated this concept in their risk assessment algorithm.

20.4.3 ACC/AHA Algorithm (Fig. 20.1)[5]

- The approach is as follows:
  1. Is the surgery emergent? (I also include urgent, meaning within 24 h)
     If so, time does not permit diagnostic testing or revascularization, and the patient should proceed to surgery. The physician should attempt to medically optimize the patient's condition in the short time period available.
  2. Assuming surgery is not emergent, does the patient have any of the "active cardiac conditions"?
     If so, these patients are at high risk, and elective surgery should be delayed for further diagnostic workup and therapy. Most patients do not have these conditions.
  3. Is the surgery low risk?
     If yes, the patient should proceed to surgery without any further testing or intervention because we cannot further reduce the low risk of complications (<1%).

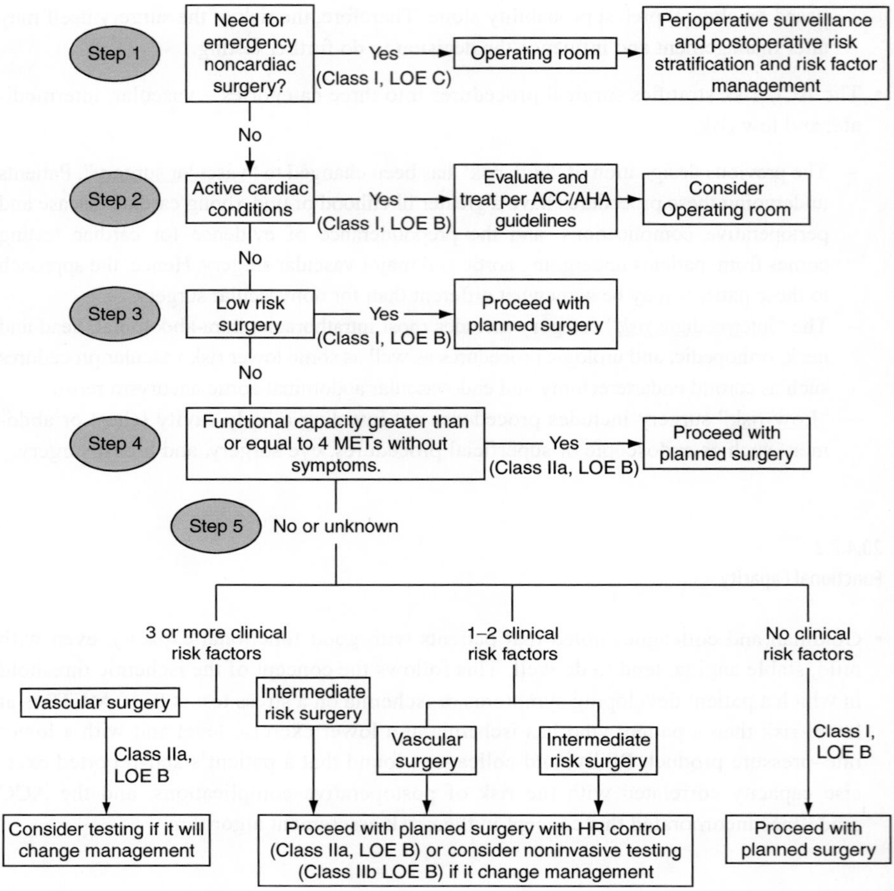

Fig. 20.1 ACC/AHA cardiac evaluation and care algorithm for noncardiac surgery (Reprinted from Fleisher et al.[9])

4. If not scheduled for low-risk surgery, does the patient have adequate exercise capacity (≥4 METS)?
   If so, for the most part, these patients do well and should proceed to surgery undergoing further cardiac testing.
5. If the answer is no to all of the previous questions, the next step is to determine the patient's clinical risk factors.

   – If there are no clinical risk factors, the patient should proceed to surgery with no further testing. (Based on the RCRI data, I include those with 1 risk factor here as well, although the ACC does not.)
   – If the patient has 1–2 risk factors, the guidelines recommend proceeding to surgery with heart rate control, but they allow you to consider NIT if the results will change management.

- The recommendations are the same for ≥3 risk factors and nonvascular surgery – proceed to surgery with heart rate control or consider NIT if the results are likely to change management; however, for ≥3 risk factors and vascular surgery, the recommendation is to consider NIT.

- This last step allows for individualizing management to a degree, but because it is vague, it may lead to significant differences in opinion and approach.

20.4.4 Diagnostic Tests

- Because stress tests were designed to diagnose CAD and myocardial ischemia and not to predict short-term perioperative events, their predictive value for complications after surgery is poor.
  - Although stress tests are good at identifying a patient with CAD, they have a low positive predictive value (PPV), usually between 15% and 20%, for predicting perioperative complications (MI and cardiac death). This means that most patients, even with an abnormal test, will not have a postoperative cardiac complication.
  - On the other hand, a normal or negative stress test is usually associated with a high negative predictive value (NPV), ranging from 95% to 99%, and may give some reassurance that these patients have a low likelihood of developing a postoperative cardiac event.
- In addition to myocardial ischemia related to coronary stenosis and an imbalance of oxygen supply and demand, the pathophysiology of perioperative MIs also includes unstable plaque rupture or coronary thrombosis which would not be predicted by stress tests.
- Because many patients with cardiac disease undergoing surgery have suboptimal exercise capacity and would be unable to achieve 85% of their target heart rate on an exercise test, pharmacologic stress testing is usually used. Furthermore, if these patients had adequate exercise capacity, they probably would not be candidates for stress testing in the first place. The tests most commonly used are dobutamine stress echocardiography (DSE) and dipyridamole or adenosine nuclear imaging (usually thallium).These tests are effective in identifying CAD, but as noted earlier, are poor at identifying patients who will develop postoperative cardiac events and should be used selectively in conjunction with the patient's pretest probability for the results to be meaningful.
- The test characteristics are influenced by patient selection and pretest probability.
  - In general, results are similar with DSE and dipyridamole thallium imaging (DTI), and test selection should be based on the local expertise available.
  - DSE tends to have fewer false positives except in the case of LBBB where DTI is preferred.
  - DSE is preferred for patients with asthma or COPD because DTI can cause bronchospasm.
  - Resting 2D echocardiography is not recommended to predict perioperative ischemic complications and should only be used to evaluate valvular heart disease or heart failure.

20.4.4.1
Stress Testing Before Surgery

- The goal of noninvasive testing (NIT) is to further refine clinical judgment and identify patients at high risk for postoperative cardiac complications. Bayes' theorem can be applied to preoperative evaluation to decide which patients might benefit from stress testing.
  - A patient with a low pretest probability will usually remain at low risk for perioperative complications even if the NIT is positive (may represent a false positive).
  - Similarly, a patient with high pretest probability will remain a relatively high-risk patient even if the stress test is negative (may represent a false negative).
  - Therefore, NIT should probably be restricted to intermediate risk patients where a positive test can move a patient into a higher risk category and a negative test can reclassify a patient as being at lower risk.
- The approach was supported by L'Italian[10] and colleagues who showed that clinical assessment correlated with outcomes for low- and high-risk patients, and stress test results only changed the probability of complications (confirmed by outcomes) for intermediate risk patients.
- Boersma[11] and colleagues also demonstrated that the clinical risk score correlated with outcomes and was rarely changed by stress testing.
  - However, Poldermans[12] and colleagues questioned the need for preoperative stress testing in intermediate risk patients. They found no difference in outcome (MI or cardiac death) regardless of whether patients had a stress test if they were adequately beta-blocked perioperatively.

20.4.4.2
Preoperative Coronary Angiography

- The ultimate goal of the preoperative evaluation process is to identify the high-risk patient and intervene to reduce the risk of postoperative complications. Assuming stress testing identifies a patient at high risk for postoperative complications, the next step should be to further define risk using cardiac catheterization with a goal of possible revascularization. Otherwise, if the patient is to be treated medically, the stress test was probably unnecessary as it did not change management.
- Potential candidates for coronary angiography include high-risk patients with ischemia on stress testing, those with unstable coronary syndromes (recent MI, severe angina, unstable angina) who meet criteria for coronary angiography independent of their need for noncardiac surgery, and patients whose pretest probability or clinical risk is high enough to bypass NIT.
  - If coronary angiography demonstrates significant anatomic lesions, a decision must be made regarding revascularization options – PCI or CABG.

20.5 Risk Reduction Strategies

Once a patient has been identified as being at high risk, either by clinical evaluation or after stress testing or coronary angiography, the next step is to employ measures to reduce that risk. The two main options include revascularization and/or medical therapy. The question is whether these therapies are effective.

20.5.1 Coronary Revascularization

20.5.1.1 Coronary Artery Bypass Grafting

- Results from the Coronary Artery Surgery Study (CASS)[13] showed that patients who had undergone CABG, were symptom free, and then went on to have noncardiac surgery at a later date had a lower risk of postoperative mortality and nonfatal MI than similar study patients treated medically. This benefit was only for high-risk surgery, and the protective effect of CABG appeared to last for 4–6 years.[14] However, the morbidity and mortality after CABG were not taken into account, and these patients had CABG for symptomatic disease rather than prophylactically in preparation for noncardiac surgery.
- These results differ from those of the Coronary Artery Revascularization Prophylaxis (CARP) trial[15] in which patients with stable cardiac symptoms scheduled to undergo elective major vascular surgery were evaluated by NIT, and those with abnormal tests went on to coronary angiography. Patients with suitable anatomy for revascularization were then randomized to medical therapy with or without revascularization (CABG or PCI). Exclusion criteria included >50% stenosis of the left main coronary artery, significant aortic stenosis, or LVEF <20%.
  - Prophylactic revascularization was associated with a mortality of 1.7%, perioperative MI of 5.8%, and reoperation rate of 2.5%. In this particular study, there were no perioperative strokes but typically this occurs in up to 2%. An additional ten patients who had successfully undergone revascularization died during the waiting period before vascular surgery.
  - Comparing the patients who had vascular surgery performed, there was no difference in 30-day mortality, postoperative MI, or long-term death between the revascularized or nonrevascularized groups. The authors concluded that prophylactic revascularization (on top of good medical therapy) in these patients was not helpful.
  - A subgroup analysis[16] of this study, as well as a recent meta-analysis[17], showed that CABG appeared to be more protective than PCI, possibly because of a more complete revascularization, and patients with left main disease benefited most.
- Because of the associated morbidity and mortality, prophylactic revascularization would only be expected to benefit patients at high risk undergoing high-risk surgery. However,

DECREASE V,[18] a small study of these very high risk patients (3 or more risk factors and extensive stress-induced ischemia on DSE undergoing major vascular surgery) in whom a previous study showed no benefit from perioperative beta-blockers, failed to demonstrate improved short- or long-term outcomes with revascularization in addition to optimal medical therapy. These patients had poor outcomes regardless of the treatment group (MI/death rates 42% vs. 32% at 30 days and 49% vs. 44% at 1 year).

- Criticisms of these studies raised concerns that the CARP trial patients did not have severe enough CAD while the DECREASE V patients were too sick. Another recent trial[19] found a benefit to routine versus selective cardiac catheterization for screening patients before elective aortic surgery. Intention-to-treat analysis showed decreased cardiac mortality and a similar trend in MACE in the routine cardiac catheterization group at 30 days and at follow-up 4 years later.

20.5.1.2 Percutaneous Coronary Interventions (PCI)

- In theory, prophylactic PCI, with its lower risk for adverse events than CABG, might be better, but there are no studies to confirm this. On the other hand, numerous studies and a meta-analysis[17] reported an increased risk associated with noncardiac surgery soon after PCI. This is primarily related to stent thrombosis (resulting in acute MI, often STEMI, and cardiac death) in patients who have prematurely discontinued the recommended course of dual antiplatelet therapy and to a lesser degree, bleeding in patients who were taking aspirin and clopidogrel.
  - The ACC/AHA guidelines[5,20] recommend delaying elective surgery for at least 2 weeks after balloon angioplasty, 4–6 weeks after placement of a bare metal stent (BMS), and 12 months after a drug-eluting stent (DES) in order to complete the course of aspirin and thienopyridine (clopidogrel or prasugrel) (Fig. 20.2).
  - Should surgery be required before these time intervals in a patient who had PCI, the recommended options, in priority order, are:

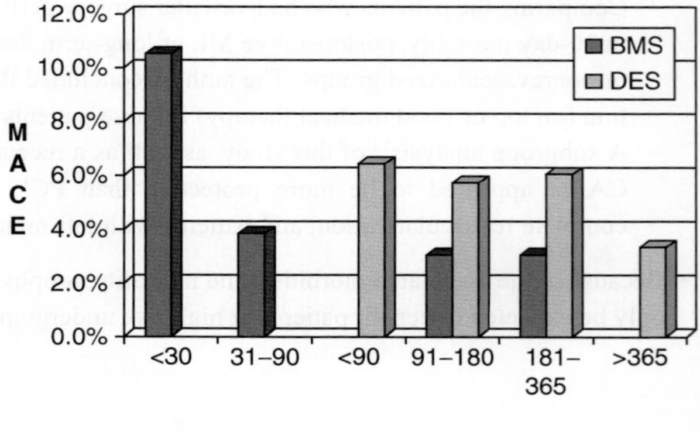

Fig. 20.2 Timing of noncardiac surgery after PCI (days) (*BMS* bare metal stent, *DES* drug eluting stent, *MACE* major adverse cardiac events) (Data from Nuttall et al.[21] and Rabbitts et al.[22])

1. Try to perform the surgery on dual antiplatelet therapy if possible,
2. Discontinue clopidogrel 5–7 days (or prasugrel 7 days) before surgery and continue aspirin, or
3. Discontinue both aspirin and clopidogrel 5–7 days before surgery.

- The antiplatelet therapy should be resumed as soon as possible after surgery, assuming adequate hemostasis has been assured. The largest observational case series from Mayo Clinic supports these recommendations for BMS[21] and DES.[22]
- A more potent antiplatelet agent, prasugrel, was recently FDA approved, but there is no clinical data yet regarding the outcomes of noncardiac surgery in patients treated with this drug. Recommendations are to discontinue it 7 days before surgery.
- Other new antiplatelet agents are in clinical trials and are expected to be submitted for FDA approval shortly. One of these drugs, ticagrelor, is a potent yet reversible antiplatelet inhibitor, which may be promising for "bridging therapy" to minimize a patient's time off antiplatelet therapy before noncardiac surgery.
- Small studies using IIB/IIIA agents for bridging had favorable results, but the numbers are too small and statistically insignificant to recommend it at this time.

20.5.2 Medical Therapy

20.5.2.1 Beta-Blockers

- Early studies with prophylactic beta-blockers demonstrated beneficial effects.
  - Mangano[23] and colleagues used atenolol, started immediately preoperatively, titrated to a heart rate of 55–65 beats per minute and continued for <7 days postoperatively, in 200 patients undergoing various operations. Perioperative ischemia was reduced in the atenolol-treated group, but there was no benefit for short-term outcomes of death or nonfatal MI. However, surviving patients in the beta-blocker group subsequently had fewer cardiovascular events by 2 years.
  - Poldermans[24] and colleagues used bisoprolol, started at least 7 days preoperatively (average 37 days before), titrated to a heart rate between 55 and 65 beats per minute, and continued for at least 30 days postoperatively, in 112 patients with abnormal DSEs undergoing major vascular surgery. The trial was stopped early because the bisoprolol-treated group had a significant reduction in postoperative MI and cardiac death (from 34% to 3%).
- Despite the small numbers of patients in these trials and methodological criticisms, various agencies and society guidelines began recommending prophylactic beta-blockers.
- Subsequent studies involving approximately 1,500 patients (POBBLE,[25] DIPOM,[26] MaVS[27]) using metoprolol, started at most 1 day before surgery and not titrated to a specific heart rate, showed no benefit in various cardiovascular outcomes.
- Lindenauer[28] and colleagues using an administrative database of over 600,000 patients reported that being on a beta-blocker within 2 days of surgery was associated with decreased in-hospital mortality in high- but not low-risk patients (stratified by RCRI score).

- The POISE trial[29] was expected to resolve this controversy but instead raised more questions. In this study, 8,351 patients with ASHD or risk factors for it who were scheduled for various surgical procedures were randomized to metoprolol succinate extended release or placebo.

  – Patients received the first dose (metoprolol ER 100 mg or placebo) 2–6 h before surgery followed by a second dose (100 mg) within 6 h after the end of surgery, and then a maintenance dose of 200 mg daily started 12 h after the postoperative dose. The drug was withheld for heart rate <45 beats per minute or systolic BP < 100 mmHg and then restarted at half the dose 12 h later if BP and pulse improved.
  – Primary outcome, a composite of cardiac death, nonfatal MI, and cardiac arrest, was significantly better in the metoprolol-treated group (5.8% vs. 6.9%) due to a statistically significant reduction in nonfatal MIs from 5.1% to 3.6%. However, this benefit came at the expense of a statistically significant increase in secondary outcome events – nonfatal stroke (0.5% to 1%) and total mortality (2.3% to 3.1%) in the treatment group, in part due to significantly more episodes of hypotension (15% vs. 9.7%) and bradycardia (6.6% vs. 2.2%).

    Mortality was increased in patients with sepsis, and stroke risk appeared to be increased in patients with prior strokes and intraoperative hypotension.

  – This study generated significant commentary and criticism, mainly related to the high dose of metoprolol that was started shortly before surgery in beta-blocker naïve patients, many of whom underwent emergency surgery or had sepsis. This tempered the enthusiasm for prophylactic beta-blockers.

- More recently, the DECREASE IV[30] study involved intermediate risk patients who were given bisoprolol, fluvastatin, both, or neither.

  – Bisoprolol was started approximately 1 month before surgery and titrated to a heart rate between 50 and 70 beats per minute.
  – Cardiac death and nonfatal MI were significantly reduced from 6% to 2.1% in the group receiving bisoprolol versus the control group.

- Van Lier[31] and colleagues performed a pooled analysis of 3,884 patients from their DECREASE trials and found the overall incidence of postoperative stroke to be 0.46% (18/3,884). There was no difference in beta-blocker users (0.5%) compared to nonusers (0.4%), and the only risk factor noted for postoperative stroke was a previous history of stroke. A case-control study[32] also showed no increased risk of postoperative stroke in patients taking chronic beta-blockers.
- If beta-blockers are to be beneficial, they probably need to be started at least 7 days before surgery[33] and titrated to a resting heart rate in the range of 55–70 beats per minute to minimize the risk of significant hypotension or bradycardia. Higher risk patients or those undergoing vascular or higher risk surgical procedures would be most likely to benefit.
- Although the final answer is not in, the ACC recently published a focused update on perioperative beta-blockers[34] that reflected results from POISE and the new DECREASE trials. Their recommendations included:

  – Class I: *continue* beta-blockers in patients already on them. (Abrupt withdrawal of beta-blockers before surgery has been associated with increased risk for ischemic events.)

- Class IIa: for patients undergoing vascular surgery, beta-blockers are *probably recommended* for patients at high cardiac risk (known CAD or ischemia on preoperative testing) and are *reasonable* for patients with two or more risk factors (besides surgery) undergoing vascular or intermediate risk surgery.
- Class IIb: usefulness of beta-blockers is *uncertain* in patients undergoing intermediate risk or vascular surgery who have only one clinical risk factor (not CAD) and in patients undergoing vascular surgery with no clinical risk factors.
- Class III: beta-blockers *should not be given* to patients with contraindications and also noted that high-dose beta-blockers started shortly before surgery without time for dose titration are not useful and may be harmful.

- Table 20.1 illustrates a comparison between the ACC update and similar but somewhat more liberal indications and recommendations for perioperative beta-blockers published by the European Society of Cardiology.[35]

Table 20.1 Recommendations for perioperative beta-blockade (ACC and ESC)

Class	Perioperative beta-blockade: indications and level of evidence	
	2009 American Heart Association/ American College of Cardiology (AHA/ACC)	European Society of Cardiology (ESC)
Class I	1. *Should be continued* if patient is already receiving BB (C)	1. *Recommended* in patients with known IHD or ischemia on preop stress testing (B) 2. *Recommended* in patients scheduled for high-risk surgery (B) 3. *Continuation recommended* in patients previously treated with BB for IHD, arrhythmias, or HTN (C)
Class IIa	BB titrated to HR and BP are: 1. *Probably recommended* for pts undergoing vascular surgery with known CAD or ischemia on preop stress testing (B); 2. *Reasonable* for patients undergoing vascular surgery with >1 clinical risk factor (C); 3. *Reasonable* for pts undergoing intermediate risk surgery with CAD or >1 clinical risk factor (C)	1. *Should be considered* for patients scheduled for intermediate-risk surgery (B); 2. *Consider continuation* in pts previously treated with BB for CHF with systolic dysfunction (C)
Class IIb	*Usefulness of BB is uncertain* for patients undergoing: 1. Intermediate-risk or vascular surgery with one clinical risk factor in the absence of CAD (C); 2. Vascular surgery with no clinical risk factors (B)	1. BB *may be considered* in patients scheduled for low-risk surgery with risk factors (B)

(continued)

Table 20.1 (continued)

Class	Perioperative beta-blockade: indications and level of evidence	
	2009 American Heart Association/ American College of Cardiology (AHA/ACC)	European Society of Cardiology (ESC)
Class III	1. *Should not be given* to patients with absolute contraindications to BB (C); 2. Routine administration of high-dose BB in the absence of dose titration *is not useful and may be harmful* to patients not currently taking BB who are undergoing noncardiac surgery (B)	1. Periop high-dose BB without titration are *not recommended* (A); 2. BB are *not recommended* in patients scheduled for low risk surgery without risk factors (B)

Adapted from Fleisher et al.[9] and Poldermans et al.[35]
Class I: benefit >>> risk
Class IIa: benefit >> risk
Class IIb: benefit ≥ risk
Class III: risk ≥ benefit

20.5.2.2
Alpha-2 Agonists

- In patients unable to take beta-blockers, the use of alpha agonists may represent an alternative.
  - A Cochrane systematic review[36] of perioperative alpha agonists, driven primarily by mivzerol (not available in the US), demonstrated a benefit in reducing MI and mortality but only in patients undergoing vascular surgery.
  - Several small studies[37] in patients undergoing noncardiac surgery have shown a reduction in perioperative ischemia in patients given clonidine.
  - The POISE-2 trial, using clonidine, aspirin, both, or neither, should provide more outcome data regarding the use of clonidine perioperatively.

20.5.2.3
Statins

- In addition to lowering cholesterol, statins have “pleotropic effects”. These include reduced platelet aggregation, improved endothelial function, and reduced inflammation. These effects may help stabilize plaques and prevent plaque rupture which might lead to an MI.
- Most observational studies report that perioperative statin use is beneficial in reducing postoperative cardiac complications and death in both cardiac and noncardiac surgery.

A meta-analysis by Kapoor[38] and colleagues confirmed this benefit; however, there are few randomized controlled trials.

– The first of these, a small study[39] of 100 patients using atorvastatin 20 mg started 14–30 days before vascular surgery, demonstrated a beneficial effect on a composite outcome of cardiovascular events after 6 months.
– The DECREASE III[40] trial randomized 497 patients to placebo or fluvastatin 80 mg extended release before vascular surgery. The statin-treated group had less ischemia and a statistically significant reduction in the composite endpoint of cardiac death and nonfatal MI. Statins reduced LDL and total cholesterol, multiple inflammatory markers including CRP and IL-6, and also were safe in that there were no cases of rhabdomyolysis or significant hepatic injury.
– In contrast to the benefit seen in vascular surgery patients, the fluvastatin arm of the DECREASE IV[30] trial in intermediate risk patients demonstrated a statistically insignificant reduction in cardiac death and nonfatal MI (from 4.9% to 3.2%) in the statin-treated group. Explanations for this difference are that a larger group is necessary to see a benefit or these lower risk patients will not benefit from statin therapy.

- Although no safety issues were found in a review[41] of statin use in vascular surgery patients, the drug manufacturers still recommend discontinuing statins before surgery due to these potential safety concerns. However, the ACC and European Society of Cardiology (ESC) guidelines recommend continuing them perioperatively as the potential benefit outweighs the theoretical risk.
- Based on the DECREASE III trial it appears that patients who are not on a statin but are scheduled for vascular surgery would benefit from starting a statin preoperatively. It is also likely that other patients with independent indications for statins (CAD, DM, PAD, hyperlipidemia) undergoing high-risk surgery might benefit as well.
- Unanswered questions regarding perioperative statin use are whether this is a class effect, what dose should be used, how long in advance to start it prophylactically for it to be effective, and which patients are most likely to benefit from them.

20.6 Other Cardiovascular Conditions

20.6.1 Hypertension

- Hypertension is at best a minor risk factor. Although various recommendations[42] mention blood pressures (diastolic BP >110 mmHg or systolic BP >180 mmHg) when cancellation of elective surgery should be considered or which might be associated with increased risk, there is no hard evidence to support them.
- Hypertensive patients, particularly if untreated or poorly controlled, are more likely to have labile blood pressure perioperatively and are at risk for intraoperative hypotension and postoperative hypertension.

- The etiology of the hypertension, especially if it is a pheochromocytoma, and presence of end organ damage are more likely to predict cardiac risk than the preoperative blood pressure itself.
- Most antihypertensive medications should be continued, including on the morning of surgery, with the possible exceptions of diuretics and ACE-inhibitors or ARBs.

20.6.2 Arrhythmias

- Hemodynamically significant arrhythmias are included in the active cardiac condition group in the ACC guidelines. These include tachyarrhythmias (AF with rapid ventricular rate, SVT, VT) as well as bradyarrhythmias (symptomatic sinus bradycardia, high degree AV block) which should be evaluated and treated before elective surgery.
- Antiarrhythmic drugs should be continued perioperatively.
- Asymptomatic sinus bradycardia and bifascicular block do not require a temporary pacemaker prophylactically as the risk of developing a complete heart block perioperatively is extremely low.
- Patients with a pacemaker or AICD should have the device interrogated preoperatively. If electrocautery will be used intraoperatively, the AICD should be inactivated.
  - Because electrocautery may interfere with pacemaker function, the rate responsive feature should be deactivated.
  - Use of a magnet will usually temporarily revert a pacemaker to a nonsensing mode or suspend detection of tachyarrhythmic events in ICDs.

20.6.3 Heart Failure

- Decompensated heart failure (HF) is an active cardiac condition requiring postponement of elective surgery in order to optimize medical therapy. Beta-blockers should not be started preoperatively in these patients, and in a subgroup analysis of the CIBIS II study,[43] patients with HF had little benefit from beta-blockers.
- Although ACEIs and ARBs have been associated with hypotension during induction of anesthesia and the need for IV fluids and pressors, they should probably be continued in patients with heart failure unless the preoperative blood pressure is low.

20.6.4 Valvular Heart Disease

- The lesion most likely to be associated with perioperative cardiac complications is symptomatic, severe aortic stenosis (AS). Patients with a systolic murmur suggestive of AS (late peaking systolic ejection murmur radiating to the carotids, associated with decreased and delayed carotid pulses), particularly if they have chest pain, dyspnea, or syncope, should have a 2D echocardiogram performed.

- If they have symptomatic severe AS and the planned noncardiac surgery is elective, the recommendation is for aortic valve replacement (AVR). Should the patient refuse or if the surgery is more urgent, it has been possible to get most of these patients through surgery successfully using medical therapy and intraoperative monitoring. Hypotension and tachycardia should be avoided by judicious use of fluids and beta-blockers. Rarely, balloon valvuloplasty is used for patients with aortic stenosis deemed to be too high risk for AVR.
- Mitral stenosis, when associated with atrial fibrillation and heart failure, may also increase risk, but most of the other valvular lesions do not require surgical intervention before noncardiac surgery.
- Pulmonary hypertension is now being recognized as a risk factor as well, but studies are limited. The patient's usual medications should be continued.
- Endocarditis prophylaxis[44] (see Chap. 6) is only indicated for patients undergoing dental and upper respiratory procedures who have a prosthetic valve, previous endocarditis, complex congenital heart disease that has not been repaired (or was repaired in the past 6 months), or valvular disease in a transplanted heart.

20.7 Summary

Using the RCRI and ACC guidelines, the patient can be classified as low, intermediate, or high risk clinically. Combining this with the risk of the planned surgery, the physician can decide not only whether further testing is indicated but also whether it is likely to change management. Prophylactic revascularization is rarely necessary just to get a patient through surgery, and the majority of the patients will be managed medically. It is important for future studies to determine optimal use of beta-blockers, statins, and other therapies in order to have patients in their optimal medical condition prior to elective noncardiac surgery to reduce postoperative complications.

References

1. Dripps RD, Lamont A, Eckenhoff JE. The role of anesthesia in surgical mortality. *JAMA*. 1961;178:261-266.
2. Goldman L, Caldera DL, Nussbaum SR, et al. Multifactorial index of cardiac risk in noncardiac surgical procedures. *N Engl J Med*. 1977;297(16):845-850.
3. Detsky AS, Abrams HB, Forbath N, Scott JG, Hilliard JR. Cardiac assessment for patients undergoing noncardiac surgery. A multifactorial clinical risk index. *Arch Intern Med*. 1986;146(11):2131-2134.
4. Lee TH, Marcantonio ER, Mangione CM, et al. Derivation and prospective validation of a simple index for prediction of cardiac risk of major noncardiac surgery. *Circulation*. 1999;100(10):1043-1049.
5. Fleisher LA, Beckman JA, Brown KA, et al. ACC/AHA 2007 guidelines on perioperative cardiovascular evaluation and care for noncardiac surgery: a report of the American College of Cardiology/American Heart Association Task Force on Practice Guidelines (Writing Committee to Revise the 2002 Guidelines on Perioperative Cardiovascular Evaluation for Noncardiac Surgery) developed in collaboration with the American Society of Echocardiography, American

Society of Nuclear Cardiology, Heart Rhythm Society, Society of Cardiovascular Anesthesiologists, Society for Cardiovascular Angiography and Interventions, Society for Vascular Medicine and Biology, and Society for Vascular Surgery. *J Am Coll Cardiol*. 2007;50(17):e159-e241.

6. Rodgers A, Walker N, Schug S, et al. Reduction of postoperative mortality and morbidity with epidural or spinal anaesthesia: results from overview of randomised trials. *BMJ*. 2000;321 (7275):1493.
7. Eagle KA, Coley CM, Newell JB, et al. Combining clinical and thallium data optimizes preoperative assessment of cardiac risk before major vascular surgery. *Ann Intern Med*. 1989; 110(11):859-866.
8. Reilly DF, McNeely MJ, Doerner D, et al. Self-reported exercise tolerance and the risk of serious perioperative complications. *Arch Intern Med*. 1999;159(18):2185-2192.
9. Fleisher LA, Beckman JA, Brown KA, et al. 2009 ACCF/AHA focused update on perioperative beta blockade incorporated into the ACC/AHA 2007 guidelines on perioperative cardiovascular evaluation and care for noncardiac surgery. American College of Cardiology Foundation/American Heart Association Task Force on Practice Guidelines; American Society of Echocardiography; American Society of Nuclear Cardiology; Heart Rhythm Society; Society of Cardiovascular Anesthesiologists; Society for Cardiovascular Angiography and Interventions; Society for Vascular Medicine; Society for Vascular Surgery. *J Am Coll Cardiol*. 2009;54(22):e13-e118.
10. L'Italien GJ, Paul SD, Hendel RC, et al. Development and validation of a Bayesian model for perioperative cardiac risk assessment in a cohort of 1,081 vascular surgical candidates. *J Am Coll Cardiol*. 1996;27(4):779-786.
11. Boersma E, Poldermans D, Bax JJ, et al. Predictors of cardiac events after major vascular surgery: role of clinical characteristics, dobutamine echocardiography, and beta-blocker therapy. *JAMA*. 2001;285(14):1865-1873.
12. Poldermans D, Bax JJ, Schouten O, et al. Should major vascular surgery be delayed because of preoperative cardiac testing in intermediate-risk patients receiving beta-blocker therapy with tight heart rate control? *J Am Coll Cardiol*. 2006;48(5):964-969.
13. Foster ED, Davis KB, Carpenter JA, Abele S, Fray D. Risk of noncardiac operation in patients with defined coronary disease: the coronary artery surgery study (CASS) registry experience. *Ann Thorac Surg*. 1986;41(1):42-50.
14. Eagle KA, Rihal CS, Mickel MC, Holmes DR, Foster ED, Gersh BJ. Cardiac risk of noncardiac surgery: influence of coronary disease and type of surgery in 3368 operations. CASS Investigators and University of Michigan Heart Care Program. Coronary artery surgery study. *Circulation*. 1997;96(6):1882-1887.
15. McFalls EO, Ward HB, Moritz TE, et al. Coronary-artery revascularization before elective major vascular surgery. *N Engl J Med*. 2004;351(27):2795-2804.
16. Ward HB, Kelly RF, Thottapurathu L, et al. Coronary artery bypass grafting is superior to percutaneous coronary intervention in prevention of perioperative myocardial infarctions during subsequent vascular surgery. *Ann Thorac Surg*. 2006;82(3):795-800. discussion 800-791.
17. Biccard BM, Rodseth RN. A meta-analysis of the prospective randomised trials of coronary revascularisation before noncardiac vascular surgery with attention to the type of coronary revascularisation performed. *Anaesthesia*. 2009;64(10):1105-1113.
18. Schouten O, van Kuijk JP, Flu WJ, et al. Long-term outcome of prophylactic coronary revascularization in cardiac high-risk patients undergoing major vascular surgery (from the randomized DECREASE-V Pilot Study). *Am J Cardiol*. 2009;103(7):897-901.
19. Monaco M, Stassano P, Di Tommaso L, et al. Systematic strategy of prophylactic coronary angiography improves long-term outcome after major vascular surgery in medium- to high-risk patients: a prospective, randomized study. *J Am Coll Cardiol*. 2009;54(11):989-996.
20. Grines CL, Bonow RO, Casey DE Jr, et al. Prevention of premature discontinuation of dual antiplatelet therapy in patients with coronary artery stents: a science advisory from the

American Heart Association, American College of Cardiology, Society for Cardiovascular Angiography and Interventions, American College of Surgeons, and American Dental Association, with representation from the American College of Physicians. *J Am Coll Cardiol.* 2007;49(6):734-739.

21. Nuttall GA, Brown MJ, Stombaugh JW, et al. Time and cardiac risk of surgery after bare-metal stent percutaneous coronary intervention. *Anesthesiology*. 2008;109(4):588-595.
22. Rabbitts JA, Nuttall GA, Brown MJ, et al. Cardiac risk of noncardiac surgery after percutaneous coronary intervention with drug-eluting stents. *Anesthesiology*. 2008;109(4):596-604.
23. Mangano DT, Layug EL, Wallace A, Tateo I. Effect of atenolol on mortality and cardiovascular morbidity after noncardiac surgery. Multicenter Study of Perioperative Ischemia Research Group. *N Engl J Med.* 1996;335(23):1713-1720.
24. Poldermans D, Boersma E, Bax JJ, et al. The effect of bisoprolol on perioperative mortality and myocardial infarction in high-risk patients undergoing vascular surgery. Dutch Echocardiographic Cardiac Risk Evaluation Applying Stress Echocardiography Study Group. *N Engl J Med.* 1999;341(24):1789-1794.
25. Brady AR, Gibbs JS, Greenhalgh RM, Powell JT, Sydes MR. Perioperative beta-blockade (POBBLE) for patients undergoing infrarenal vascular surgery: results of a randomized double-blind controlled trial. *J Vasc Surg.* 2005;41(4):602-609.
26. Juul AB, Wetterslev J, Gluud C, et al. Effect of perioperative beta blockade in patients with diabetes undergoing major non-cardiac surgery: randomised placebo controlled, blinded multicentre trial. *BMJ.* 2006;332(7556):1482.
27. Yang H, Raymer K, Butler R, Parlow J, Roberts R. The effects of perioperative beta-blockade: results of the Metoprolol after Vascular Surgery (MaVS) study, a randomized controlled trial. *Am Heart J.* 2006;152(5):983-990.
28. Lindenauer PK, Pekow P, Wang K, Mamidi DK, Gutierrez B, Benjamin EM. Perioperative beta-blocker therapy and mortality after major noncardiac surgery. *N Engl J Med.* 2005; 353(4):349-361.
29. Devereaux PJ, Yang H, Yusuf S, et al. Effects of extended-release metoprolol succinate in patients undergoing non-cardiac surgery (POISE trial): a randomised controlled trial. *Lancet.* 2008;371(9627):1839-1847.
30. Dunkelgrun M, Boersma E, Schouten O, et al. Bisoprolol and fluvastatin for the reduction of perioperative cardiac mortality and myocardial infarction in intermediate-risk patients undergoing noncardiovascular surgery: a randomized controlled trial (DECREASE-IV). *Ann Surg.* 2009;249(6):921-926.
31. van Lier F, Schouten O, Hoeks SE, et al. Impact of prophylactic beta-blocker therapy to prevent stroke after noncardiac surgery. *Am J Cardiol.* 2010;105(1):43-47.
32. van Lier F, Schouten O, van Domburg RT, et al. Effect of chronic beta-blocker use on stroke after noncardiac surgery. *Am J Cardiol.* 2009;104(3):429-433.
33. Flu W, van Kuijk J, Chonchol M, et al. Timing of pre-operative beta-blocker treatment in vascular surgery patients. *J Am Coll Cardiol.* 2010;56:1922-1929.
34. Fleischmann KE, Beckman JA, Buller CE, et al. 2009 ACCF/AHA focused update on perioperative beta blockade. *J Am Coll Cardiol.* 2009;54(22):2102-2128.
35. Poldermans D, Bax JJ, Boersma E, et al. ESC Committee for Practice Guidelines (CPG). Guidelines for pre-operative cardiac risk assessment and perioperative cardiac management in non-cardiac surgery: the Task Force for Preoperative Cardiac Risk Assessment and Perioperative Cardiac Management in Non-cardiac Surgery of the European Society of Cardiology (ESC) and European Society of Anaesthesiology (ESA). *Eur Heart J.* 2009; 30(22):2769-2812. Epub 2009 Aug 27.
36. Wijeysundera DN, Bender JS, Beattie WS. Alpha-2 adrenergic agonists for the prevention of cardiac complications among patients undergoing surgery. *Cochrane Database Syst Rev.* 2009;(4):CD004126.

37. Wallace AW, Galindez D, Salahieh A, et al. Effect of clonidine on cardiovascular morbidity and mortality after noncardiac surgery. *Anesthesiology*. 2004;101(2):284-293.
38. Kapoor AS, Kanji H, Buckingham J, Devereaux PJ, McAlister FA. Strength of evidence for perioperative use of statins to reduce cardiovascular risk: systematic review of controlled studies. *BMJ*. 2006;333(7579):1149.
39. Durazzo AE, Machado FS, Ikeoka DT, et al. Reduction in cardiovascular events after vascular surgery with atorvastatin: a randomized trial. *J Vasc Surg*. 2004;39(5):967-975, discussion 975-966.
40. Schouten O, Boersma E, Hoeks SE, et al. Fluvastatin and perioperative events in patients undergoing vascular surgery. *N Engl J Med*. 2009;361(10):980-989.
41. Schouten O, Kertai MD, Bax JJ, et al. Safety of perioperative statin use in high-risk patients undergoing major vascular surgery. *Am J Cardiol*. 2005;95(5):658-660.
42. Fleisher LA. Preoperative evaluation of the patient with hypertension. *JAMA*. 2002; 287(16):2043-2046.
43. Bohm M, Maack C, Wehrlen-Grandjean M, Erdmann E. Effect of bisoprolol on perioperative complications in chronic heart failure after surgery (Cardiac Insufficiency Bisoprolol Study II (CIBIS II)). *Z Kardiol*. 2003;92(8):668-676.
44. Wilson W, Taubert KA, Gewitz M, et al. Prevention of infective endocarditis: guidelines from the American Heart Association: a guideline from the American Heart Association Rheumatic Fever, Endocarditis, and Kawasaki Disease Committee, Council on Cardiovascular Disease in the Young, and the Council on Clinical Cardiology, Council on Cardiovascular Surgery and Anesthesia, and the Quality of Care and Outcomes Research Interdisciplinary Working Group. *Circulation*. 2007;116(15):1736-1754.

21 Pulmonary Disease

Steven L. Cohn

21.1 Introduction

- Postoperative pulmonary complications (PPCs) are a major source of morbidity among patients undergoing surgery and occur as often as cardiac complications. Although not necessarily having as high mortality, PPCs are more likely to be associated with an increased hospital length of stay and higher costs than postoperative cardiac complications.
- When attempting to interpret the perioperative pulmonary literature, problems arise because of the various definitions of what constitutes a PPC and studies confined to a specific medical condition or surgical procedure that may not be applicable to other situations. There are also fewer randomized controlled trials and multivariate analyses in the pulmonary literature so confounders further complicate the process of defining risk factors.
- Major PPCs that will be considered here are those resulting in morbidity or mortality and include pneumonia, respiratory failure, exacerbation of chronic obstructive pulmonary disease (COPD), and atelectasis requiring intervention (e.g., bronchoscopy for lobar collapse).
- Patient-related risk factors, procedure-related risk factors, laboratory testing, and interventions to reduce PPC risk in patients undergoing noncardiothoracic surgery will be discussed. Lung resection surgery is discussed in Chap. 10.

S.L. Cohn
Internal Medicine-Medical Consultation Service,
SUNY Downstate - Kings County Hospital Center,
450 Clarkson Ave, Box 68, Brooklyn, NY 11203, USA
e-mail: steven.cohn@downstate.edu

S.L. Cohn (ed.), *Perioperative Medicine*,
DOI: 10.1007/978-0-85729-498-2_21,

21.2 Postoperative Pulmonary Pathophysiology

- PPCs may result from exaggerated responses of the normal postoperative pulmonary physiology or the usual expected changes superimposed on a patient with already compromised pulmonary function.
- Lung volume reduction after surgery and anesthesia is the underlying mechanism that increases the risk for atelectasis and other PPCs.
  - 50% reduction after intrathoracic and upper abdominal surgery; 25% reduction after lower abdominal surgery
  - These lung volumes do not return to baseline until several weeks postoperatively
- Breathing patterns are altered.
  - Tidal volume (TV) decreases, respiratory rate (RR) increases to compensate, and minute ventilation is maintained with no significant change.
  - Diaphragmatic dysfunction occurs and sighs decrease.
  - PO_2 decreases by 10–20%.
- Defense mechanisms are suppressed.
- Decreased cough, ciliary activity, and mucus clearance leading to increased risk for colonization.

21.3 Risk Factors

- Potential patient-related risk factors to be considered include general health status (age, functional status, American Association of Anesthesiologists (ASA), Goldman, or Charlson classification), nutritional status (low albumin, obesity), neurologic status (impaired sensorium, CVA), fluid status (CHF, CRF, BUN), immune status (steroids, alcohol, DM, cancer), and the respiratory status (COPD, asthma, cigarette smoking, sputum, infection (pneumonia, upper respiratory infection), obstructive sleep apnea (OSA), unexplained dyspnea).
- Much of the following discussion is based on the ACP guidelines published in 2006 as an executive summary[1] of two systematic reviews[2,3] for preoperative risk assessment and strategies to reduce PPCs for patients undergoing noncardiac surgery. (The guidelines are to be updated in 2012.)
- Risk factors (Table 21.1) were classified as patient related or procedure related, and the strength of recommendation for each risk factor was graded as follows:
  - A = good evidence supporting risk factor
  - B = fair evidence supporting risk factor
  - C = fair evidence against risk factor

Table 21.1 Summary of risk factors associated with PPCs ACP guidelines: good (A) or fair (B) supporting evidence

Patient-related risk factors	# of studies	Odds ratio (OR)	Strength of recommendation
Advanced age (increasing from age 50)	14	2.09–3.04	A
ASA class ≥ II	17	2.55–4.87	
Congestive heart failure	3	2.93	
Functional dependence	4	1.65–2.51	
Chronic obstructive pulmonary disease	8	1.79	
Weight loss	2	1.62	B
Impaired sensorium	2	1.39	
Cigarette use	5	1.26	
Alcohol use	2	1.21	
Procedure-related risk factors			
Surgical site:			
• Aortic surgery	2	6.90	A
• Thoracic surgery	3	4.24	
• Abdominal surgery	6	3.01	
(especially upper)	2	2.53	
• Neurosurgery	2	2.21	
• Head and neck surgery	2	2.10	
• Vascular surgery	6	2.21	
Emergency surgery	5	2.26	
Prolonged surgery (>2.5–4 h)	6	1.83	
General anesthesia			
Perioperative transfusion	2	1.47	B
Laboratory Tests			
Serum albumin <3.5 g/dL	5	2.53	A
Chest x-ray	8	4.81	B
BUN>21 mg/dL	2		

Modified from Smetana et al.[2]
ASA = American Society of Anesthesiologists
BUN = blood urea nitrogen
Evidence against risk for: diabetes, obesity, asthma; hip, gynecologic, urologic surgery
Insufficient evidence for: obstructive sleep apnea, corticosteroid use, HIV infection, arrhythmia, poor exercise capacity, esophageal surgery, spirometry

- D = good evidence against risk factor
- I = insufficient evidence

- It was noted that most of these risk factors were not modifiable, and that procedure-related risk factors (surgical site) were more important predictors of PPCs in contrast to cardiac complications where patient-related risk factors predominated.

21.3.1 Patient-Related Risk Factors

21.3.1.1 Age

- Although the impact of *age* on the risk of PPCs has been controversial, the ACP meta-analysis established that age is an independent risk predictor of PPCs even after adjustment for medical comorbidities. The pooled odds ratios (OR) for PPCs increased with each decade beginning after age >50, with a 50% increase in risk in the 50–59 year old group to more than a five-fold increase after age 80.
- Age is probably a marker of decreased cardiopulmonary reserve and possibly subclinical disease. However, by itself, the risk is not prohibitive, and elderly patients should not be denied necessary surgery due to concern for PPCs based on advanced age alone, in the absence of other important risk factors.

21.3.1.2 Functional Status

- Various measures of overall health and functional status predict PPC rates in addition to overall perioperative mortality.
  - The *American Association of Anesthesiologists (ASAr)'s functional status classification* was derived to predict perioperative mortality. In addition, it predicts PPC rates. ASA class ≥ 2 confers a 4–5 fold increase in risk of PPCs. Other risk indices, including the *Charlson co-morbidity index* and *Goldman cardiac risk index*, also predicted PPCs.
  - Both *self-reported and directly observed exercise capacity* identify patients at higher risk of PPCs.

    Self-reported inability to climb at least 2 flights of stairs or walk at least 4 blocks on level ground confers a modest increase in PPC rates.
    Directly observed stair climbing also predicts risk for patients undergoing high-risk surgeries. Patients who can climb at least 4 flights of stairs without resting have a low risk of PPCs.
    Partial or total functional dependence was also associated with an increased risk in PPCs.

21.3.1.3 Nutritional Status

- *Obesity* may be associated with restrictive lung disease, increased work of breathing, and alteration in closing volumes as well as potential for aspiration, airway problems, and more frequent microatelectasis. However, despite these factors, the ACP guidelines did not find obesity, even morbid obesity, to be associated with an increased risk in meaningful pulmonary complications after surgery. Additionally, among patients undergoing gastric bypass surgery for obesity, PPC rates are similar to nonobese patients and did not differ even when stratified by degree of obesity (BMI).

- *Malnutrition*, as reflected by a low serum albumin, predicts postoperative morbidity and mortality.

21.3.1.4
Neurologic Status

- *Impaired sensorium*, defined as mental status changes, confusion, and delirium, is associated with an increased risk of PPCs. These patients may be confined to bed and unable to cooperate with postoperative instructions for cough and deep breathing exercises.
- *Stroke* patients with residual neurologic deficits may be bedbound as well and have swallowing difficulties that increase risk of aspiration.

21.3.1.5
Fluid Status

- Cardiac risk factors may also predict pulmonary risk. *Congestive heart failure* was identified as a risk factor for PPCs in the ACP guidelines and in the respiratory risk index.
- *Dehydration* (prerenal azotemia) as reflected by an elevated BUN and hypernatremia may also predict PPCs.

21.3.1.6
Immune Status

- The ACP guidelines did not find *diabetes mellitus* to be a risk factor for PPCs. They noted insufficient evidence for *corticosteroid use* and *HIV infection* as risk factors. However, the postoperative pneumonia index noted chronic steroid use as a risk factor.
- *Alcohol intake* (>2 drinks/day in the past 2 weeks) was a modest risk predictor for postoperative PPCs in both the ACP guidelines and postoperative pneumonia index.

21.3.1.7
Respiratory Status/Pulmonary Disease

- *Cigarette smoking* increase bronchial secretions and airway reactivity and is associated with an increased risk of PPCs, even for patients without chronic obstructive pulmonary disease. Wound infections, oxygen desaturation, laryngospasm, and coughing with anesthesia are more likely in smokers. The risk depends on the patient's current smoking status, amount and duration of cigarette use (>20 pack-years), and associated pulmonary disease (cough, dyspnea, abnormal chest exam, established COPD).

- Current smokers and recent quitters are more likely to develop PPCs than are non-smokers or smokers who quit more than 8 weeks before surgery.
- Although smoking cessation shortly before surgery does not decrease risk of PPCs, it appears that there is no paradoxical increase in risk as reported in an earlier study.

- Well-controlled *asthma* does not seem to be a risk factor for PPCs although patients who are wheezing at the time of surgery may have a higher risk. Many of these complications, however, are minor such as bronchospasm requiring treatment.
- *Chronic obstructive pulmonary disease (COPD)* on the other hand is a risk factor for PPCs but not as significant as previously thought (OR was only 1.79). An abnormal chest exam (decreased breath sounds, rales, rhonchi, or wheezing, or prolonged expiration) and a positive cough test may predict a higher risk of complications. Patients with COPD are also at higher risk for nonpulmonary complications including wound infections and atrial arrhythmias.
- While obesity itself is not a PPC risk factor, *obstructive sleep apnea (OSA)* may increase risk, even for patients who have not been previously diagnosed. In the immediate postoperative period there is a higher incidence of airway management problems such as hypoxia, hypercarbia, the need for reintubation, and unplanned transfers to the intensive care unit. It is unclear whether traditional PPCs, such as pneumonia and atelectasis, are more common among patients with OSA although a recent study found patients with an oxygen desaturation index (ODI4) ≥5 to have an increased risk.

  - The gold standard for diagnosis is sleep laboratory polysomnography although home nocturnal oximetry is a simpler screening tool. The STOP-BANG questionnaire can be used clinically to screen for OSA.[4]
  - (1) ***S***noring, (2) ***T***ired, (3) ***O***bserved apnea, (4) high blood ***P***ressure, (5) ***B***MI >35 kg/m^2, (6) ***A***ge >50, (7) ***N***eck circumference >40 cm, (8) ***G***ender (male)
  - High risk of OSA is indicated if 3 or more items are answered "yes."

- *Pulmonary hypertension (PH)* has been associated with increased risk of postoperative arrhythmias, heart failure, and death although not mentioned in the ACP guidelines. Two recent studies reported an increased risk in prolonged intubation (with pulmonary artery pressure >70 mmHg) and postoperative respiratory failure and death (with moderate to severe PH and right axis deviation, right ventricular hypertrophy, and RV systolic pressure/systolic BP ≥0.66).
- Any incremental risk of *chronic restrictive lung disease* or restrictive physiology related to neuromuscular disease or chest wall deformities is unknown.

21.3.2
Surgery-Related Risk Factors

21.3.2.1
Surgical Site

- The surgical site is the single most important risk factor for the development of PPCs.
- *PPCs are more common as the incision approaches the diaphragm* due to splinting of the abdominal muscles and diaphragmatic dysfunction resulting in decreased postoperative lung volumes.
  - *Thoracic and upper abdominal surgeries* carry the highest risk (20–35%), and within these groups, aortic and esophageal surgery are associated with the highest rate of PPCs.
  - Head and neck surgery carried an intermediate risk of complications (15%).
  - Low-risk procedures include hip, gynecologic, and urologic surgeries. PPCs are rare for low-risk procedures (<5%), even for high-risk patients.

21.3.2.2
Type of Anesthesia

- Controversy exists as to whether a particular anesthetic technique influences morbidity or PPC rates. Although laryngoscopy and intubation may precipitate bronchospasm, general anesthesia subsequently has the advantage of airway control. General anesthesia may affect pulmonary function more than neuraxial (spinal or epidural) anesthesia.
  - The largest meta-analysis to date of randomized controlled trials of anesthetic technique reported lower rates of PPCs with neuraxial blockade than with general anesthesia.
- The ACP guidelines noted that *general anesthesia* confers a higher risk of PPCs than neuraxial blockade but commented that the evidence was conflicting. The choice of anesthesia involves many other factors and is really beyond the expertise of the medical consultant. Rather than recommending any particular anesthetic technique, the medical consultant should collaborate with the anesthesiologist to determine the optimal strategy for a given patient.

21.3.2.3
Neuromuscular Blockers

- *Long acting neuromuscular blockers* (pancuronium) lead to more residual neuromuscular blockade after surgery than intermediate-acting agents (atracurium, vecuronium). This could lead to postoperative hypoventilation and an increased risk of PPCs.
  - Patients who received *pancuronium* and had residual blockade were three times more likely to develop PPCs than those without residual block.

21.3.2.4
Surgical Technique

- There is no difference in PPC rates between *midline and transverse incisions* for patients undergoing abdominal surgery.
- *Laparoscopic surgery* may confer a lower risk for PPCs than open abdominal surgery but the evidence is conflicting. Newer studies with bariatric surgery suggest that laparoscopic technique in this setting may reduce PPCs.
  - Laparoscopic techniques are associated with less postoperative pain, quicker return to normal functioning, and a less conspicuous scar.
- Perioperative use of *pulmonary artery catheters* does not reduce the risk of mortality or postoperative pneumonia.
- *Prolonged surgical procedures* (duration>3–4 h) have higher PPC rates than briefer operations.
- *Emergency surgery* is a moderate risk factor for the development of PPCs.

21.4
Preoperative Evaluation and Testing to Stratify Risk[5]

21.4.1
Clinical Assessment

- A thorough *history and physical examination* with special attention to potential risk factors is always important. Remember that the most important consideration when stratifying PPC risk is to determine the planned procedure and surgical site.
  - The history for patients with obstructive airway disease should include the frequency and duration of attacks, precipitating factors, medications (and compliance), recent exacerbations, most recent emergency room visit, last hospitalization, need for intubation or ICU, and recent symptoms (dyspnea, cough, sputum, fever, wheezing). Ask the patient about their baseline peak flow and most recent values.
  - Physical examination should include assessment for fever, tachypnea, and abnormal chest exam findings (wheezes, rhonchi, rales).

21.4.2
Chest Radiography

- Routine preoperative *chest radiography* in healthy individuals rarely adds useful information to the preoperative evaluation nor does it predict PPCs or change perioperative management.
  - Although chest x-rays may find abnormalities, only a minority are unexpected, and they rarely change perioperative management.

- Only obtain chest radiographs to further evaluate unexplained dyspnea or better characterize underlying cardiac or pulmonary disease that is not at baseline.

21.4.3 Laboratory Testing

- Selected laboratory abnormalities are risk factors for the development of PPCs.
  - *Hypoalbuminemia* (serum albumin <3.0 g/dL-ACP; <3.5 respiratory risk index) and BUN > 30 mg/dL were associated with increased risk for PPCs.
  - *Renal function:*

    BUN <8 mg/dL or >22 mg/dL increased the risk for the development of postoperative pneumonia.
    Serum creatinine >1.5 mg/dL may also be a risk factor.
- Consider obtaining these tests in patients at high risk for PPCs either due to patient-related risk factors or a planned high-risk procedure (e.g., elderly patients undergoing major thoracic or abdominal procedures) although the results rarely change management.

21.4.4 Arterial Blood Gas Analysis

- Older studies concluded that *hypoxemia and hypercarbia* (P_aCO_2>45 mmHg) predicted PPCs; however, these patients probably would have been identified as high risk for developing PPCs simply from the clinical history and physical examination alone.
- Avoid ordering routine arterial blood gas analysis to assist in predicting PPCs following noncardiothoracic surgery except in patients with severe lung disease who require home oxygen supplementation or in those with chronic CO_2 retention.

21.4.5 Pulmonary Function Testing (Spirometry)

- *Spirometric testing* (FEV_1 and FEV_1/FVC) is helpful in predicting PPCs following lung resection and is part of the standard preoperative evaluation for this procedure (see Chap. 10).
- Controversy exists as to whether or not routine spirometry accurately predicts the development of PPCs following noncardiothoracic surgery. In general, spirometry adds little to the risk estimate established by clinical evaluation for these procedures. The majority of the literature fails to support routine spirometry as an independent predictor of PPCs following noncardiothoracic surgery, even among patients with severe COPD.
- While values <50% predicted may be associated with increased risk, no prohibitive cut-off levels exist for FEV_1 and FVC, so do not order routine spirometry for patients

awaiting noncardiothoracic surgery. Consider preoperative spirometry for the evaluation of dyspnea that remains unexplained after clinical evaluation or for patients with asthma or COPD who are wheezing if it is uncertain whether the patient is at his or her optimal baseline before surgery.

21.4.6
Risk Indices

- Two *risk indices,*[6,7] developed and validated across a large number of Veterans Affairs Medical Centers, identified patients at risk for postoperative pneumonia and respiratory failure (Tables 21.2 and 21.3.) The respiratory failure index was updated in 2007.[8]
- These risk indices confirmed previously established risk factors for the development of PPCs including surgical site, tobacco use, COPD, functional status, and age as well as identifying additional risk factors not previously well defined in the literature. These included other surgical sites (e.g., neck, neurosurgery, and vascular procedures), blood transfusion, additional comorbidities (e.g., cerebrovascular disease and low or elevated BUN), and other markers of general health status, including weight loss, steroid use, and alcohol intake.
- Due to the complex nature of these multifactorial risk indices, they are typically used more as a research tool than in day-to-day clinical practice. Unfortunately, most of the risk factors in these indices cannot be modified.

21.5
Perioperative Management to Reduce Risk (See Table 21.4)

21.5.1
Preoperative Interventions

- Delay elective surgery to treat any significant acute illness.
- Consider delaying elective surgery in a patient with an acute viral upper respiratory infection, especially one of recent onset or with worsening symptoms. However, this is only based on data from the pediatric literature, which suggests there may be an increased incidence of laryngospasm, bronchospasm, and oxygen desaturation, and the associated morbidity in adults may be minimal.
- *Optimize existing treatment for airflow limitation* for patients with COPD or asthma. In general, these patients should be treated as they would be if they were not going for surgery. Long-acting anticholinergics, beta-agonists, and inhaled corticosteroids can improve pulmonary function in symptomatic patients. The goal before elective surgery is that these patients are free of wheezes, cough, or dyspnea and have peak expiratory flows >80% predicted or near their personal best.

Table 21.2 Comparison of the risk factors included in the postoperative pneumonia and respiratory failure risk indices and the update resp failure index

Risk factors	Postop pneumonia risk index point value	Postop resp failure risk index point value	Updated respiratory failure risk factors	Updated resp fail risk index point value
Type of surgery			Type of surgery (vs. hernia)	
AAA repair	15	27	Integumentary	1
Thoracic	14	21	Respiratory	3
Upper abdominal	10	14	Heart	2
Neck	8	11	Aneurysm	2
Neurosurgery	8	14	Mouth	7
Vascular	3	14	Stomach	2
			Endocrine	2
Emergency surgery	3	11	Emergency surgery	2
General anesthesia	4	–	ASA class 3	3
			ASA class 4–5	5
Age			Age	
≥80 years	17	–	40–65	2
70–79 years	13	–	>65	2
60–69 years	9	–	Gender (male)	1
50–59 years	4	–	Work RVU 10–17	2
≤50 years	–	–	Work RVU >17	4
≥70 years	–	6		
60–69 years	–	4		
≤60 years	–	–		
Functional status			Wound class	
Totally dependent	10	7	Clean/	1
Partially dependent	6	7	contaminated	1
Independent	–	–	Contaminated	1
			Infected	
Albumin			Albumin <3.5	1
<3.0 g/dl	–	9	SGOT >40	1
≥3.0 g/dl	–	–	Bilirubin >1.0	1
Weight loss>10% (Within 6 months)	7	–	Weight loss >10%	1
Chronic steroid use	3	–	Sepsis	2
Alcohol >2 drinks/day (Within 2 weeks)	2	–	>2 drinks (past 2 week)	1
			Ascites	2
Diabetes – insulin treated	–	–	CHF	1

(continued)

Table 21.2 (continued)

Risk factors	Postop pneumonia risk index point value	Postop resp failure risk index point value	Updated respiratory failure risk factors	Updated resp fail risk index point value
History of COPD	5	6	History of severe COPD	2
Current smoker			Smoker	1
Within 1 year	3	–	Dyspnea	1
Within 2 weeks	–	–		
Impaired sensorium	4	–	Impaired sensorium	1
History of CVA	4	–	CVA	1
Blood urea nitrogen			Preop acute renal failure	2
<8 mg/dl	4	–	Preop creatinine	2
8–21 mg/dl	–	–	≥1.5	2
22–30 mg/dl	2	–	Preop sodium >145	1
>30 mg/dl	3	8	Preop WBC <2.5	1
			Preop WBC >10	
Preoperative transfusion (>4 units)	3	–	Preop Hct≤38	1
			Preop	1
			platelets≤150	1
			Bleeding disorder	

Adapted from Arozullah et al.[6,7] and Johnson et al.[8]
AAA Abdominal aortic aneurysm, *COPD* Chronic obstructive pulmonary disease, *CVA* Cerebrovascular accident, *CHF* Congestive heart failure

Table 21.3 Risk class assignment in the postoperative pneumonia and respiratory failure risk indices

Risk class	Postoperative pneumonia risk index (point total)	Predicted probability of pneumonia	Respiratory failure risk index (point total)	Predicted probability of respiratory failure
1	0–15	0.2%	0–10	0.5%
2	16–25	1.2%	11–19	2.2%
3	26–40	4.0%	20–27	5.0%
4	41–55	9.4%	28–40	11.6%
5	>55	15.3%	>40	30.5%
Risk Level			Updated respiratory failure index	
Low			<8	0.1–0.2%
Medium			8–12	1%
High			>12	6.5–6.64%

Adapted from Arozullah et al.[6,7,9] and Johnson et al.[8]

Table 21.4 Risk reduction strategies

Preoperative	Intraoperative	Postoperative
Discuss plan with surgeon and anesthesiologist regarding surgical site, technique, and type of anesthesia.	Minimize duration of surgery.	Initiate lung expansion maneuvers (deep breathing exercises, incentive spirometry). [A]
Treat acute illness and delay surgery if necessary.	Consider neuraxial (spinal or epidural) anesthesia instead of general anesthesia in high-risk patients. [I]	Continue CPAP in patients with OSA. [A]
Optimize existing airflow limitation (asthma/COPD) using beta-agonists, steroids, tiotropium.	Consider laparoscopic versus an open procedure if possible. [C]	Provide adequate pain control. Use epidural analgesia instead of parenteral analgesia when possible. Consider intercostal nerve blocks. [I]
Initiate smoking cessation, ideally at least 8 weeks prior to surgery, if possible. [I]	Avoid long-acting muscle relaxants (pancuronium). [B]	Use a nasogastric tube selectively (only if necessary and remove as soon as possible). [B]
Initiate patient education on lung expansion maneuvers.		

The grading system is from the *ACP* guidelines
COPD chronic obstructive pulmonary disease, *CPAP* continuous positive airway pressure, OSA obstructive sleep apnea

- Preoperative *systemic corticosteroids* may shorten hospital and intensive care units stays and do not appear to increase wound complications or pulmonary infection.
- Preoperative *corticosteroids and inhaled beta-agonists* decrease the incidence of bronchospasm after tracheal intubation. The combination of corticosteroids and salbutamol attenuates this bronchospasm to a greater degree than inhaled beta-2 agonists alone.
- *Tiotropium* (compared with a short-acting inhaled anticholinergic bronchodilator) in combination with a long-acting beta-2 agonist and a pulmonary rehabilitation program was associated with a lower incidence of pulmonary infection and acute respiratory failure.
- Chest physiotherapy, including inspiratory muscle training, can decrease rates of PPCs.
- Routine preoperative broad-spectrum antibiotics do not reduce PPCs in patients with COPD and should only be used for lower respiratory infections.

- Encourage *smoking cessation* for at least 8 weeks prior to elective surgery if possible to achieve maximum benefit in reducing PPCs.
  - The ideal duration of preoperative abstinence remains controversial. After quitting, the following changes occur:

    Carbon monoxide levels decrease within 12 h, improving oxygen delivery and utilization.

Cyanide levels decrease benefiting mitochondrial oxidative metabolism.
Ciliary function improves.
Sputum production increases during the first 1–2 months which is the reason postulated for why there was a paradoxical increase in PPCs in recent quitters. However, there were various criticisms of these studies and more recent studies demonstrate that although smokers who are recent quitters do not show a reduction in PPCs, there is no increase in complications.

– Physicians should encourage patients to quit smoking before surgery and provide resources and options including nicotine replacement therapy, varenicline, and individual or group counseling. The lifelong benefit clearly outweighs any short-term theoretical risk.

- Begin patient education on *lung expansion maneuvers*.

21.5.2 Intraoperative Interventions

- Anesthesiologists and surgeons direct intraoperative risk reduction strategies, but the medical consultant should be knowledgeable enough to participate in the decision-making process.
- If the risk of PPCs is deemed prohibitive, then consider cancellation of surgery or changing to a lower risk procedure (e.g., laparoscopic surgery) if possible.
- Other intraoperative interventions include *minimizing the duration of surgery*, the use of *neuraxial blockade* instead of general anesthesia, and *avoiding long-acting muscle relaxants* (e.g., pancuronium).

21.5.3 Postoperative Interventions

21.5.3.1 Lung Expansion Maneuvers

- Lung expansion maneuvers, which include deep breathing exercises, chest physiotherapy, incentive spirometry, intermittent positive pressure breathing, and continuous positive airway pressure (CPAP), can maximize alveolar inflation.
- In high-risk patients, particularly following upper abdominal surgery, lung expansion maneuvers can decrease PPCs by 50%. Although the ACP guidelines found good evidence to support these measures as a risk reduction strategy, a more recent qualitative review questioned their benefit. The difference relates to methodology, with the newer review including smaller studies, others with no explicit definition of PPCs, and studies using physiologic (changes in vital capacity or hypoxemia) rather than clinical complications. Since the higher quality evidence seems to suggest a benefit and deep breathing exercises and incentive spirometry carry no risk, this strategy is still recommended.

- No particular lung expansion maneuver has been found to be superior; however, IPPB may be associated with abdominal distension. One recommended deep breathing regimen is to take 8–10 breaths with a 3–5 s inspiratory hold every 1–2 h while awake followed by forced expirations and coughing. Use CPAP in patients who cannot perform deep breathing exercises or use an incentive spirometer, and continue it postoperatively in patients with OSA who use home CPAP.

21.5.3.2
Postoperative Pain Control

- Postoperative abdominal and chest pain may cause splinting and interfere with deep breathing and cough. This results in decreased lung volumes leading to microatelectasis and possibly more severe PPCs.
- Postoperative pain control with parenteral narcotic analgesia can provide effective pain management and improve deep breathing; however, if oversedated, the patient's respiratory drive may be blunted and increase risk of PPCs.
- Postoperative epidural analgesia provides superior pain relief compared with parenteral narcotic analgesia and can reduce PPCs. Several systematic reviews found that epidural opioids reduced the risk of atelectasis and pneumonia compared with systemic opioids. Epidural local anesthetics reduced rates of pulmonary infection and all PPCs, and thoracic epidural analgesia decreased respiratory failure after open aortic surgery. The evidence base for patient-controlled intravenous opioid analgesia is insufficient to draw any conclusions.
- Manage postoperative pain following high-risk procedures with postoperative epidural analgesia when feasible.

21.5.3.3
Postoperative Nasogastric Tube Placement

- Use of a nasogastric tube postoperatively can impair the cough reflex, increase risk of aspiration, and contribute to the development of PPCs.
- Routine use (inserted perioperatively and maintained until bowel function returns) versus selective use (not used, removed within 24 h, or only inserted for nausea, vomiting, ileus, or abdominal distension) of a nasogastric tube was associated with a higher incidence of pneumonia and atelectasis.
- Selective use of a nasogastric tube after abdominal surgery is preferred.

21.5.3.4
Nutritional Support

- Although hypoalbuminemia and malnutrition increase postoperative complications, there is no evidence that total parenteral nutrition (TPN) or total enteral nutrition (TEN) decreases pneumonia or PPCs although they may reduce other complications. Routine TPN has no advantage over TEN or no hyperalimentation except perhaps for patients with severe malnutrition or for long periods of inadequate oral nutrition.

References

1. Qaseem A, Snow V, Fitterman N, et al. Clinical Efficacy Assessment Subcommittee of the American College of Physicians. Risk assessment for and strategies to reduce perioperative pulmonary complications for patients undergoing noncardiothoracic surgery: a guideline from the American College of Physicians. *Ann Intern Med.* 2006;144(8):575-580.
2. Smetana GW, Lawrence VA, Cornell JE. American College of Physicians. Preoperative pulmonary risk stratification for noncardiothoracic surgery: systematic review for the American College of Physicians. *Ann Intern Med.* 2006;144(8):581-595.
3. Lawrence VA, Cornell JE, Smetana GW. American College of Physicians. Strategies to reduce postoperative pulmonary complications after noncardiothoracic surgery: systematic review for the American College of Physicians. *Ann Intern Med.* 2006;144(8):596-608.
4. Chung F, Yegneswaran B, Liao P, et al. STOP questionnaire: a tool to screen patients for obstructive sleep apnea. *Anesthesiology.* 2008;108(5):812-821.
5. Bapoje SR, Whitaker JF, Schulz T, et al. Preoperative evaluation of the patient with pulmonary disease. *Chest.* 2007;132(5):1637-1645.
6. Arozullah AM, Daley J, Henderson WG, Khuri SF. Multifactorial risk index for predicting postoperative respiratory failure in men after major noncardiac surgery. The National Veterans Administration Surgical Quality Improvement Program. *Ann Surg.* 2000;232:242.
7. Arozullah AM, Khuri SF, Henderson WG, et al. Development and validation of a multifactorial risk index for predicting postoperative pneumonia after major noncardiac surgery. *Ann Intern Med.* 2001;135:847.
8. Johnson RG, Arozullah AM, Neumayer L, et al. Multivariable predictors of postoperative respiratory failure after general and vascular surgery: results from the patient safety in surgery study. *J Am Coll Surg.* 2007;204(6):1188-1198.
9. Arozullah AM, Conde MV, Lawrence VA. Preoperative evaluation for postoperative pulmonary complications. *Med Clin North Am.* 2003;87:153-173.

Endocrine Disease 22

Amish Ajit Dangodara and Visala S. Muluk

22.1 Perioperative Diabetes

22.1.1 Introduction

- Surgery and anesthesia stimulate a "stress-response" resulting in production of counter-regulatory hormones, including glucagon, epinephrine, and cortisol, while decreasing endogenous insulin. This in turn increases gluconeogenesis, glycogenolysis, peripheral insulin resistance, and ketogenesis culminating in hyperglycemia.
- Hyperglycemia in hospitalized patients with or without diagnosed diabetes mellitus (DM) has been associated with poor outcomes including increased infections, length of stay, cognitive defects, and mortality.[1-5]
- On the other hand, perioperative fasting and exogenous insulin administration may result in hypoglycemia which has also been associated with adverse patient outcomes.
- Perioperative management, particularly of the patient with DM, involves anticipating and preventing significant hyperglycemia and hypoglycemia.

22.1.2 Patient-Specific Risk Factors

- Patients with DM have a higher prevalence of cardiovascular, renal, gastrointestinal, and neurologic disease placing them at increased risk for perioperative morbidity and mortality.

A.A. Dangodara (✉)
UCI Medical Center, UCI Hospitalist Program, University of California,
Irvine, College of Medicine, 101 The City Drive South, Building 26,
Room 1006, Orange, CA 92868, USA
e-mail: aadangod@uci.edu

S.L. Cohn (ed.), *Perioperative Medicine*,
DOI: 10.1007/978-0-85729-498-2_22,

  - Ischemic heart disease, DM, stroke, and chronic kidney disease are factors in the Revised Cardiac Risk Index (RCRI)[6] which is incorporated into the ACC algorithm for preoperative cardiac evaluation (see Chap. 20).
  - Diabetic nephropathy with renal insufficiency may be associated with fluid and electrolyte abnormalities, acute kidney injury (AKI), and increased insulin sensitivity.
  - Diabetic neuropathy may lead to perioperative hypotension, arrhythmias, decreased recognition of angina, gastroparesis, and decubitus ulcers.

- Diabetic patients are more likely to experience perioperative lability of their blood glucose placing them at risk for developing diabetic ketoacidosis, a nonketotic hyperosmolar state, wound infections, hypoglycemia, seizures, coma, and death.
- Hyperglycemia is a risk factor for impaired wound healing and wound infections. Hyperglycemia impairs neutrophil function and C3 complement function,[4,5] especially at glucose levels greater than 200 mg/dL.

22.1.3 Surgery-Specific Risk Factors

- Major surgery is associated with increased postoperative hyperglycemia. The more prolonged, invasive, and complicated the surgery, the greater the degree of hyperglycemia.
  - Major abdominal, thoracic (particularly CABG), vascular, and neurosurgery procedures are more likely to cause hyperglycemia than are minor, short duration, or superficial procedures.
  - Diabetic patients undergoing CABG are at higher risk of developing sternal wound infections and mediastinitis.[2-4]
- Hyperglycemia will cause osmotic shifts of fluid and electrolytes, which can lead to dehydration, acute renal insufficiency, metabolic acidosis, pseudohyponatremia, and transient hyperkalemia, followed by hypokalemia with glucose correction. In theory, this can impact hemodynamics, respiratory function and drug clearance or membrane transport, including that of anesthetics.

22.1.4 Glucose Target

- Numerous studies have linked hyperglycemia to adverse outcomes,[1-5] but there is significant controversy over how tightly to control glucose.[7-10] Although an earlier study of ICU patients showed a benefit of intensive control (glucose 80–110 mg/dL),[3] subsequent studies have failed to demonstrate similar benefits, while some have actually shown that tighter control is detrimental.[7-9]
- Patients who are more likely to benefit from lower glucose levels include those undergoing going CABG,[2-4] trauma surgery, or those who are septic.[7-9] There are no randomized control trials evaluating tight control of surgical patients in a noncritical care setting.

- The American Association of Clinical Endocrinologists (AACE) and American Diabetes Association (ADA) issued a consensus statement[10] on inpatient glycemic control in 2009. Their recommendations included the following:
  - For critically ill patients, initiate insulin therapy for persistent hyperglycemia starting at ≤180 mg/dL. Maintain glucose in a range of 140–180 mg/dL, preferably using an intravenous (IV) insulin protocol with frequent glucose monitoring.
  - For most noncritically ill patients, the fasting target should be <140 mg/dL with random glucoses <180 mg/dL. Scheduled subcutaneous administration of insulin with basal, nutritional, and correction components is the preferred method. Noninsulin antihyperglycemic agents are not appropriate in most hospitalized patients who require therapy for hyperglycemia.
- Numerous factors will affect achieving the target glucose.
  - Nutritional intake or NPO status: Bolus feeding will result in a postprandial elevation of blood sugar. Continuous feeding or TPN will result in a constant elevation of blood sugar. Unpredictable postprandial elevations of blood sugar occur when NPO status lasts more than 12-24 h or with variable feeding (TPN is being titrated up or off, or tube feeding rate is being advanced or held periodically).
  - Intravenous (IV) fluid type: IV fluid with D5 at 100 mL/h or D10 at 50 mL/h is necessary to prevent hypoglycemia and ketosis if the NPO status is more than 12 h or if the patient is being treated with a long-acting insulin. If not NPO, dextrose-containing fluids, including IV piggyback solutions, can contribute to hyperglycemia.
  - Medications such as corticosteroids can worsen insulin resistance and cause hyperglycemia. As the steroid dose is changed, insulin requirements will change.
  - Acute illness causes a stress response that releases cortisol, which can worsen insulin resistance and cause hyperglycemia. Conditions such as acute myocardial infarction and infection in particular worsen insulin resistance.
  - Consider renal clearance when selecting diabetic medications or the insulin dose since these drugs all have renal excretion.

22.1.5 Preoperative Evaluation and Management

- Patients with diabetes are more likely to have cardiac, renal, and neurologic disease. History and physical examination should focus on these systems.
  - Preoperative cardiac risk assessment should follow the ACC guidelines (see Chap. 20).
- Evaluate glycemic control by history, patient's home glucose monitoring, and preoperative blood tests, including glycosylated hemoglobin (HbA1C).
- Review the patient's medication regimen and adjust the treatment plan for surgery (see Table 22.1), including starting dextrose-containing IV fluids for prolonged fasting.

Table 22.1 Perioperative medication adjustment

Treatment type	Preoperative adjustment	Postoperative adjustment
Biguanides (Metformin)	Hold 24 h before	Hold 24–48 h after, resume when tolerating diet
Sulfonylureas		
First generation	Hold 24 h before	Resume when tolerating diet
Newer sulfonylureas	Hold on day of surgery	
Other oral hypoglcemics: Glinides, incretins, Alpha-Glucosidase inhibitors	Hold on day of surgery	Resume when tolerating diet
Amylin, Analog insulin	Hold on day of surgery	Resume when tolerating diet
Consolidated insulin		
NPH/regular (70/30 or 75/25)	Use full dose the night before Use half of the long-acting portion (NPH) on day of surgery	Resume full dose when tolerating diet
Corrective insulin	Continue while NPO	Continue while NPO or when eating
Basal-bolus insulin	Use full basal dose the night before surgery and on the day of surgery Hold bolus insulin on day of surgery	Continue full basal dose while NPO or when eating; Resume bolus insulin when tolerating diet
Basal-continuous insulin	Use full basal dose the night before surgery and on the day of surgery Hold continuous insulin only when continuous nutrition source is stopped, otherwise continue preoperatively	Continue full basal dose while NPO or on continuous nutrition source Hold continuous insulin only when continuous nutrition source is stopped, otherwise continue postoperatively
Continuous IV insulin drip	Continue before surgery with hourly adjustment	Continue after surgery with hourly adjustment

- Baseline preoperative tests should include fasting glucose, BUN/creatinine, potassium, and EKG. Consider obtaining a glycosylated hemoglobin (HbA1C) to evaluate recent glucose control as newer studies are looking at correlating this with postoperative outcome.

22.1.6 Treatment Strategies (See Table 22.1)

- Oral hypoglycemic medications and noninsulin injections should generally be held either on the day of surgery, or one day before, and restarted postoperatively once the patient is tolerating a stable diet and able to consume more than 50% of their meals.
- Consolidated insulin therapy
  - This consists of using combined long-acting insulin such as NPH insulin and short-acting insulin such as Regular insulin mixed together simultaneously and administered twice daily before breakfast and dinner, usually with 2/3 of the total daily dose given in the morning and 1/3 given in the evening.
- Corrective insulin
  - This involves using a short-acting insulin such as Regular or Analog insulin[11] administered in a sliding scale that starts at glucose values above the treatment goal. However, using this form of treatment by itself will only work if the fasting glucose is less than 200 mg/dL and if moderate or tight control is not desired.[12]

  Corrective scales should differ for insulin sensitive, such as type 1 diabetic, and for insulin resistant, such as type 2 diabetic, patients[12] (see Table 22.2).
  For patients with normal renal clearance, the corrective scale schedule should be every 4 h while the patient is NPO or before every meal and bedtime (qAC and qHS)

Table 22.2 Corrective insulin therapy for usual treatment/type II DM

Glucose level	Correction insulin dose (units)
Glucose at treatment goal	0
Glucose >goal – 180	4
181–220	6
221–260	8
261–300	10
301–350	12
351–400	14
>400	16

Adapted from Umpierrez et al.[12]
For insulin sensitive/type I patients: Give 2 units less than the usual correction dose
For insulin resistant patients: Give 2 units more than the usual correction dose

Table 22.3 Insulin pharmacokinetics

Insulin	Onset	Peak	Duration
Apidra Humalog Novolog	10–15 min	60–90 min	4–5 h
Regular	30–60 min	2–4 h	5–8 h
NPH	1–3 h	5–8 h	12–18 h
Levemir	90 min	Relatively peakless	12–24 h
Lantus	90 min	Peakless	24 h

Adapted from Hirsch, IB[11]

if the patient is eating. With impaired renal function, the schedule should be every 6 h while NPO.

This strategy can be used in *addition* to all other treatment strategies and should rarely be used as the sole treatment method.

- Basal-bolus insulin
  - This targets the fasting basal requirement with a long-acting insulin that is given every 12–24 h, depending on the type of insulin (see Table 22.3) and the bolus meal requirement with a short-acting insulin that is given every meal.[12] Basal insulin does not need adjustment for a fasting state, but IV fluid containing dextrose should be started if the patient is expected to fast for more than 12–24 h. Bolus insulin should be held while the patient is not getting bolus feeding.

  The fasting basal insulin requirement is estimated as 50% of the total daily insulin requirement, but should be reduced by 30–50% of the initial estimation in patients with renal impairment with a GFR of less than 50.
  Assuming normal renal function, estimated total daily insulin requirements are:

  - Type 1 diabetic – 0.3 units/kg/day.[13]
  - Type 2 diabetic – 0.4 units/kg/day[12] for a fasting blood sugar<200 mg/dL or 0.5 units/kg/day if the fasting blood sugar is ≥200 mg/dL.
  - NPH insulin can be used for basal therapy by dividing 50% of the total daily insulin requirement by 3 and giving it every 8 h. In renal impairment, the daily basal dose should be divided by 2 and given every 12 h.
  - Glargine (Lantus®) and detemir (Levemir®) insulin offer advantages over NPH because of their much more physiological effect. These can be dosed either daily or BID at 50% of the total daily insulin requirement.

  The bolus requirement is estimated to be 50% of the total daily insulin requirement divided by the number of meals per day.[12] Any type of short-acting insulin such as Regular, Humalog, Glulisine, or Aspart insulin can be used, but the Analog insulins are more physiological. The total daily dose should be reduced by 30–50% in patients with renal impairment.

- Basal-continuous insulin strategy

  - This is used when there is a continuous nutritional source such as TPN or continuous tube feeding and consists of using a long-acting insulin to meet the fasting basal insulin requirement and a separate long-acting insulin dose to meet the additional continuous insulin requirement.

    The basal dose can be calculated as in the basal-bolus recommendations above and should be continued even while NPO or if the continuous nutrition source is stopped. The continuous insulin dose is approximately 10–30% of the total daily insulin requirement[14] and should be administered as a separate long-acting insulin dose that can be held if the continuous source of nutrition is stopped.

    - Use NPH for overnight tube feeding or cyclic overnight TPN and time the dose 1 h before the start of the nutrition source.
    - Use Glargine or Detemir insulin for continuous tube feeding or TPN.

- Continuous IV insulin drip is typically a short-acting insulin such as Regular insulin and is ideal for variable nutritional intake or glycemic stress and can also be added directly to the TPN, although that makes it difficult to adjust. This is usually titrated based on predetermined protocols by monitoring the blood sugar hourly. Converting from IV to subcutaneous insulin is anywhere from 60% to 80% of the total daily insulin requirement.[14]

22.1.7 Selecting Treatment Strategies[12-15] (See Table 22.4)

- For patients who have bolus feeding and are undergoing procedures where the patient is expected to resume bolus feeding soon after surgery, the ideal treatment strategy depends on whether or not the diabetes was controlled prior to surgery.

  - If the fasting blood sugar is <200 mg/dL, then the patient should be treated with their home diabetic medications and a corrective insulin sliding scale with perioperative adjustments as indicated in Table 22.1.
  - If the fasting blood sugar is ≥200 mg/dL, then the ideal strategy is to use basal-bolus insulin and a corrective insulin sliding scale, either in addition to the patient's home oral diabetic medications or in place of the patient's home therapy. Perioperative adjustments should be made as indicated in Table 22.1. When nearing discharge, this strategy may be continued at home or it can be converted to a consolidated insulin strategy.

- For patients who have variable nutritional intake or glycemic stress, the ideal strategy is basal-bolus insulin or continuous IV insulin drip with perioperative adjustments as indicated in Table 22.1. This strategy is ideal for patients who are not expected to resume nutritional intake for more than 24 h after surgery or for those who may need multiple procedures during the course of hospitalization. Intravenous fluid with dextrose should be started while NPO.

Table 22.4 Selecting the appropriate treatment strategy

Nutrition type & glycemic stress	Ideal treatment strategy	Adjustment for GFR <50
	Adjust perioperatively as in Table 22.1	Adjust perioperatively as in Table 22.1
Stable bolus intake expected to resume post-op within 24 h, with stable glycemic stress	• Continue home therapy if controlled previously • Use basal-bolus if not controlled on home therapy • Add a corrective scale every 4 h if NPO or qAC/qHS if eating	• Hold oral medications until GFR normalizes and convert to basal-bolus with 30–50% reduced dosing • Add an insulin-sensitive corrective scale q 6 h if NPO or qAC/qHS if eating
Variable nutritional intake (frequent NPO, prolonged fasting, titrating tube feeding or TPN) or Variable glycemic stress (titrating steroid dose, worsening or improving infection or renal function)	• Hold home therapy and convert to basal-bolus with a corrective scale every 4 h if NPO or qAC/qHS if eating • IV insulin drip is an alternative	• Hold oral medications until GFR normalizes and convert to basal-bolus with 30–50% reduced dosing • Add an insulin-sensitive scale q 6 h if NPO or qAC/qHS if eating • IV insulin drip is an alternative
Continuous intake or Continuous glycemic stress	• Hold home therapy and convert to Basal-Continuous with a corrective scale every 4 h • IV insulin drip is an alternative	• Hold home therapy and convert to Basal-Continuous with 30–50% reduced dosing • Add an insulin-sensitive corrective scale q 6 h • IV insulin drip is an alternative

Adapted from Umpierrez,[12] Braithwaite,[13] Schmeltz,[14] and Inzucchi[15]

- For patients who have continuous nutritional intake or glycemic stress, the ideal strategy is basal-continuous insulin or continuous IV insulin drip with perioperative adjustments as indicated in Table 22.1.

In summary, marked hyperglycemia and hypoglycemia should be avoided. Using one of the strategies described with frequent glucose monitoring will help achieve the recommended target level.

22.2 Adrenal Insufficiency

22.2.1 Introduction

- Adrenal insufficiency is the inability of the adrenal gland, either due to primary or secondary causes, to respond appropriately to stress including surgical stress.
- The hypothalamic-pituitary-adrenal (HPA) axis plays a pivotal role in maintaining hemodynamic stability during stressful situations.
- The adrenal cortex secretes cortisol (a glucocorticoid), aldosterone (a mineralocorticoid), and androgens (primarily dehydroepiandrosterone and androstenedione). The adrenal medulla secretes the catecholamines epinephrine and norepinephrine.
- ACTH stimulates secretion of all adrenal cortical hormones but predominantly cortisol.
- Aldosterone, regulated by renin angiotensin system, causes sodium and water retention and increases extracellular fluid volume to maintain perfusion.
- A patient with an intact HPA axis under surgical stress increases cortisol production. The hypothalamus is stimulated to release ACTH secretogogues, corticotropin releasing hormone (CRH), and arginine vasopressin (AVP) which in turn increase ACTH release from the anterior pituitary which in turn stimulates the adrenal glands to increase cortisol production.
- With adrenal insufficiency, there is suppression at the level of the hypothalamus, pituitary, or adrenals resulting in an inability to appropriately increase cortisol production (see Fig. 22.1).
- Cortisol is essential to maintain cardiovascular tone and thereby prevent hypotension in the perioperative period, and it plays a role in mobilizing the energy sources by gluconeogenesis, lipolysis, and proteolysis.

22.2.2 Etiology of Adrenal Insufficiency

- Primary
  - Destruction of the adrenal cortex: autoimmune; granulomatous diseases (histoplasmosis, tuberculosis, sarcoidosis); infiltrative diseases (AIDS, amyloidosis, hemochromatosis, lymphoma, metastatic carcinoma)[16]

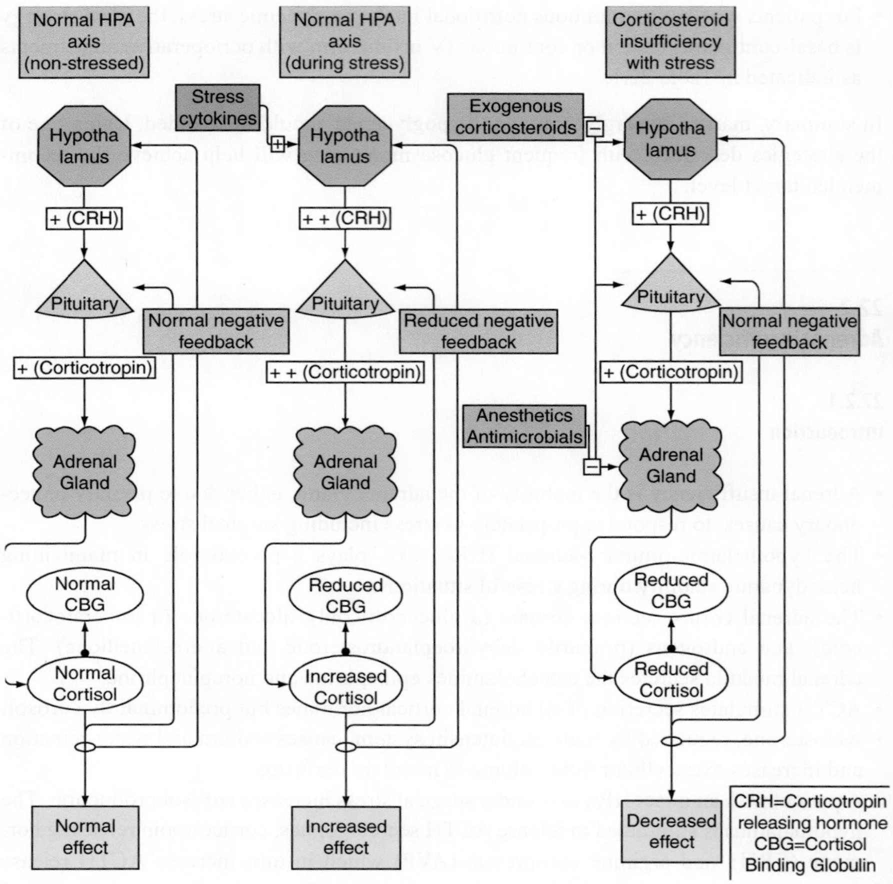

Fig. 22.1 Hypothalamic-pituitary-adrenal axis under various conditions

- Secondary
  - Exogenous steroids in supraphysiologic doses can suppress HPA axis
  - Adrenocortical atrophy secondary to ACTH deficiency

    Pituitary: tumors, necrosis or infarction, inflammatory disease (meningitis), hemochromatosis, stalk destruction (surgery, trauma, or mass), empty sella syndrome
    Hypothalamic: sarcoidosis, eosinophilic granuloma

- Differentiating features:
  - In primary adrenal insufficiency, ACTH is increased whereas it is decreased in secondary adrenal insufficiency.

- Cortisol and urinary metabolites are decreased in both forms.
- Sodium is decreased and potassium is increased in both but more in primary adrenal insufficiency. Both increase glucose.

22.2.3 Patient-Specific Risks

- Exogenous steroids in physiologic or supraphysiologic doses can suppress the HPA axis, and during surgery this can result in hemodynamic instability, hypotension, and death.[17]
  - Supplemental steroids in the perioperative period can increase postoperative morbidity by multiple mechanisms: poor wound healing, poor glycemic control, mental status changes, fever suppression, and masking of infection.

22.2.4 Surgery-Specific Risks

- The ACTH and cortisol secretion increase rapidly at the time of incision and during surgery, and remain elevated during reversal of anesthesia, extubation, and immediate recovery period (primarily in response to pain) for 48–72 h after surgery.[18]
  - Daily cortisol production will increase up to 150 mg of hydrocortisone equivalent after major surgery and 50 mg of hydrocortisone equivalent after minor surgery.
- In a patient in whom HPA axis is suppressed, if supplemental steroids are not provided, there is a potential danger for cardiovascular collapse and death. Risk is greater with major surgery.
  - The most common cause of HPA axis suppression is exogenous steroids, depending on the dose and duration of steroid use.
- The relationship between HPA axis suppression and dosage and duration of steroid use is typically described as follows:
  - **Not suppressed**: <5 mg/day of prednisone or its equivalent for any duration or steroids at any dose for<3 weeks
  - **Most likely suppressed**: >20 mg/day of prednisone or its equivalent for≥3 weeks or Cushingoid appearance
  - **Suppression uncertain**: 5–20 mg/day of prednisone or its equivalent for >3 weeks or≥5 mg/day for 3 weeks or more anytime during one year prior to surgery
- The dose of supplemental steroids as recommended by Salem and colleagues[19] should be based on the degree of stress anticipated with the surgical procedure (see Table 22.5). However, the current evidence does not fully support or oppose the use of supplemental steroids in a surgical patient who is suspected to have adrenal insufficiency.[20-25]

Table 22.5 Degree of surgical stress and recommended steroid dose

Surgical stress	Anticipated cortisol secretion	HPA axis not suppressed	HPA axis most likely suppressed	HPA axis suppression uncertain
Minor (inguinal herniorrhaphy, endoscopies)	25 mg of HC equivalent per day for 1 day	Usual daily dose with no supplementation	Usual daily dose with no supplementation	Usual daily dose with no supplementation
Moderate (open cholecystectomy, peripheral vascular surgery, hip and knee replacements)	50–75 mg of HC equivalent per day for 1–2 days	Usual daily dose with no supplementation	HC 50 mg IV preoperatively, then 25 mg IV every 8 h for 48 h and resume usual daily dose	[a]Consider corticotropin stimulation test. If positive: HC 50 mg IV preoperatively, then 25 mg IV every 8 h for 48 h and resume usual daily dose
Major (coronary bypass surgery, intra-abdominal procedures done over prolonged duration like Whipple's procedure)	100–150 mg of HC equivalent per day for 2–3 days	Usual daily dose with no supplementation	HC 100 mg IV preoperatively, then 50 mg IV every 8 h for 48–72 h and resume usual daily dose	[a]Consider corticotropin stimulation test. If positive: HC 100 mg IV preoperatively, then 50 mg IV every 8 h for 48–72 h and resume usual daily dose

[a]Steroid supplementation for the brief period may be more cost-effective and time efficient than obtaining a corticotropin stimulation test. Although the test is highly sensitive, it may not be an accurate predictor of adrenal crisis. Hence, testing should be recommended cautiously

- Patients who have responded normally to ACTH stimulation test may have subnormal response to surgical stress and still go through perioperative period without complications, suggesting that cortisol secretion beyond basal amounts is not necessary to tolerate surgical stress.
- More recent studies concluded that patients with secondary adrenal insufficiency undergoing surgery do not experience hypotension in the absence of supplemental steroids as long as they receive their usual dose of steroids in the perioperative period.

22.2.5
Preoperative Evaluation

- A thorough history and physical is useful in identifying patients at risk for adrenal insufficiency.
  - Note chronic medical conditions that require long-term corticosteroids such as COPD, asthma, organ transplants, and inflammatory and autoimmune diseases.
  - Review the medication history, specifically current or recent use of systemic steroids.
  - Ask about fatigue, depression, orthostasis, dizziness, nausea, vomiting, and diarrhea.
  - Hyperpigmentation is associated with primary adrenal insufficiency. Scant axillary and pubic hair, small testicles, amenorrhea, and decreased libido are associated with secondary insufficiency.
  - Serum electrolytes may be suggestive (hyponatremia, hyperkalemia).
- Consider testing in patients with high clinical suspicion or uncertain situations if going for intermediate or high risk surgery. Tests include serum cortisol level, ACTH stimulation – standard or low dose, insulin-induced hypoglycemia, metyrapone, and CRH stimulation tests.[16]
- Steroids should be held for at least 48 h prior to testing. Otherwise, they should be switched to an equivalent dose of dexamethasone and the test performed after 48 h.
- Serum cortisol level:
  - Adrenal insufficiency can be ruled out if random serum cortisol level is >20 mcg/dl.
  - Serum cortisol peaks in the morning and hence 8 A.M. serum cortisol <3 mcg/dl is suggestive of adrenal insufficiency.
  - In stressful situations, a serum cortisol of <20 mcg/dl is highly suggestive of adrenal insufficiency.
- ACTH stimulation test:[26,27]
  - Standard dose test:

    250 mcg of cosyntropin is given intramuscularly or intravenously.
    Serum cortisol is measured at baseline, 30 min and 60 min.
    Normal response is considered to be a peak cortisol of 18–20 mcg/dl.

- Low dose test:

  1 mcg of cosyntropin is given intravenously.
  1 mcg/1.73 m2 body surface area is considered more of a physiologic dose. As patients with larger body surface area as the response may have a subnormal response with a smaller dose.
  Serum cortisol measured at baseline and 30 min.
  Normal response is considered to be a peak cortisol value of 17–22.5 mcg/dl.

- A subnormal response to either test confirms adrenal insufficiency. A normal response to the standard dose test rules out primary adrenal insufficiency; however, some cases of secondary adrenal insufficiency, such as chronic partial pituitary ACTH deficiency or recent pituitary resection, where the adrenals are not completely atrophied, might response to high-dose ACTH.
- A meta-analysis of 28 studies reported for the standard dose test, at 95% specificity, a sensitivity for primary adrenal insufficiency of 97.5% and 57% for secondary adrenal insufficiency.
- Low dose ACTH test may be more reliable in diagnosing secondary and tertiary adrenal insufficiency. Basal ACTH level might also help in distinguishing primary versus secondary adrenal insufficiency, but due to longer turnaround time for the results may not be useful in deciding treatment options.

• Insulin-induced hypoglycemia test[27]

  - Rarely used due to the difficulty involved as well as cost.
  - Can assess the whole HPA axis, as hypoglycemia is a potent stimulant of CRH as well as ACTH secretion.
  - Hypoglycemia to a level of 40 mg/dl is produced by administering insulin and cortisol levels are measured at baseline, 30 min and 60 min.
  - A response of serum cortisol at 18–22 mcg/dl is considered normal.
  - Appropriate test in secondary adrenal insufficiency with ACTH deficiency, as in recent pituitary surgery.
  - Should be avoided in patients with seizure disorder, cerebrovascular disease, and cardiovascular disease.

• Metyrapone test

  - Effectively decreases cortisol level and thereby provokes ACTH secretion.
  - In secondary adrenal insufficiency, ACTH rise is not seen after overnight metyrapone administration.
  - Can cause adrenal crisis and hence cannot be done as an outpatient.

• CRH stimulation test

  - Can be used to differentiate secondary and tertiary adrenal insufficiency.
  - When CRH is administered, both ACTH and cortisol levels rise in tertiary insufficiency, and both remain suppressed in secondary insufficiency.
  - Safe to perform as an outpatient.

- When HPA axis suppression is established supplemental steroids should be considered.
  - Dosage of steroids is based on the degree of stress associated with the surgery (Table 22.5).

22.2.6 Perioperative Management and Risk Reduction Strategies

22.2.6.1 Preoperative

- Identify patients at risk for HPA axis suppression.
- Choose the right patients for supplemental steroids either by historical or laboratory data.
- Tailor steroid dosage to the stress associated with the planned surgery (see Table 22.5).[19,21,24]
- Check electrolytes, specifically sodium and potassium, and correct abnormalities. Continue mineralocorticoid supplementation until the day of surgery, and when patient cannot take oral medications, supplement with isotonic saline.

22.2.6.2 Intraoperative

- Certain anesthetic agents like etomidate, due to its suppressive effect on cortisol production, may cause deleterious effects during surgery. This effect is particularly pronounced in patients who have suppressed HPA axis undergoing moderate to high stress surgeries.
- Opiates tend to blunt the HPA axis response to surgical stress and thereby decrease cortisol secretion. This may pose a problem in a patient in whom HPA axis suppression is not suspected.
- Promptly correct hypotension with isotonic fluid supplementation. In majority of the cases, hypotension responds to intravenous fluids without requiring glucocorticoids.

22.2.6.3 Postoperative

- The first 48–72 h after surgery is the most stressful period during which the cortisol secretion is at its maximum when the HPA axis is intact. This is primarily in response to pain.
- In primary adrenal insufficiency, hypotension is most likely due to hypovolemia associated with mineralocorticoid deficiency and therefore should be corrected with fluid replacement until patient can resume oral mineralocorticoid supplementation. When hydrocortisone is administered at higher doses, it has mineralocorticoid effect.

- In secondary adrenal insufficiency when patient is receiving supplemental steroids, hypotension is less likely to be due to cortisol deficiency. Such a patient should be evaluated for cardiac causes, sepsis, or bleeding (gastrointestinal or surgical site).
- Because steroids can blunt the fever response, maintain a high degree of surveillance so as not to miss an infection.
- Treat hyperglycemia associated with glucocorticoids (see section on DM targets and management).

22.2.7 Summary

- Patients with absolute or relative adrenal insufficiency are potentially at increased risk for perioperative complications. Classic teaching has recommended stress-dose steroids in patients felt to be at risk although more recent opinion is challenging that concept. We need larger RCTs to determine which patients, for what type of surgery, and for what length of time are supplemental steroids indicated.

22.3 Hyperthyroidism

22.3.1 Introduction

- Hyperthyroidism is more common in women than in men (5:1) with increased prevalence in older age groups.[28,29]
- Thyrotoxicosis in the younger age group is almost always due to Grave's and in the older age group could be due to toxic multinodular goiter as well.
- Thyrotoxicosis, which constitutes the clinical and physiological effects of excess thyroid hormone, can be due to:
  - Increased de novo synthesis of the hormone by the gland
  - Release of preformed hormone into circulation due to inflammation and destruction of the gland
  - Ingestion of excess thyroid hormone
- Causes of hyperthyroidism (Table 22.6).
- Grave's disease affects 0.5% of the population and is the most common cause of hyperthyroidism.
- Thyroid storm is an acute event that can be precipitated in patients undergoing thyroid or nonthyroid surgery, and is characterized by hyperpyrexia, palpitations, agitation, delirium, and coma.
- Surgically induced thyroid storm can be prevented by adequate preparation of the hyperthyroid patient preoperatively.

Table 22.6 Causes of hyperthyroidism

Increased synthesis of hormone (increased radioiodine uptake)	Increased release of preformed hormone (decreased radioiodine uptake)
Grave's disease	Thyroiditis
Hashitoxicosis	De quervain's thyroiditis (sub acute)
Toxic adenoma	Painless or lymphocytic thyroiditis
Toxic multinodular goiter	Amiodarone induced
Iodine induced	Radiation thyroiditis
Trophoblastic disease and germ cell tumors	Interferon alpha
TSH mediated	Struma ovarii (ectopic production of hormone)
Epoprostenol (PG I2)	Levothyroxine overdose

22.3.2 Patient-Specific Risk Factors (Table 22.7)

- Signs and symptoms of thyroid hormone excess are mainly due to sympathetic overactivity and increased metabolism.
- Untreated hyperthyroidism will increase perioperative morbidity.
- Most common presenting symptoms and signs include:
  - Symptoms: generalized weakness, increased appetite, weight loss, fatigue, irritability, insomnia, heat intolerance, oligomenorrhea, decreased libido, and palpitations.
  - Signs: tachycardia, lid lag, proptosis, enlarged thyroid (painful if thyroiditis), gynecomastia, hyperreflexia, tremor and muscle weakness.
- Some patients, especially elderly, may be asymptomatic or have vague symptoms like weight loss and asthenia. This presentation is described as apathetic or masked hyperthyroidism.
- Even if the symptoms are vague, associated conditions like atrial fibrillation and osteoporosis and lab abnormalities like elevated calcium, alkaline phosphatase, and urinary calcium may suggest underlying hyperthyroidism, and it is important to identify these patients during preoperative evaluation.
- Subclinical hyperthyroidism, defined as normal levels of T4 and T3 and suppressed TSH, is associated with threefold increase in incidence of atrial fibrillation especially in elderly.

22.3.3 Surgery-Specific Risks

- Precipitation of thyroid storm is always of concern in hyperthyroid patients who are undergoing surgery.
- Although more common during emergency surgery, thyroid storm can be precipitated during minor procedures as well.

Table 22.7 Clinical manifestations of hyperthyroidism

Skin	• Increased sweating • Hyperpigmentation • Thinning of hair • Onycholysis and thinning of nails • Infiltrative dermatopathy/pretibial myxedema (Grave's)
Eyes	• Stare and lid lag • Exophthalmos (Grave's) • Corneal ulcerations
Cardiovascular	• Elevated heart rate • Systolic hypertension • Wide pulse pressure • High or normal output CHF • Atrial fibrillation • Mitral valve prolapse/regurgitation
Endocrine	• Low total cholesterol/HDL • Hyperglycemia
Pulmonary	• Dyspnea due to respiratory muscle weakness and decreased lung volumes • Hypoxemia and hypercapnia
Gastrointestinal	• Hyperphagia and weight loss • Anorexia (in elderly) • Diarrhea and vomiting due to hypermotility • Liver dysfunction with cholestatic picture
Bone	• Increased serum and urine calcium • Increased serum alkaline phosphatase • Osteoporosis
Genitourinary	• Increased urinary frequency • Decreased libido • Erectile dysfunction
Hematologic	• Normochromic normocytic anemia • Elevated ferritin level

- Other conditions that can precipitate thyroid storm besides surgery are trauma, stroke, infection, and diabetic ketoacidosis.
- Prominent clinical features of thyroid storm include:
  - Hyperpyrexia with temperatures to 104–106 F.
  - Tachycardia >140 beats/min and congestive heart failure.
  - Delirium, agitation, stupor, and coma.
  - Severe vomiting, diarrhea, and liver dysfunction associated with jaundice.
- Most perioperative complications in hyperthyroid patients are due to sympathetic and metabolic effects associated with excess hormone.[30]

22.3.4 Preoperative Evaluation

- A thorough history and physical is required to identify patients with undiagnosed hyperthyroidism.
- In addition to the obvious presenting signs and symptoms of hyperthyroidism, one should look for less obvious signs like atrial fibrillation and osteoporosis which may be due to subclinical or apathetic hyperthyroidism.
- Laboratory studies
  - Hyperthyroidism: suppressed or undetectable TSH and elevated free T4 and/or T3.
  - Subclinical hyperthyroidism: normal free T4 and T3 and suppressed TSH. This thyroid function pattern is also seen in central hyperthyroidism, nonthyroidal illness, and recovery from hyperthyroidism.
  - Overt ophthalmopathy seen in Grave's disease does not need any further lab investigation.
  - Women of child bearing age should always be screened for pregnancy as treatment varies in pregnant women.
- When diagnosis is uncertain, radioactive iodine uptake study should be performed, as uptake will be high in hyperthyroidism and low in thyroiditis.
- Patients with hyperthyroidism should be treated prior to elective surgery to achieve euthyroid state to prevent thyroid storm.
- Treatment of hyperthyroidism[31-34]
  - Beta-blockers

    Used to quickly ameliorate the symptoms like palpitations, tachycardia, tremors, and heat intolerance which are due to increased beta adrenergic activity of the excess thyroid hormone.
    Atenolol is the preferred agent due to once a day dosing as well as beta-1 selectivity; however all beta blockers are equally effective.
    Longer acting beta-blockers can give sustained effect through the intra and postoperative period.
  - Antithyroid medications (methimazole and propylthiouracil (PTU)) are thioamides.

    They block the production of thyroid hormone by inhibiting thyroid peroxidase.
    PTU also blocks the peripheral conversion of T4 to T3.
  - Iodide

    Blocks the release of thyroid hormone by inhibiting the proteolysis of colloid
    In supraphysiologic doses can act to block the synthesis of new thyroid hormone as well
    Usually given along with antithyroid drugs to prevent accumulation of thyroid hormone
  - Radioiodine therapy:

    Results in ablation of the gland within 6–12 weeks resulting in hypothyroidism.
    Primary choice of treatment in mild, well-tolerated hyperthyroidism.

In severe hyperthyroidism especially in elderly population, thionamides are given as pretreatment prior to radioactive iodine ablation.

– Surgery

Usually less preferred
Indicated in cases of large obstructive goiter, pregnant women who are allergic to thionamides, and patients who refuse radioiodine ablation

22.3.5 Perioperative Management and Risk Reduction Strategies

22.3.5.1 Preoperative Period

- Patient with hyperthyroidism should continue taking antithyroid medications throughout the perioperative period whenever possible.
  - If a patient is in NPO status, PTU can be crushed and administered via nasogastric tube.
  - PTU is also the preferred agent over methimazole in pregnant women.
- If a patient has uncontrolled hyperthyroidism or newly diagnosed hyperthyroidism, elective surgery should be postponed until euthyroid state is achieved.
- If an emergency surgery has to be performed in a patient with uncontrolled hyperthyroidism, the following measures need to be undertaken:
  - Iodine

    Preferred agent in preparing a patient for surgery, due to its fairly rapid onset of action, but should be given only after (1 h later) giving thioamides first – iodine supplementation may result in more thyroid hormone synthesis and release, resulting in thyroid storm (the jod-basedow effect or iodine-induced hyperthyroidism)
  - Glucocorticoids

    Patients with thyrotoxicosis are also at risk for adrenal insufficiency and should receive stress doses of steroids.[35]
    They also decrease peripheral conversion of thyroxine to T3.
  - Beta-blockers

    Long-acting beta-blockers like atenolol are preferred agents to initiate preoperatively.

22.3.5.2 Intraoperative Period

- Intraoperatively short-acting beta-blockers like esmolol are preferred agents to reduce beta adrenergic activity.
- Glucocorticoids should be administered every 6 h.

- Fluids, glucose, and vitamin supplementation should be continued.
- Heart failure and arrhythmias should be managed appropriately.

22.3.5.3 Postoperative Period

- Continue antithyroid medications to block thyroid hormone synthesis.
- Continue long-acting beta-blockers.
- Management of thyroid storm:
  - Monitor the patient in an ICU setting.
  - Use acetaminophen and cooling blankets to control the fever.

    Avoid aspirin as it may increase free thyroid hormone level by interfering with protein binding of T3 and T4.
  - Administer beta-blockers, iodine, antithyroid drugs, and glucocorticoids.
  - Provide glucose and vitamin supplementation.
  - Manage cardiac complications, atrial fibrillation, and high output cardiac failure.
  - Facilitate thyroid hormone clearance.

    Cholestyramine
    Charcoal hemoperfusion
    Rarely hemodialysis and plasmapheresis

22.4 Hypothyroidism

22.4.1 Introduction

- Hypothyroidism is more prevalent in women and older patients. Despite the high prevalence there is no indication for preoperative screening for thyroid disease.[28]
- Critically ill and hospitalized patients, including postsurgical patients, can have abnormal thyroid function tests in the absence of underlying thyroid disease.
- Subclinical hypothyroidism is a clinical entity with elevated TSH without overt symptoms of hypothyroidism.[36]
- Hypothyroid patients when exposed to certain precipitants like infection, hypothermia, and drugs like sedatives can rarely develop myxedema coma, which is associated with high perioperative morbidity and mortality.
- Hypothyroidism can be primary (thyroid) or central (pituitary or hypothalamic).
  - Primary: accounts for 95% of the cases

    Etiologies include thyroprivic (loss of thyroid tissue from surgical removal of the gland or radioactive ablation), goitrous (low hormone production leading to increased TSH secretion as in Hashimoto's autoimmune thyroiditis), transient causes (other thyroiditis), congenital causes, or others (nutritional, medications).

- Central: The thyroid gland is normal but TSH or TRH secretion is low.

  Pituitary causes (secondary, low TSH) include Sheehan's syndrome or postpartum pituitary necrosis, pituitary tumor, carotid tumor.

  Hypothalamic causes (tertiary, low TRH) include idiopathic, traumatic, and infiltrative.

22.4.2 Patient-Specific Risks (Table 22.8)

- Thyroid hormone deficiency can affect multiple systems that can lead to poor outcomes in the perioperative period.
- Hashimoto's thyroiditis may be associated with other autoimmune disorders like SLE, RA, pernicious anemia, and DM.
- Hypothyroidism has an insidious onset and sometimes can remain undetected for a long time.
- General signs and symptoms that makes one consider thyroid hormone deficiency are due to:
  - Decreased metabolism: fatigue, cold intolerance, constipation, weight gain, slow movement, bradycardia, delayed relaxation phase of deep tendon reflexes.
  - Accumulation of matrix substances: coarse/dry skin and hair, hair loss, brittle nails, hoarseness, macroglossia, and periorbital and pretibial edema.

22.4.3 Surgery-Specific Risks[37,38]

- Hypothyroid patients may have a prolonged recovery and rehabilitation period.
- Decreased heart rate and stroke volume result in decreased cardiac output and increased systemic vascular resistance resulting in decreased total blood volume. This leads to prolonged circulation time and narrow pulse pressure due to elevated diastolic pressure.
- Hypothyroid patients are more prone to intraoperative hypotension during noncardiac surgery and CHF during cardiac surgery.
- Delayed gastric emptying increases risk for aspiration.
- Due to impaired hepatic and renal clearance, sensitivity to anesthetic agents is increased.
- Blunted fever response may delay the diagnosis of infection.
- System-related symptoms and signs and surgery-specific risks are listed in Table 22.8.

22.4.4 Preoperative Evaluation

- Clinically assess the severity of thyroid disease based on history and physical examination.
- Review the patient's medications. It may be advisable to check thyroid hormone status in patients taking the following medications which may cause hypothyroidism:
  - Lithium, amiodarone, and interferon
  - Iron, carbamazepine, and cholestyramine (can decrease absorption of T4)

Table 22.8 Risk factors with hypothyroidism

System	Symptoms	Signs	Surgery-specific risks
Cardiovascular	• Decreased exercise capacity • Dyspnea on exertion	• Bradycardia • Low voltage on EKG • Prolonged QT interval • Pericardial effusion • Elevated diastolic BP and narrow pulse pressure • Hypercholesterolemia	• Hemodynamic instability • CHF
Pulmonary	• Dyspnea on exertion • Increasing oxygen requirements • Obstructive sleep apnea	• Hypoventilation due to respiratory muscle weakness • Decreased response to hypoxia and hypercarbia	• Inability to wean from mechanical ventilation • Inability to mount a fever response may delay the diagnosis of infections
Gastrointestinal	• Anorexia • Constipation • Decreased taste sensation	• Paralytic ileus • Ascites (rarely)	• Increased sensitivity to anesthetic agents due to impaired hepatic metabolism • Increased risk for GI bleed • Increased risk for aspiration due to delayed gastric emptying
Hematology	• Fatigue • Increased bleeding (due to acquired von Willebrand syndrome I and decreased platelet adhesiveness)	• Normocytic anemia • Pernicious anemia in 10% • Iron deficiency anemia due to menorrhagia • Requires higher doses of warfarin due to prolonged half-life of some coagulation factors (II,VII and X)	• Difficulty achieving desired INR level • Increased bleeding complications
Neuromuscular	• Muscle weakness and myalgias • Decreased mentation and short-term memory deficits	• Cerebellar ataxia • Cognitive impairment • Delayed response to DTRs • Proximal muscle weakness • Carpal tunnel syndrome	• Prolonged recovery time from anesthesia • Muscle weakness might prolong postoperative rehabilitation

(continued)

Table 22.8 (continued)

System	Symptoms	Signs	Surgery-specific risks
Endocrine	• Decreased libido • Decreased fertility • Symptoms from coexisting disease: anorexia and weight loss with adrenal insufficiency, excessive sweating with acromegaly, excessive thirst with diabetes insipidus	• Amenorrhea or menorrhagia • Loss of pregnancies • Hyponatremia. • Co-existing Addison's disease with primary hypothyroidism and decreased adrenal reserve with secondary hypothyroidism	• Hemodynamic instability with co-existing adrenal insufficiency • In severe hypothyroidism and myxedema coma, stress dose steroids may need to be administered • Electrolyte abnormalities predominantly hyponatremia
Psychiatric	• Depression • Loss of memory	• Decreased compliance with medications • Lack of motivation and anhedonia	• Postoperative delirium and psychosis • Depression affecting postoperative recovery and rehabilitation

- Hypothyroid patients who are well compensated with thyroid hormone supplements do not need special consideration prior to surgery.
- Checking TSH (+/−free T4) level is indicated when:
  - Thyroid dysfunction is suspected based on symptoms and signs.
  - The patient does not appear euthyroid on current hormone replacement dose.
- Thyroid function tests may be abnormal in hospitalized or seriously ill patients due to nonthyroidal illness or euthyroid sick syndrome, and thyroid hormone supplementation is not indicated.
- Mild to moderate hypothyroidism does not increase perioperative morbidity or mortality. However, severe hypothyroidism can increase risk, and elective surgery should be postponed pending further treatment.

22.4.5 Perioperative Management and Risk Reduction Strategies

- Perioperative risk and management strategies depend on the degree of hypothyroidism.
- In newly diagnosed or chronic mild to moderate hypothyroidism, there is no consensus on the timing of surgery, but most data confirm that these patients are not at an increased risk for perioperative morbidity and mortality, and hence surgery need not be delayed.
- In patients with severe hypothyroidism, elective noncardiac surgery should be postponed.
  - T4 supplementation should be started orally and may take 2–3 weeks to achieve a steady state.

  - Emergency surgery can be performed but with close monitoring for anticipated problems associated with hypothyroidism including myxedema coma.
  - The patient with hypothyroidism undergoing cardiac surgery is challenging.[39]

    Thyroid hormone supplementation prior to revascularization can precipitate acute coronary event, and an untreated hypothyroid patient is at a higher risk for perioperative hypotension and cardiac failure.

    There is no general consensus, but the most prudent management is to postpone supplementation until after CABG or consider partial supplementation with titration after surgery.

    In the postoperative period, T4 should be started at a low dose and titrated up slowly to achieve a euthyroid state.

  - T4 has a long half-life, and IV thyroid hormone supplements for hypothyroid patients on oral replacement therapy are indicated if the NPO state is prolonged beyond 7 days, there are signs of hypothyroidism like paralytic ileus or severe depression interfering with rehabilitation, or myxedema coma is suspected.
- Myxedema coma is state of severe hypothyroidism associated with high mortality.
  - Clinical characteristics include decreased mental status leading to coma, congestive heart failure, depressed respiratory drive, hypothermia, hyponatremia, hypotension, and hypoglycemia.
  - Precipitating factors include infection, exposure to sedatives, hypothermia, and inadequate thyroid hormone supplementation.
  - It should be suspected in hypothyroid patients when they are having difficulty waking up or weaning off of the ventilator.
  - When suspected, intravenous thyroid supplements should be started immediately, without waiting for laboratory confirmation.
  - T3 may be preferable to T4 because of its 100% absorption and shorter half life, hence quicker recovery.
  - Co-existing adrenal insufficiency should always be considered, and supplemental glucocorticoids should be given prior to thyroid supplementation, which otherwise could precipitate adrenal crisis.

22.5 Pheochromocytoma

22.5.1 Introduction

Pheochromocytoma is a rare tumor (<0.7% prevalence) of catecholamine-secreting chromaffin cells and is most commonly found in the adrenal medulla. Its diagnosis is difficult and must be confirmed prior to surgery to distinguish it from other benign neuroendocrine tumors that do not pose the same risks. This section will review the special perioperative preparation of pheochromocytoma to manage the catecholamine surges that can result in significant cardiovascular complications and mortality.

22.5.2
Diagnosis of Pheochromocytoma (see Fig. 22.2)

- Pheochromocytoma should be suspected if:
  - Patients have classic symptoms of sweating, tachycardia, and intermittent headaches. Other presentations include hypertension at young age (less than 20 years old), refractory hypertension, or paroxysmal hypertension, especially in response to stress such as surgery or anesthesia.[40] These are high-risk features.
  - Patients have a positive family history of pheochromocytoma, familial paragangliomas, multiple endocrine neoplasia type 2 (MEN2), neurofibromatosis type 1 (NF-1), or von Hippel-Lindau (VHL) disease.[40]
  - Asymptomatic adrenal incidentaloma is noted on CT or MRI imaging with high-risk features.[40-42]
- Suspicion of pheochromocytoma should always be confirmed with biochemical testing prior to surgery[40,43] (see Table 22.9).
- Once confirmed with biochemical testing, the tumor should be localized with imaging (CT, MRI, PET) (see Table 22.9).

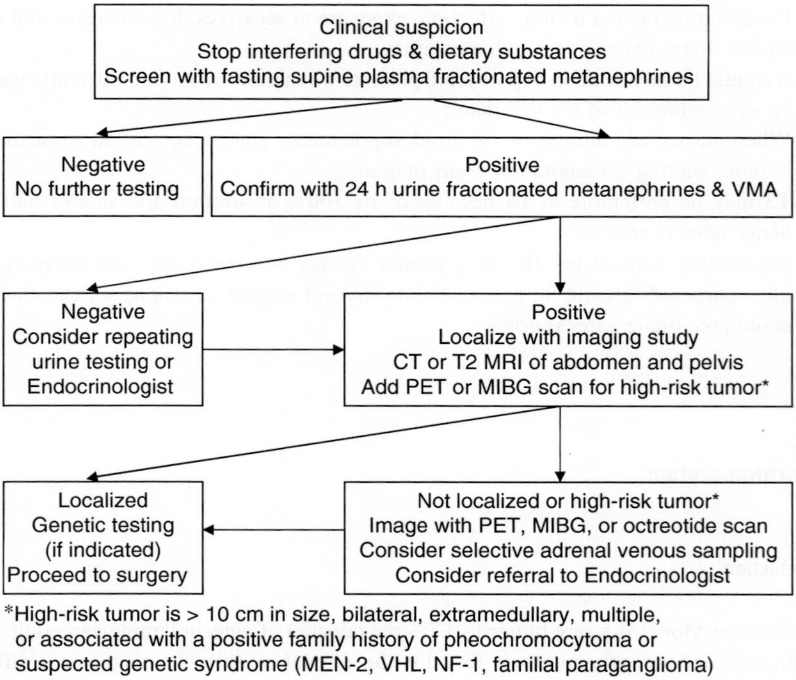

Fig. 22.2 Approach to the diagnosis of pheochromocytoma

Table 22.9 Diagnostic tests for pheochromocytoma

Test	Sensitivity (negative predictive value)	Negative test	Specificity (positive predictive value)	Positive test**
Plasma fractionated metanephrines: Normetanepherine Metanepherine	99%	 <0.6 nmol/L <0.3 nmol/L	89%	 >1.4 nmol/L >0.42 nmol/L
Plasma catecholamines: Noradrenaline Adrenaline	84%	 <3 nmol/L <0.45 nmol/L	81%	 >7.7 nmol/L >1.2 nmol/L
Chromogranin A	Poor	–	Poor	–
Urine VMA	64%	<40 μmol/24 h	95%	>55 μmol/24 h
Urine metanephrines: Normetanepherine Metanepherine Total metanephrines	Fractionated: 97% Total: 77%	 <3,000 nmol/24 h <1,000 nmol/24 h <6 μmol/24 h	Fractionated: 69% Total: 93%	 >6,550 nmol/24 h >2,880 nmol/24 h >12.7 μmol/24 h
Urine catecholamines: Norepinepherine (NE) Epinepherine (Epi)	86%	 <500 nmol/24 h <100 nmol/24 h	88%	 >1,180 nmol/24 h >170 nmol/24 h
**Consider repeat testing for values less than the positive cutoff but greater than negative cutoff since these values are possibly positive				
CT with and without IV contrast	90–100%	Tumor not localized	70–80%	Tumor localized
MRI T2 weighted with gadolinium contrast	90–100%	Tumor not localized	70–80%	Tumor localized
PET scans with CT: ^{18}F-fluorodopamine ^{18}F-fluorodopa ^{11}C-hydroxyephedrine ^{18}F-fluorodeoxyglucose	 78–90% 81% >80 76–88%	 Tumor not localized	Best ↓ Worst	 Tumor localized
MIBG scans: 123-MIBG 131-MIBG	78–90% Better Worse	 Tumor not localized	84–99% Better Worse	 Tumor localized
Octreotide scan: ^{111}In-pentetreotide	Head and neck: 77–94% Other areas: 25%	Tumor not localized	Head and neck: 75% Other areas: ?	Tumor localized

Adapted from Lenders,[40,43] Fiebrich,[44] Timmers,[45] Shapiro,[46] Telischi,[47] and van der Harst[48]

- Referral to an endocrinologist is warranted to assess for malignant potential, bilateral disease, extramedullary disease, or metastatic disease in order to adequately plan the operative approach.
- Consider genetic testing for high-risk tumors.[40]

22.5.3 Preoperative Preparation

- The preoperative approach for cardiovascular complications should be per the latest ACC-AHA guidelines[49] for preoperative cardiac evaluation of noncardiac surgery (see Chap. 20).
  - Myocardial infarction is rarely due to pheochromocytoma itself but occurs in the setting of pre-existing coronary artery disease. Pheochromocytoma itself may cause nonspecific ST-T wave changes and wall motion abnormalities from cardiomyopathy. Additionally, provocative stress testing with exercise or dobutamine may precipitate a pheochromocytoma crisis.
  - Congestive heart failure can occur preoperatively due to cardiomyopathy caused by pheochromocytoma, but is rare.
  - Stroke can occur due to paroxysmal malignant hypertension, so preoperative blood pressure control below 160/90 is imperative.
  - Aortic dissection can rarely occur due to paroxysmal malignant hypertension.
- The goals of preoperative preparation are to control blood pressure and heart rate and replete volume. Hypertension should be controlled for at least 1 week prior to surgery. There are several strategies, all of which are equally acceptable with respect to outcomes and mortality[40,50] and each has its merits and disadvantages (see Table 22.10).
  - The traditional approach is to pretreat with a nonselective alpha antagonist followed by a beta-blocker. The vasoconstrictive effects of pheochromocytoma are countered by beta-mediated vasodilation. Therefore, beta-blockers should never be used first because this will lead to unopposed alpha effect and precipitate a pheochromocytoma crisis. Beta-blocker treatment after adequate alpha-blockade is used for heart rate control.
  - Newer approaches include pretreatment with a selective alpha-1 antagonist or alpha-2-agonist without a preoperative beta-blocker.[50]
  - The most recent approach is to pretreat with a dihydropyridine calcium-channel blocker without any preoperative antiadrenergic therapy, or use only intraoperative treatment strategies (see Sect. 22.5.4) with any means of preoperative blood pressure control.[50]
  - Second-line agents that can be used in addition to any of the above strategies include alpha-methyl-paratyrosine (metyrosine), urapidil, or labetalol.
  - Salt loading or preoperative volume repletion may be an adjunct to any of the above preoperative strategies to correct the intravascular volume depletion that occurs with pheochromocytoma. This helps to minimize intra- and postoperative fluid volume and associated edema or heart failure, but is not necessarily indicated in every case of pheochromocytoma surgery. Ensure that the orthostatic upright blood pressure does not drop below 80/45.

Table 22.10 Preoperative preparation for pheochromocytoma surgery

Preoperative strategy	Advantage	Disadvantage
Non-selective Alpha-Beta Blockade		
Phenoxybenzamine 10 mg BID, titrate every 2–3 days by 10–20 mg/day to maximum of 80–100 mg/day (1 mg/kg) to achieve goal BP <160/90 mmHg without orthostatic hypotension <80/45 mmHg for total of 10–14 days of pre-treatment.	Non-competitive alpha-1 and alpha-2 blockade prevents drug displacement by catecholamine surges and ensures good preoperative blood pressure control	Postoperative hypotension Reflex tachycardia Postoperative edema and CHF Central sedation
Beta-blockade only *after* alpha-blockade: • Propranalol 40 mg TID, or • Atenolol 25–50 mg daily, or • Metoprolol 50–100 mg BID to target <1 PVC per every 5 min.	Control of tachyarrhythmias and extra-systoles	Unopposed alpha effect if initiated prior to alpha-blockade Negative inotropic effect
Selective Alpha-1 Blockade:		
• Doxazosin 1 mg/day, titrate every 2–3 days by 2–4 mg/day to maximum of 16 mg/day, or	Competitive alpha-1 blockade has a shorter duration of action and avoids postoperative hypotension	Competitive alpha-1 blockade can cause drug displacement during catecholamine surges and lead to poor blood pressure control
• Prazosin 1 mg BID – TID, titrate every 2–3 days by 3–15 mg/day to maximum of 40 mg/day, or	Less reflex tachycardia and orthostatic hypotension	Tachyarrhythmias not controlled preoperatively
• Alpha-2 Agonist: Clonidine 0.1 mg BID to TID, titrate every 2–3 days by 0.3 mg/day to maximum of 1.2 mg/day	Less need for preoperative volume expansion results in less postoperative edema	
Di-hydro-pyridine Ca^{++} Channel Blocker:		
IV Nicardipine drip 5 mg/h, titrate to maximum of 15 mg/h	Rapid surgical preparation with less postoperative orthostatic hypotension	Tachyarrhythmias not controlled preoperatively

(continued)

Table 22.10 (continued)

Preoperative strategy	Advantage	Disadvantage
Second-line drugs (in addition to above):		
• alpha-methyl-paratyrosine (metyrosine) 0.5–4 g/day, or	Additional blood pressure control if above strategies are unsuccessful with less postoperative hypotension	Fatigue, anxiety, diarrhea, depression, crystalluria
• Urapidil, or		
• Labetalol 100 mg PO TID – QID, titrate by 300–800 mg/day to maximum of 2,400 mg/day, or	Control of tachyarrhythmias and extra-systoles	Negative inotropic effect
• IV Labetalol drip 0.5–2 mg/min to maximum of 300 mg/day		

Adapted from Lenders[40] and van der Horst-Schrivers[50]
Volume expansion with salt loading using NaCl 1–2 g TID for 3 days before surgery or IV NS infusion preoperatively may be indicated if there is orthostatic hypotension to <80/45 mmHg. This reduces the need for intra- or postoperative fluid and reduces postoperative edema and CHF

22.5.4 Intraoperative Treatment

- Intraoperative strategies are similar to preoperative strategies for control of blood pressure, heart rate, and volume, and offer the advantage of rapid titration. Medications used intraoperatively may include:
  - Alpha blockade with continuous IV phentolamine drip.
  - Beta-blockade with continuous IV esmolol or labetalol drips.
  - Calcium-channel blockade with a continuous IV nicardipine drip.
  - Continuous IV nitroprusside drip.
  - Intraoperative hypotension is normally treated with IV saline bolus infusion rather than pressors because it is predominantly caused by preoperative volume contraction.

22.5.5 Postoperative Complications

- Hypertension persists in up to 50% of patients after surgical resection of the pheochromocytoma[40] and is usually due to idiopathic hypertension. Other causes include residual effects of circulating catecholamines, fluid overload, or residual tumor. Recurrence of the tumor may occur in up to 17% of patients, especially if they have high-risk features and about half of the recurrences are malignant.[40] Phenoxybenzamine may be continued in this setting.

- Hypotension can occur after removal of the pheochromocytoma in those who do not have underlying hypertension, especially if they were prepared with nonselective alpha-1 and alpha-2 antagonists pre- or intraoperatively or did not have adequate preoperative volume expansion. Replacement of intravascular volume and withdrawal of antihypertensive medications are needed.
- Postoperative edema and decompensated heart failure occur more commonly in patients who did not have adequate preoperative volume expansion and then needed intraoperative fluid boluses for management of hypotension. Those with pheochromocytoma cardiomyopathy or underlying heart failure are also at risk, especially if they were treated with pre- or intraoperative beta-blockers. Treat with diuretics and the usual chronic therapies for heart failure, including ACE inhibition or angiotensin receptor blockade, and a beta-blocker, if necessary.
- Hypoglycemia may occur from rebound hyperinsulinism as the inhibitory effects of catecholamines resolve.

References

Diabetes References

1. Malmberg K, Rydén L, Efendic S, et al. Randomized trial of insulin-glucose infusion followed by subcutaneous insulin treatment in diabetic patients with acute myocardial infarction (DIGAMI study): effects on mortality at 1 year. *J Am Coll Cardiol*. 1995;26(1):57-65.
2. Furnary AP, Gao G, Grunkemeier GL, et al. Continuous insulin infusion reduces mortality in patients with diabetes undergoing coronary artery bypass grafting. *J Thorac Cardiovasc Surg*. 2003;125(5):1007-1021.
3. van den Berghe G, Wouters P, Weekers F, et al. Intensive insulin therapy in the critically ill patients. *N Engl J Med*. 2001;345(19):1359-1367.
4. Zerr KJ, Furnary AP, Grunkemeier GL, Bookin S, Kanhere V, Starr A. Glucose control lowers the risk of wound infection in diabetics after open heart operations. *Ann Thorac Surg*. 1997;63(2):356-361.
5. Golden SH, Peart-Vigilance C, Kao WH, Brancati FL. Perioperative glycemic control and the risk of infectious complications in a cohort of adults with diabetes. *Diab Care*. 1999;22(9):1408-1414.
6. Lee TH, Marcantonio ER, Mangione CM, et al. Derivation and prospective validation of a simple index for prediction of cardiac risk of major noncardiac surgery. *Circulation*. 1999;100(10):1043-1049.
7. NICE-SUGAR Study Investigators, Finfer S, Chittock DR, Su SY, et al. Intensive versus conventional glucose control in critically ill patients. *N Engl J Med*. 2009;360(13):1283-1297.
8. Wiener RS, Wiener DC, Larson RJ. Benefits and risks of tight glucose control in critically ill adults: a meta-analysis. *JAMA*. 2008;300(8):933-944.
9. Van den Berghe G, Wilmer A, Hermans G, et al. Intensive insulin therapy in the medical ICU. *N Engl J Med*. 2006;354(5):449-461.
10. Moghissi ES, Korytkowski MT, DiNardo M, et al. American Association of Clinical Endocrinologists and American Diabetes Association consensus statement on inpatient glycemic control. *Diab Care*. 2009;32(6):1119-1131.

11. Hirsch IB. Insulin analogues. *N Engl J Med*. 2005;352:174-183.
12. Umpierrez GE, Smiley D, Zisman A, et al. Randomized study of basal-bolus insulin therapy in the inpatient management of patients with type 2 diabetes (RABBIT 2 trial). *Diab Care*. 2007;30(9):2181-2186.
13. Braithwaite SS. Inpatient insulin therapy. *Curr Opin Endocrinol Diabetes Obes*. 2008;15: 159-166.
14. Schmeltz LR, DeSantis AJ, Schmidt K, et al. Conversion of intravenous insulin infusions to subcutaneously administered insulin glargine in patients with hyperglycemia. *Endocr Pract*. 2006;12(6):641-650.
15. Inzucchi SE. Clinical practice management of hyperglycemia in the hospital setting. *N Engl J Med*. 2006;355(18):1903-1911.

Adrenal References

16. Oelkers W. Adrenal insufficiency. *N Engl J Med*. 1996;335:1206-1212.
17. Krasner AS. Glucocorticoid-induced adrenal insufficiency. *JAMA*. 1999;282:671-676.
18. Lamberts SW, Bruining HA, de Jong FH. Corticosteroid therapy in severe illness. *N Engl J Med*. 1997;337:1285-1292.
19. Salem M, Tainsh REJ, Bromberg J, et al. Perioperative glucocorticoid coverage. A reassessment 42 years after emergence of a problem. *Ann Surg*. 1994;219:416-425.
20. Glowniak JV, Loriaux DL. A double-blind study of perioperative steroid requirements in secondary adrenal insufficiency. *Surgery*. 1997;121:123-129.
21. Coursin DB, Woods KE. Corticosteroid supplementation for adrenal insufficiency. *JAMA*. 2002;287:236-240.
22. Poulter S, Morris S. Perioperative steroid supplementation. *Anaesthesia*. 1999;54:507.
23. Brown CJ, Buie WD. Perioperative stress dose steroids: do they make a difference? *J Am Coll Surg*. 2001;193:678-686.
24. Marik PE, Varon J. Requirement of perioperative stress doses of corticosteroids: a systematic review of the literature. *Arch Surg*. 2008;143:1222-1226.
25. Yong SL, Marik P, Esposito M, Coulthard P. Supplemental perioperative steroids for surgical patients with adrenal insufficiency. *Cochrane Database Of Systematic Reviews (Online)* 2009;CD005367
26. Mayenknecht J, Diederich S, Behr V, et al. Comparison of low and high dose corticotropin stimulation tests in patients with pituitary disease. *J Clin Endocrinol Metab*. 1998;83:1558-1562.
27. Weintrob N, Sprecher E, Josefsberg Z, et al. Standard and low-dose short adrenocorticotropin test compared with insulin-induced hypoglycemia for assessment of the hypothalamic-pituitary-adrenal axis in children with idiopathic multiple pituitary hormone deficiencies. *J Clin Endocrinol Metab*. 1998;83:88-92.

Thyroid References

28. Davies TF, Larsen PR. The thyroid gland. In: Larsen PR, Kronenbord HM, eds. *Williams Textbook of Endocrinology*. Philadelphia: W.B. Saunders; 2003.
29. Davies TF, Larsen PR. Thyrotoxicosis. In: Larsen PR, Kronenbord HM, eds. *Williams Textbook of Endocrinology*. Philadelphia: W.B. Saunders; 2003:413-414.
30. Osman F, Gammage MD, Franklyn JA. Hyperthyroidism and cardiovascular morbidity and mortality. *Thyroid*. 2002;12:483-487.

31. Feek CM, Sawers JS, Irvine WJ, Beckett GJ, Ratcliffe WA, Toft AD. Combination of potassium iodide and propranolol in preparation of patients with Graves' disease for thyroid surgery. *N Engl J Med.* 1980;302:883-885.
32. Franklyn JA. The management of hyperthyroidism. *N Engl J Med.* 1994;330:1731-1738.
33. Singer PA, Cooper DS, Levy EG, et al. Treatment guidelines for patients with hyperthyroidism and hypothyroidism. Standards of Care Committee, American Thyroid Association. *JAMA.* 1995;273:808-812.
34. Woeber KA. Update on the management of hyperthyroidism and hypothyroidism. *Arch Intern Med.* 2000;160:1067-1071.
35. Udelsman R, Ramp J. Gallucci WT, et al: Adaptation during surgical stress A reevaluation of the role of glucocorticoids. *J Clin Invest.* 1986;77:1377-1381.
36. Surks MI, Ortiz E, et al. Subclinical thyroid disease: scientific review and guidelines for diagnosis and management. *JAMA.* 2004;291(2):228-238.
37. Ladenson PW, Levin AA, Ridgway EC, Daniels GH. Complications of surgery in hypothyroid patients. *Am J Med.* 1984;77:261.
38. Weinberg AD, Brennan MD, Gorman CA. Outcome of anesthesia and surgery in hypothyroid patients. *Arch Intern Med.* 1983;143:893.
39. Drucker DJ, Burrow GN. Cardiovascular surgery in the hypothyroid patient. *Arch Intern Med.* 1985;145:1585.

Pheochromocytoma References

40. Lenders JW, Eisenhofer G, Mannelli M, Pacak K. Phaeochromocytoma. *Lancet.* 2005;366:665-675.
41. Hamrahian AH, Ioachimescu AG, Remer EM, et al. Clinical utility of noncontrast computed tomography attenuation value (Hounsfield units) to differentiate adrenal adenomas/hyperplasias from nonadenomas: Cleveland Clinic experience. *J Clin Endocrinol Metab.* 2005;90(2):871-877.
42. Hennings J, Hellman P, Ahlström H, Sundin A. Computed tomography, magnetic resonance imaging and 11 C-metomidate positron emission tomography for evaluation of adrenal incidentalomas. *Eur J Radiol.* 2009;69(2):314-323.
43. Lenders JW, Pacak K, Walther MM, et al. Biochemical diagnosis of pheochromocytoma: which test is best? *JAMA.* 2002;287(11):1427-1434.
44. Fiebrich HB, Brouwers AH, Kerstens MN, et al. 6-[F-18]Fluoro-L-dihydroxyphenylalanine positron emission tomography is superior to conventional imaging with (123) I-metaiodobenzylguanidine scintigraphy, computer tomography, and magnetic resonance imaging in localizing tumors causing catecholamine excess. *J Clin Endocrinol Metab.* 2009;94(10):3922-3930.
45. Timmers HJ, Chen CC, Carrasquillo JA, et al. Comparison of 18 F-fluoro-L-DOPA, 18 F-fluoro-deoxyglucose, and 18 F-fluorodopamine PET and 123I-MIBG scintigraphy in the localization of pheochromocytoma and paraganglioma. *J Clin Endocrinol Metab.* 2009;94(12):4757.
46. Shapiro B, Copp JE, Sisson JC, et al. Iodine-131 metaiodobenzylguanidine for the locating of suspected pheochromocytoma: experience in 400 cases. *J Nucl Med.* 1985;26(6):576-585.
47. Telischi FF, Bustillo A, Whiteman ML, et al. Octreotide scintigraphy for the detection of paragangliomas. *Otolaryngol Head Neck Surg.* 2000;122(3):358-362.
48. van der Harst E, de Herder WW, Bruining HA, et al. [(123)I]metaiodobenzylguanidine and [(111)In] octreotide uptake in benign and malignant pheochromocytomas. *J Clin Endocrinol Metab.* 2001;86:685-693.

49. Fleisher LA, Beckman JA, Brown KA, et al. ACC/AHA 2007 guidelines on perioperative cardiovascular evaluation and care for noncardiac surgery: executive summary: a report of the American College of Cardiology/American Heart Association Task Force on Practice Guidelines (Writing Committee to Revise the 2002 Guidelines on Perioperative Cardiovascular Evaluation for Noncardiac Surgery): Developed in Collaboration With the American Society of Echocardiography, American Society of Nuclear Cardiology, Heart Rhythm Society, Society of Cardiovascular Anesthesiologists, Society for Cardiovascular Angiography and Interventions, Society for Vascular Medicine and Biology, and Society for Vascular Surgery. *Circulation*. 2007;116(17):1971-1996.
50. van der Horst-Schrivers AN, Kerstens MN, Wolffenbuttel BH. Preoperative pharmacological management of phaeochromocytoma. *Neth J Med*. 2006;64(8):290-295.

Hematologic Disease

23

Shuwei Gao and Sunil K. Sahai

23.1 Introduction

Many patients have hematologic issues before and/or after undergoing surgery. Hematologic disorders (such as anemia, bleeding diathesis, or hypercoagulability) can affect perioperative management and outcomes. Therefore, recognizing and correcting these hematologic conditions can significantly reduce perioperative complications. This chapter will focus on the evaluation and management of hematologic issues commonly encountered in surgical patients.

23.2 Red Blood Cell Disorders

23.2.1 Anemia

- Anemia is the most common hematologic issue in surgical patients.
- Broadly speaking, anemia is defined as decreased red cell count compared with normal levels.
- The percentage of individuals with preoperative anemia varies greatly, ranging from 5% to 75%, depending on the patient population studied and the diagnostic criteria used.[1]
- Both preoperative and postoperative anemias independently increase the risk of mortality and morbidity. The extent of preexisting comorbidities, specifically cardiovascular disease, substantially affects the patient's tolerance for perioperative anemia and morbidity.[2]
- The presence of anemia increases mortality independent of transfusion, but increased transfusions also are associated with increased mortality.

S.K. Sahai (✉)
Department of General Internal Medicine, The University of Texas
MD Anderson Cancer Center, 1515 Holcombe Blvd, Houston, TX, USA
e-mail: ssahai@mdanderson.org

S.L. Cohn (ed.), *Perioperative Medicine*,
DOI: 10.1007/978-0-85729-498-2_23, © Springer-Verlag London Limited 2011

23.2.1.1 Patient-Related Risk Factors Associated with Anemia

- Older age and the presence of comorbid illnesses (such as diabetes, cardiovascular disease, pulmonary disease, renal disease, or cancer) increase a patient's likelihood of being anemic.[1]
- When evaluating a patient with anemia for surgery, the etiology of the anemia has not been demonstrated to be associated with an increased risk of morbidity or mortality. Rather, the severity and chronicity of the anemia as well as compromised cardiopulmonary function play more important roles in determining perioperative outcomes.
- Patients with cardiovascular disease seem to be at the highest risk: morbidity and mortality increase with a hemoglobin concentration below 10 g/dL. As the hemoglobin concentration decreases, the patient's risk of mortality increases.[2]
- Although pulmonary disease has not been established to increase the risk of anemia, tissue extraction and delivery of oxygen may be compromised in these patients.

23.2.1.2 Surgery-Related Risk Factors Associated with Anemia

- Independent risk factors that contribute to increased perioperative morbidity and mortality include the type and length of surgery and the expected or estimated blood loss.
- The risk of mortality increases as the preoperative hemoglobin concentration decreases and as the amount of blood lost increases.[2]
- Despite the use of various techniques to reduce blood loss, it is inevitable in major surgeries. Bleeding during and/or after surgical procedures can be extremely difficult to quantify and is often underestimated.

23.2.1.3 Preoperative Evaluation for Anemia

- A complete history and physical examination should be performed to identify patients who are anemic or at risk for it.
- The baseline hemoglobin concentration and hematocrit value should be checked in patients who are elderly, have comorbidities, or will have a major surgery or a surgery with anticipated blood loss. Anemia screening is not indicated for young, healthy patients undergoing low-risk surgeries.
- A peripheral blood smear should be examined, and additional tests should be guided by these initial findings.
- The three main causes of anemia are decreased red blood cell production, increased red blood cell destruction, and blood loss. The most common causes of anemia in perioperative patients are listed in Table 23.1.

Table 23.1 Common causes of anemia

Decreased red blood cell production	Increased red blood cell destruction	Blood loss
Lack of nutrients Iron deficiency Vitamin B12 deficiency Folate deficiency Bone marrow disorders Aplastic anemia Myelodysplasia Tumor infiltration Bone marrow suppression Drugs Chemotherapy Irradiation Lack of trophic hormones Decreased erythropoietin in renal insufficency Hypothyroidism Hypogonadism Chronic disease Infections Inflammation Malignancy	Inherited hemolytic anemia Hereditary spherocytosis Sickle cell disease Thalassemia major Acquired hemolytic anemia Autoimmune hemolytic anemia Thrombotic thrombocytopenic purpura Hemolytic uremic syndrome Malaria	Obvious bleeding Surgery Trauma Melena Hematemesis Menometrorrhagia Occult bleeding Slowly bleeding ulcers Carcinoma Induced bleeding Phlebotomy Hemodialysis Excessive blood donation

- The decision to pursue a diagnostic evaluation for anemia must be weighed against the severity and urgency of surgery. While it may be appropriate to investigate anemia prior to an elective procedure, it may not be appropriate in a patient with cancer set to undergo urgent curative surgery if the anemia evaluation would delay surgery (Fig. 23.1).

23.2.1.4
Perioperative Management to Reduce the Risks Associated with Anemia

- Management of perioperative anemia is driven by the etiology of the anemia.
- Any nutritional deficiencies (including low levels of iron, folic acid, and B12) should be treated.
- Bleeding and coagulopathies should be identified and treated.
- If a causative factor (such as a drug-related effect or an autoimmune condition) is identified, appropriate action should be taken.

23.2.1.5
Blood Transfusion in Anemic Patients

- Blood transfusion is the mainstay of therapy for intraoperative and postoperative anemia. However, evidence from several large, prospective randomized studies has been inconsistent regarding the potential of blood transfusion for reducing postoperative morbidity and mortality.[3-6]

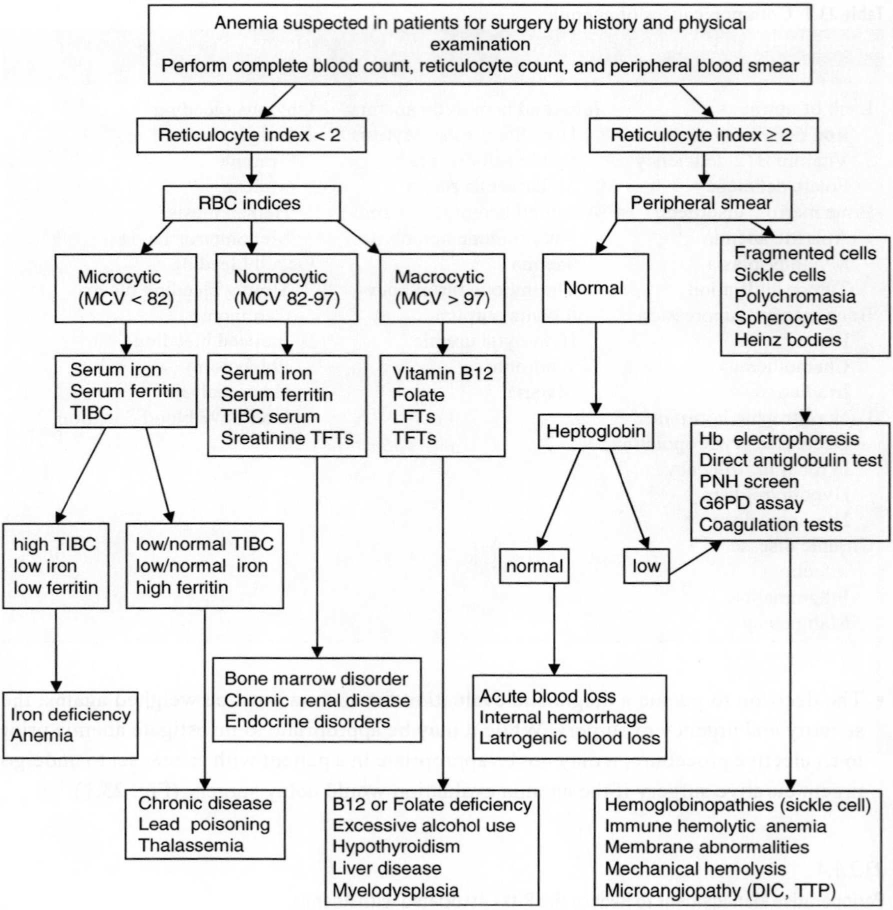

Fig. 23.1 Laboratory evaluation of anemia. Reticulocyte index: reticulocyte count × (hematocrit/normal hematocrit). *MCV* mean corpuscular volume, *TIBC* total iron binding capacity, *TFTs* thyroid function tests, *LFTs* liver function tests

- The decision to transfuse should be individualized based on the patient's symptoms and signs, underlying comorbidities, type of surgery, anticipated blood loss, and preoperative hemoglobin concentration.
- A restrictive transfusion trigger of 7–8 g/dL hemoglobin concentration is appropriate for most patients; a higher transfusion trigger of 9–10 g/dL hemoglobin concentration might be indicated for symptomatic patients with cardiovascular disease. Anemic patients with hemoglobin concentration above 10 g/dL generally do not require transfusion prior to surgery.

23.2.1.6
Use of Erythropoiesis-Stimulating Agents in Anemic Patients

- Although erythropoiesis-stimulating agents are approved for the treatment of anemic patients scheduled to undergo elective, noncardiac, nonvascular surgeries to reduce the need for allogeneic blood transfusions, erythropoiesis-stimulating agents should be used with caution.
- The Food and Drug Administration has issued a warning that erythropoiesis-stimulating agents may have serious and life-threatening side effects, including increased risks of death, blood clots or stroke, heart failure, or heart attack. Therefore, the use of erythropoietin remains controversial.[7]
- The use of erythropoiesis-stimulating agents should only be considered in patients at high risk for significant blood loss, especially patients who are anemic but who for various reasons (including religious reasons) are unable to receive blood transfusions.

23.2.2
Sickle Cell Disease

- Patients with a sickle cell disease are more likely to undergo surgery than are healthy individuals.
- Sickle cell anemia is associated with higher surgical morbidity and mortality rates. Even with meticulous care, approximately 14% to 35% of patients with sickle cell anemia experience postoperative complications.[8]
- Various strategies to reduce risk (such as administration of oxygen, a prophylactic blood transfusion, or an exchange transfusion) have been tried with mixed results.
- A conservative transfusion regimen designed only to increase hemoglobin concentration to 10 g/dL has been proved to be as effective and safe as an aggressive exchange transfusion regimen designed to reduce the sickle cell hemoglobin concentration to less than 30%. The incidence of serious complications (35% and 31%) and acute chest syndrome (10%) did not differ between the conservative and aggressive regimens, respectively.[8]

23.2.3
Polycythemia

- Polycythemia vera, a myeloproliferative disorder characterized by an absolute increase in red blood cell mass, may be associated with thrombocytosis, leukocytosis, and splenomegaly.
- Hematocrit values greater than 52% in men or 48% in women are abnormal and require further evaluation. It is essential to establish a clear-cut diagnosis of polycythemia vera, since secondary polycythemia and relative erythrocytosis have a low risk of postoperative complications while polycythemia vera has a high risk of postoperative complications.

- Secondary polycythemia can be classified as either physiologically appropriate or inappropriate.[9]
  - Secondary polycythemia is classified as physiologically inappropriate when erythropoietin overproduction occurs in response to an exogenous source (such as renal cell carcinoma, which produces an erythroid-stimulating substance, or doping in competitive sports).
  - Secondary polycythemia is classified as physiologically appropriate when erythropoietin overproduction occurs in response to high altitude or cardiopulmonary disease, resulting in chronic hypoxia.
- Patients with uncontrolled polycythemia vera prior to surgery have the highest rate of perioperative hemorrhagic and thrombotic complications as well as increased risk of mortality.[10,11]
- In polycythemia vera patients, the hematocrit value should be reduced by phlebotomy to less than 45% prior to surgery.[12]

23.3 White Blood Cell Disorders

23.3.1 Leukocytosis

- Leukocytosis – whether neutrophilic or lymphocytic – may be an indicator of infection, inflammation, or steroid use. Leukocytosis can also occur when the regulation of white blood cell development is disrupted and immature or abnormal cells are released into the blood, as in myelocytic leukemia, lymphocytic leukemia, and lymphoma.
- The leukemic patient with significant leukocytosis (white blood cells greater than 100,000/μL) should receive treatment (chemotherapy or leukapheresis) to reduce the leukocyte count, since leukocytosis is associated with a high rate of mortality and morbidity in surgery patients.
- The cause of leukocytosis in nonleukemic patients should be investigated before elective surgery. If an infection is suspected, specific antibiotics should be administered and elective surgery should be postponed (unless the surgery is part of the treatment of infection, such as debridement or abscess draining).

23.3.2 Leukopenia

- Leukopenia, a decrease in the number of white blood cells to less than 4,000/μL, can be further classified as neutropenia or lymphocytopenia.
- Neutropenia can be caused by cancer treatments, including chemotherapy, radiation therapy, or bone marrow suppression. In some bacterial infections, allergic disorders,

and drug treatments, neutrophils are destroyed faster than they are produced. In autoimmune diseases, antibodies destroy neutrophils, resulting in neutropenia. In splenomegaly, the enlarged spleen traps and destroys neutrophils.

- An absolute neutrophil count greater than 1,500/mL is not associated with a significantly increased risk of infection.
- An absolute neutrophil count of 1,000–1,500/mL is associated with a slight risk of infection.
- An absolute neutrophil count less than 500/mL is associated with vulnerability for an opportunistic infection.

- Lymphocytopenia can be caused by viral infections (such as the human immunodeficiency virus) or malnutrition. Other causes include chemotherapy, radiation therapy, and hereditary immunodeficiency disorders.
- The effects of preoperative administration of granulocyte colony-stimulating factor are controversial,[13,14] as is the role of pre- and postoperative granulocyte transfusion; however, granulocyte transfusions may reduce the risk of infections in neutropenic patients.[15] Fever might be the only manifestation of postoperative wound infection because a neutropenic patient may not form pus or manifest leukocytosis.

23.4 Platelet Disorders

- Platelet disorders (including thrombocytopenia, thrombocytosis, and platelet dysfunction) impose a significant risk of postoperative hemorrhagic and thrombotic complications.

23.4.1 Thrombocytopenia

- A reduced platelet count is mainly due to decreased production or increased destruction (Table 23.2) and may also be caused by dilutional or distributional mechanisms.
- Before evaluating the mechanism of thrombocytopenia, it is imperative to validate the platelet count to exclude the possibility of pseudothrombocytopenia.

- Pseudothrombocytopenia is due to inadequate anticoagulation of the blood sample or administration of a murine monoclonal antibody (such as abciximab), resulting in platelet clumps. The platelet count should be repeated using a citrated tube (blue top). Dilutional thrombocytopenia can occur after a massive red cell transfusion without the addition of platelet concentrates.

- The patient with mild to moderate thrombocytopenia is often asymptomatic.
- Surgical bleeding rarely occurs when the platelet count exceeds 50,000/μL.
- Spontaneous bleeding usually does not occur until the platelet count falls below 10,000/μL.

Table 23.2 Etiology of thrombocytopenia

Decreased platelet production	Increased platelet destruction	Other mechanisms
Bone marrow suppression (due to chemotherapy or radiation therapy)	Idiopathic thrombocytopenic purpura	Pseudothrombocytopenia (clumping)
Aplastic anemia	Systemic lupus erythematosus	Dilutional (after massive red blood cell transfusion)
Myelodysplastic syndrome	Disseminated intravascular coagulopathy	Distributional (splenic sequestration)
Viral infection (rubella, varicella, parvovirus, hepatitis C, Epstein–Barr virus, human immunodeficiency virus)	Thrombocytopenic purpura/hemolytic uremic syndrome	
Direct alcoholic toxicity	Hemolysis, elevated liver enzymes, low platelets	
Vitamin B12 and folate deficiency	Drugs (heparin-induced thrombocytopenia, valproic acid)	
	Infections (infectious mononucleosis, cytomegalovirus, human immunodeficiency virus)	
	Physical destruction of platelets	

- Bleeding due to thrombocytopenia (or platelet dysfunction) is usually mucosal (such as epistaxis or gingival bleeding) or cutaneous (such as petechiae or superficial ecchymosis). Unlike clotting factor disorders, bleeding from platelet disorders usually occurs immediately after a minor trauma or superficial cut and is not a delayed deep bleeding into tissues, muscles, or joints.

23.4.1.1 Perioperative Management of Thrombocytopenia

- An accurate patient history, focusing on personal and familial bleeding history, previous diagnosis of hematologic or oncologic disorders, medications taken, previous and recent transfusions, and recent viral infections, should be obtained.
- Reported thrombocytopenia should be confirmed. The peripheral blood smear should be examined for platelet numbers, morphology, absence of platelet clumping, and associated white and red cell changes.
- A bone marrow aspiration biopsy may be indicated in virtually all patients with severe thrombocytopenia of which the cause (such as chemotherapy, obvious offending drugs, or mass infusion) is not known.
- The etiology of thrombocytopenia dictates management during the perioperative period.

- Patients with idiopathic thrombocytopenic purpura can be given prednisone, intravenous immunoglobulin, or methylprednisolone to reduce autoimmune platelet destruction and raise platelet counts preoperatively.
- In patients with suspected drug-induced thrombocytopenia, the offending drugs should be discontinued.

- Regardless of the cause of thrombocytopenia, a perioperative platelet count greater than 50,000/μL is required for most surgeries except neurosurgery and ophthalmic surgery, in which counts greater than 100,000/μL are recommended.[16] A platelet count of 100,000/μL is often required by anesthesiologists administering epidural anesthesia.
- A platelet transfusion is often required 24 h before an elective surgery if the platelet count is lower than 50,000/μL and may be required postoperatively as well.
- Regardless of the etiology of the thrombocytopenia, urgent management of a perioperative patient with severe thrombocytopenia and critical bleeding requires immediate transfusion. Platelet transfusions are contraindicated in patients with thrombotic thrombocytopenic purpura; hemolytic uremic syndrome; hemolysis, elevated liver enzymes, and low platelets; heparin-induced thrombocytopenia; idiopathic thrombocytopenic purpura; and/or posttransfusion purpura.

23.4.2 Thrombocytosis

- Although thrombocytosis is defined as a platelet count greater than 550,000/μL, a platelet count less than 1,000,000/μL (extreme thrombocytosis) is rarely clinically significant in perioperative patients.
- Thrombocytosis can be autonomous (primary) but is more often a reactive phenomenon (secondary).
  - Reactive thrombocytosis can be caused by a variety of conditions, such as infection, surgery, trauma, blood loss, postsplenectomy, or malignancy. The platelet count usually normalizes after resolution of those conditions. Reactive thrombocytosis usually is not associated with perioperative bleeding or thrombosis.
  - Autonomous thrombocytosis refers to an elevated platelet count in a chronic myeloproliferative or myelodysplastic disorder.

- Regardless of the cause, a high platelet count has the potential to be associated with vasomotor (headache, visual disturbance, chest pain), thrombotic, and bleeding complications.
- Patients are considered at high risk for morbidity and mortality if they have autonomous thrombocytosis, are over 60 years old, and have a platelet count greater than 1,000,000/μL.
- Although extreme thrombocytosis occurs more often in reactive conditions, it is autonomous thrombocytosis that is more often associated with hemorrhagic and thrombotic complications.
- When a patient's platelet count is greater than 1,000,000/μL, patients with autonomous thrombocytosis have significantly higher rates of significant thrombosis (24%) and hemorrhage (24%) than do patients with reactive thrombocytosis.[17]

- Patients with chronic myeloid leukemia, primary myelofibrosis, polycythemia vera, myelodysplastic syndrome, and acute myeloid leukemia can sometimes present with thrombocytosis as a prominent feature.
- Essential thrombocythemia is usually diagnosed by excluding all causes of reactive thrombocytosis as well as all causes of autonomous thrombocytosis. There are no laboratory findings which are pathognomonic for essential thrombocythemia.
- A preoperative reduction of the platelet count is recommended in patients with autonomous thrombocytosis if the platelet count is greater than 1,000,000/μL.
  - In elective surgery, the platelet count can be lowered by administering myelosuppressive agents, such as anagrelide or hydroxyurea.[18]
  - In emergent surgery, platelet apheresis can be used before surgery and after surgery to reduce and maintain platelet levels below 1,000,000/μL.

23.4.3 Platelet Dysfunction (Qualitative Platelet Disorders)

- Qualitative platelet disorders are suggested by a prolonged bleeding time or clinical evidence of bleeding in the setting of a normal platelet count and coagulation studies.
- Platelet dysfunction may be associated with normal, reduced, or elevated platelet counts.
- Platelet dysfunction may involve platelet adherence, platelet activation, platelet aggregation, or platelet interaction with coagulation factors.
- Although platelet dysfunction can be caused by inherited disorders (such as von Willebrand disease, Glanzmann thrombasthenia, or Bernard-Soulier syndrome), platelet dysfunction is more often due to common acquired medical conditions (such as drug-induced effects, uremia, dysproteinemia, or myeloproliferative disorder).
- Drugs are the most common cause of acquired platelet dysfunction.
  - Aspirin is the most common drug responsible for platelet dysfunction, either as a desired therapeutic effect or an adverse medication effect.
  - Other antiplatelet agents include nonaspirin nonsteroidal anti-inflammatory drugs, dipyridamole, ticlopidine, clopidogrel, prasugrel, glycoprotein IIb–IIIa receptor antagonists (such as abciximab or eptifibatide), and heparin.

23.4.3.1 Hepatic Insufficiency (See Chap. 27)

- Liver disease causes impairment of hemostasis through a variety of mechanisms, including decreased coagulation factors, thrombocytopenia, and platelet dysfunction. Both acute and chronic liver diseases are associated with platelet dysfunction.
- Patients with hepatic insufficiency should be given vitamin K orally to assist in vitamin K-dependent factor production. In urgent situations or in situations where vitamin K has been ineffective, a transfusion of fresh frozen plasma is indicated.

23.4.3.2
Renal Insufficiency

- Patients with renal disease also have platelet dysfunction. As the severity of renal insufficiency and uremia worsen, the risk of bleeding increases.
- Uremia due to chronic renal failure can increase clinical bleeding caused by coexisting coagulopathies, the use of heparin with dialysis, anatomic abnormalities, decreased platelet aggregation, and impaired platelet adhesiveness.
- Desmopressin administered intravenously is effective in some uremic patients. The improvement in bleeding time begins within 1 h and lasts 4–24 h. The combination of desmopressin along with the correction of anemia may have an additive effect on lowering the bleeding time in uremic platelet dysfunction. If the bleeding time is prolonged, dialysis prior to surgery can partially correct the bleeding time to minimize bleeding.

23.4.3.3
Von Willebrand Disease

- Von Willebrand disease, the most common inherited bleeding diathesis, is caused by either deficiency (in types 1 and 3) or dysfunction (in type 2) of the von Willebrand factor.
- Most cases of von Willebrand disease (types 1 and 2) are relatively mild except for type 3.
- The bleeding manifestations are predominantly skin related and mucocutaneous (such as bruising easily, epistaxis, or gastrointestinal hemorrhage) and are reflective of platelet dysfunction. Most bleeding episodes occur following trauma or surgery.
- Factor VIII levels should be checked preoperatively and followed during and after surgery. Recombinant factor VIII should be given to keep the levels above 50% of the normal range. For patients with type 1 von Willebrand disease who are undergoing minimally invasive procedures, desmopressin may be given.[19,20]

23.4.3.4
Perioperative Management of Platelet Dysfunction

- The correction of platelet dysfunction is recommended in patients who are actively bleeding or who are about to undergo a surgical procedure. The correction of anemia will improve platelet aggregation and adhesion to endothelial cells.
- Platelet transfusions are the mainstay of perioperative platelet management, but they are not useful in patients with dysproteinemia or uremia.
- If possible, any drugs that interfere with platelet function should be discontinued before surgery and avoided in the perioperative period. Management of antiplatelet therapy during the perioperative period in a patient with coronary stents should follow the recommendations of evidence-based guidelines.[21]
- Other treatment options to correct platelet dysfunction during the perioperative time period include desmopressin, estrogen, cryoprecipitate, antifibrinolytics, dialysis, and

platelet transfusion. Platelet transfusions may be required in bleeding patients with disordered platelet function when prior treatments (such as desmopressin or estrogen) have been unsuccessful during the perioperative period.

23.5 Coagulation Disorders

- Evaluation of coagulation disorders is complicated by the fact that a patient may have both hypercoagulability and bleeding (such as a cancer patient who is undergoing chemotherapy). The physician must consider the patient's overall risk in determining a perioperative plan. Common coagulation disorders are listed in Table 23.3.

23.5.1 Inherited Bleeding Diatheses

- With the exception of von Willebrand disease, inherited bleeding disorders are usually known to both the patient and physician prior to surgery. For these situations, the assistance of a hematologist in the perioperative period may prove invaluable.
- Von Willebrand disease may be undetected until the first surgery and, even then, excessive bleeding may be attributed to another cause, such as aspirin or sepsis.
- Hemophilia A (factor VIII deficiency) is an X-linked recessive disorder caused by mutation of the factor VIII gene. The severity of illness is proportional to the factor VIII level and activity.
- Hemophilia B (factor IX deficiency) is an X-linked recessive disorder caused by mutation of the factor IX gene. Again, the severity of illness is proportional to factor IX level and activity.
- Deficiency of factor XI is an less common disorder, mainly seen in Ashkenazi Jews but otherwise rare. This deficiency is an autosomal dominant disorder that may be clinically asymptomatic until the patient is challenged by surgical trauma. Bleeding is usually not significant in minor procedures.[22]
- Deficiencies of factors II, V, VII, X, XIII, and fibrinogen that may increase perioperative bleeding are rare.

23.5.2 Acquired Hemostatic Deficiencies

- Normal coagulation mechanisms may be disrupted by a variety of causes ranging from illnesses to treatments (Table 23.3).

Table 23.3 Common coagulation disorders

Bleeding	Thrombosis
Inherited	Inherited
Von Willebrand disease	Factor V Leiden
Hemophilia A (factor VIII deficiency)	Prothrombin gene mutation
Hemophilia B (factor IX deficiency)	Antithrombin III deficiency
Factor XI deficiency	Protein C deficiency
Afibrinogenemia (rare)	Protein S deficiency
Hypofibrinogenemia (rare)	Hyperhomocysteinemia
Prothrombin deficiency (very rare)	Dysfibrinogenemia (rare)
Factor V deficiency (rare)	
Factor VII deficiency (rare)	
Factor X deficiency (rare)	
Factor XIII deficiency (rare)	
Acquired	Acquired hypercoagulable states/risk factors
Coagulation factor inhibitors	Malignancy
Vitamin K deficiency	Pregnancy
Malnutrition	Oral contraceptives/hormone replacement therapy
Renal insufficiency	Antiphospholipid antibody syndrome
Hepatic insufficiency	Immobilization
Anticoagulants administration	Previous venous thromboembolism
Platelet-inhibiting medications	Surgery
Idiopathic thrombocytopenic purpura	Trauma
Disseminated intravascular coagulation	Presence of a central venous catheter
	Congestive heart failure
	Chronic obstructive pulmonary disease
	Inflammatory bowel disease
	Nephrotic syndrome
	Myeloproliferative disorders
	Paroxysmal nocturnal hematuria
	Heparin-induced thrombocytopenia
	Erythropoiesis-stimulating agents
	Tamoxifen, bevacizumab, thalidomide

23.5.3 Anticoagulant and Thrombolytic Medications

- Patients receiving thrombolytic therapy are at risk of excessive bleeding, and the decision to undergo surgery needs to be made after careful consideration of the risks of withholding thrombolytic therapy.
- Anticoagulants (such as warfarin, unfractionated heparin, low-molecular-weight heparin, fondaparinux, lepirudin, and argatroban) also increase the risk of bleeding. In cases of urgent surgery, it may be necessary to interrupt treatment with anticoagulants or to proceed to the operating room with a reduced dose (such as in the case of a recent pulmonary embolus in a patient with a brain malignancy).

- Nonsteroidal anti-inflammatory drugs inhibit cyclooxygenase reversibly. However, aspirin causes irreversible inhibition. Medications that affect the cyclooxygenase-2 pathway have minimum to no effects on platelets. However, most perioperative centers encourage the discontinuation of such agents prior to surgery.
- Adenodiphosphate inhibitors (such as clopidogrel, prasugrel, and ticlopidine) irreversibly inhibit platelet aggregation whereas cilostazol causes reversible platelet inhibition through its phosphodiesterase inhibition. Dipyridamole is rarely used alone and causes mild reversible platelet dysfunction.
- A minority of hemophilia patients (A and B) will develop antibody inhibitor factors VIII and IX after repeated exposure to blood products. These inhibitors complicate treatment of bleeding by acting against the factors used to treat the disease itself. If the presence of such an inhibitor is suspected, a hematologist should be consulted prior to surgery.
- Autoantibody-mediated destruction of platelets is usually treated with steroids and intravenous immunoglobulin. Platelet transfusion may exacerbate the condition.[23]
- Disseminated intravascular coagulation is due to the failure of the normal homeostatic coagulation mechanism. Both profound thrombosis and bleeding may be present concurrently. Disseminated intravascular coagulation is frequently encountered in trauma, sepsis, and obstetric complications. Treatment consists of treating the underlying condition and judicious use of packed red blood cells, platelets, and cryoprecipitate.[24]
- Dilution coagulopathy, also known as massive transfusion syndrome, is usually seen in cases of severe trauma and is a result of the transfusion of packed red blood cells out of proportion to cryoprecipitate and platelets.[25]

23.5.4 Inherited Thrombophilias

- Inherited hypercoagulable disorders place patients at an increased risk for thrombosis and, subsequently, for postoperative thrombosis. Most hereditary thrombophilias go undiagnosed or are masked by other hypercoagulable states (such as pregnancy or cancer), thus reducing clinical suspicion of an inherited disorder.
- Factor V Leiden is the most prevalent form of inherited hypercoagulable states and is found in up to 50% of cases of familial thrombosis. While prevalent, the thrombosis risk conferred appears to be lower than other risk factors and may only pose significant clinical effects in concert with other risk factors (such as malignancy). Homozygous patients carry a higher risk than heterozygous patients.[26]
- Mutation of the prothrombin gene (G20210A) results in increased levels of prothrombin. As with factor V Leiden, the relative risk is lower than that of natural anticoagulant deficiencies.[26]
- Risk is also increased by abnormalities of the proteins involved in the coagulation cascade, including deficiency of protein C, protein S, or antithrombin.
- Although hyperhomocysteinemia has been associated with an increased risk for venous thromboembolism, reducing levels of homocysteine has not resulted in a subsequent reduction in the incidence of venous thromboembolism. There is an association with the methylene tetrahydrofolate reductase gene mutation, which may lead to thrombosis during pregnancy.

- Other rare inherited thrombophilias include plasminogen deficiency, heparin cofactor II deficiency, factor XIII mutations, dysfibrinogenemia, and excess plasminogen activator inhibitor-1.

23.5.5 Acquired Hypercoagulable States

- Acquired hypercoagulable states, such as pregnancy, cancer, medication-induced states (estrogens and thalidomide), and antiphospholipid antibody syndrome interact with inherited prothrombotic states and thereby increase the risk of venous or arterial thromboembolism.

23.5.6 Preoperative Evaluation and Testing

- Clinical history remains the cornerstone of the preoperative assessment of hemostasis, but laboratory screening tests may play important roles in assessment in some patients if history alone is not sufficient owing to a forgetful physician, unreliable patient, unchallenged patient, or recently acquired hemostatic defect. Table 23.4 lists clinical findings from history and physical examination and the hemostatic abnormalities they suggest.
- In the absence of a history of bleeding diathesis in elective surgery patients, abnormal bleeding time, prothrombin time, and activated partial thromboplastin time results are estimated to be less than 1%.

Table 23.4 Clinical findings of bleeding disorders

Clinical characteristic	Coagulation abnormality	
	Platelet defect	Clotting factor deficiency
Mild immediate bleeding after surgery or dental extraction	Common	
Petechiae or small superficial ecchymosis	Common	
Prolonged bleeding with minor trauma	Common	Uncommon
Skin, mucous membrane bleeding (gingiva, nares)	Common	
Severe delayed bleeding after surgery or dental extraction		Common
Hemarthroses or muscle hematoma	Rare	Common
Large palpable ecchymosis		Common
Recent antibiotic use		Possible
Prolonged or excessive menses	Yes	Yes
Family history of bleeding	Yes	Yes
Prior blood product transfusions	Yes	Yes

  - In patients who are deemed low risk according to their history and physical examination, activated partial thromboplastin time does not predict the risk of perioperative bleeding.
  - Similarly, the bleeding time has no predictive value on the incidence of perioperative bleeding in healthy patients set to undergo elective surgery.

- Accordingly, prothrombin time, activated partial thromboplastin time, and bleeding time are not recommended for routine preoperative testing (screening).[27]
- However, when a bleeding diathesis is suspected, the initial laboratory evaluation should include a platelet count, prothrombin time, and partial thromboplastin time (and bleeding time). Further evaluation of a potential bleeding disorder should proceed based on these results (see Fig. 23.2).
- An abnormal preoperative clotting study should be repeated for verification, and administration of anticoagulants should be ruled out.
- When abnormal prothrombin time or activated partial thromboplastin time is confirmed, the test should be repeated after a 1:1 dilution with normal plasma.

  - The correction of an abnormality may indicate a clotting factor deficiency because less than 50% (only about 25%) of the normal level of each factor is required to produce a normal prothrombin time or activated partial thromboplastin time.
  - Noncorrection of an abnormal prothrombin time or activated partial thromboplastin time by 1:1 mixture suggests the presence of an inhibitor directed against the clotting factor (usually an antibody or drug).

- In patients with idiopathic thrombocytopenic purpura, hemophilia, and other coagulation deficiencies, measuring levels of the deficient hemostasis component guides preoperative risk-reduction measures.

23.5.7 Perioperative Management

- Perioperative medication management of antiplatelet and anticoagulant drugs is discussed in Chaps. 2 and 4. The risk of bleeding or of having a thromboembolism needs to be considered in deciding whether or not to continue or temporarily discontinue these drugs perioperatively.

23.5.8 Management of Specific Coagulation Abnormalities

- Previously documented or newly diagnosed coagulopathies require specialized preoperative management to reduce the risk of perioperative bleeding. These therapies and other perioperative risk-reduction methods are listed in Table 23.5. Cooperation with hematology and blood bank consultants in the management of coagulopathies is strongly advised.

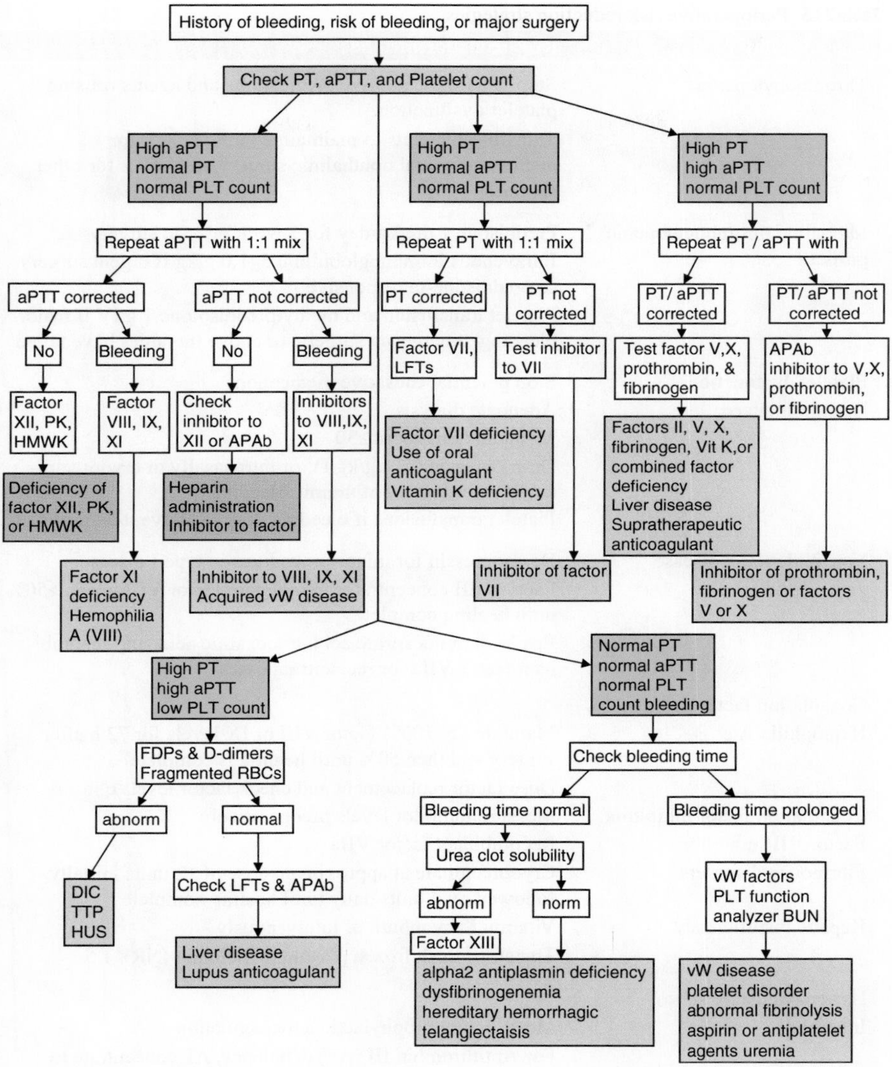

Fig. 23.2 Evaluation of abnormal coagulation. *aPTT* activated partial thromboplastin time, *PT* prothrombin time, *PLT* platelets, *PK* prekallikren, *vW* von Willebrand, *LFTs* liver function tests, *APAb* antiphospholipid antibody, *Ab* antibody, *FDPs* fibrin degradation products, *DIC* disseminated intravascular coagulation, *HUS* hemolytic uremic syndrome, *TTP* thrombotic thrombocytopenic purpura, *HMWK* high molecular weight kininogen, *Vit* vitamin, *RBC* red blood cell, *BUN* blood urea nitrogen

Table 23.5 Perioperative risk reduction strategies

Coagulopathy	Risk-reduction methods
Thrombocytopenia	Stop potential causative medications and agents causing platelet dysfunction Transfuse platelets to maintain counts >100 k for neurosurgery and ophthalmic surgery and >50 k for other surgeries
Idiopathic thrombocytopenic purpura	Prednisone 1 mg/kg/day for 1 week prior to surgery Intravenous immunoglobulin 0.5–1.0 g/kg if urgent surgery or prednisone-unresponsive Platelet transfusion and methylprednisolone 1 g IV if major bleeding, emergency surgery, or above therapies have failed
Platelet dysfunction Uremia-induced	Stop potential causative medications Adequate dialysis Maintain hematocrit ≥30 Desmopressin 0.3 μg/kg IV or intranasally or cryoprecipitate if prior history of uremic bleeding Platelet transfusions if bleeding despite above therapies
Von Willebrand disease	Desmopressin for minor procedures in type I disease Factor VIII concentrates to maintain factor VIII levels >50% until healing complete Epsilon-aminocaproic acid, tranexamic acid, and recombinant factor VIIa for recalcitrant cases
Coagulation factor deficiencies	
Hemophilia A & B	Maintain 75–100% factor VIII or IX levels for 72 h after surgery and then 50% until healing is complete Dose factor replacement and check factor levels q8h
Coagulation factor inhibitors	Measure inhibitor levels preoperatively
Factor VIII inhibitor	Recombinant factor VIIa
Fibrinogen disorders	Cryoprecipitate at approximate dose of 12 units initially followed by 4 units daily until healing complete
Hepatic insufficiency	Vitamin K by mouth or intravenously Transfuse fresh frozen plasma to maintain INR < 1.5
Hypercoagulable states	
Inherited	Most require prophylactic anticoagulation For Antithrombin III (AT) deficiency, AT concentrate to maintain AT activity at 100–120% for several days postop, until INR is in target range in those receiving warfarin
Acquired	Perform comprehensive venous thromboembolism risk assessment and initiate prophylactic measures as appropriate

From Pfeifer and Abu-Hajir[28] (Table 31-3), with permission

References

1. Shander A, Knight K, Thurer R, Adamson J, Spence R. Prevalence and outcomes of anemia in surgery: a systematic review of the literature. *Am J Med.* 2004;116(Suppl 7A):58S-69S.
2. Carson JL, Duff A, Poses RM, et al. Effect of anaemia and cardiovascular disease on surgical mortality and morbidity. *Lancet.* 1996;348(9034):1055-1060.
3. Hebert PC, Wells G, Blajchman MA, et al. A multicenter, randomized, controlled clinical trial of transfusion requirements in critical care. Transfusion requirements in critical care investigators, Canadian Critical Care Trials Group. *N Engl J Med.* 1999;340(6):409-417.
4. Vincent JL, Baron JF, Reinhart K, et al. Anemia and blood transfusion in critically ill patients. *JAMA.* 2002;288(12):1499-1507.
5. Corwin HL, Gettinger A, Pearl RG, et al. The CRIT study: anemia and blood transfusion in the critically ill–current clinical practice in the United States. *Crit Care Med.* 2004;32(1):39-52.
6. Vincent JL, Sakr Y, Sprung C, Harboe S, Damas P. Are blood transfusions associated with greater mortality rates? Results of the sepsis occurrence in acutely Ill patients study. *Anesthesiology.* 2008;108(1):31-39.
7. Testa U. Erythropoietic stimulating agents. *Expert Opin Emerg Drugs.* 2010;15(1):119-138.
8. Vichinsky EP, Haberkern CM, Neumayr L, et al. A comparison of conservative and aggressive transfusion regimens in the perioperative management of sickle cell disease. *N Engl J Med.* 1995;333(4):206-214.
9. McMullin MF. The classification and diagnosis of erythrocytosis. *Int J Lab Hematol.* 2008;30(6):447-459.
10. Ruggeri M, Rodeghiero F, Tosetto A, et al. Postsurgery outcomes in patients with polycythemia vera and essential thrombocythemia: a retrospective survey. *Blood.* 2008;111(2):666-671.
11. Wasserman LR, Gilbert HS. Surgery in polycythemia vera. *N Engl J Med.* 1963;269(23):1226-1230.
12. Solberg LA Jr. Therapeutic options for essential thrombocythemia and polycythemia vera. *Semin Oncol.* 2002;29(3 Suppl 10):10-15.
13. Schaefer H, Engert A, Grass G, et al. Perioperative granulocyte colony-stimulating factor does not prevent severe infections in patients undergoing esophagectomy for esophageal cancer: a randomized placebo-controlled clinical trial. *Ann Surg.* 2004;240(1):68-75.
14. Schneider C, von Aulock S, Zedler S, Schinkel C, Hartung T, Faist E. Perioperative recombinant human granulocyte colony-stimulating factor (Filgrastim) treatment prevents immunoinflammatory dysfunction associated with major surgery. *Ann Surg.* 2004;239(1):75-81.
15. Massey E, Paulus U, Doree C, Stanworth S. Granulocyte transfusions for preventing infections in patients with neutropenia or neutrophil dysfunction. *Cochrane Database Syst Rev.* 2009;(1):CD005341.
16. Liumbruno G, Bennardello F, Lattanzio A, Piccoli P, Rossetti G. Recommendations for the transfusion of plasma and platelets. *Blood Transfus.* 2009;7(2):132-150.
17. Finazzi G, Barbui T. Evidence and expertise in the management of polycythemia vera and essential thrombocythemia. *Leukemia.* 2008;22(8):1494-1502.
18. Emadi A, Spivak JL. Anagrelide: 20 years later. *Expert Rev Anticancer Ther.* 2009;9(1):37-50.
19. Michiels JJ, van Vliet HH, Berneman Z, Schroyens W, Gadisseur A. Managing patients with von Willebrand disease type 1, 2 and 3 with desmopressin and von Willebrand factor-factor VIII concentrate in surgical settings. *Acta Haematol.* 2009;121(2–3):167-176.
20. Nichols WL, Hultin MB, James AH, et al. von Willebrand disease (VWD): evidence-based diagnosis and management guidelines, the National Heart, Lung, and Blood Institute (NHLBI) expert panel report (USA). *Haemophilia.* 2008;14(2):171-232.

21. Grines CL, Bonow RO, Casey DE Jr, et al. Prevention of premature discontinuation of dual antiplatelet therapy in patients with coronary artery stents: a science advisory from the American Heart Association, American College of Cardiology, Society for Cardiovascular Angiography and Interventions, American College of Surgeons, and American Dental Association, with representation from the American College of Physicians. *J Am Dent Assoc*. 2007;138(5):652-655.
22. Gomez K, Bolton-Maggs P. Factor XI deficiency. *Haemophilia*. 2008;14:1183-1189.
23. The American Society of Hematology ITP Practice Guideline Panel. Diagnosis and treatment of idiopathic thrombocytopenic purpura: recommendations of the American Society of Hematology. The American Society of Hematology ITP Practice Guideline Panel. *Ann Intern Med*. 1997;126(4):319-326.
24. Kitchens CS. Thrombocytopenia and thrombosis in disseminated intravascular coagulation (DIC). *Hematology Am Soc Hematol Educ Program*. 2009;240–246.
25. Sihler KC, Napolitano LM. Massive transfusion: new insights. *Chest*. 2009;136(6): 1654-1667.
26. Coppola A, Tufano A, Cerbone AM, Di Minno G. Inherited thrombophilia: implications for prevention and treatment of venous thromboembolism. *Semin Thromb Hemost*. 2009;35(7): 683-694.
27. Chee YL, Crawford JC, Watson HG, Greaves M. Guidelines on the assessment of bleeding risk prior to surgery or invasive procedures. *Br J Haematol*. 2008;140(5):496-504.
28. Pfeifer K, Abu-Hajir M. Coagulation disorders. In: Cohn SL, Smetana GW, Weed HG, eds. *Perioperative Medicine-Just the Facts*. New York: McGraw Hill; 2006.

Cancer

24

Sunil K. Sahai and Ellen F. Manzullo

24.1 Introduction

- Cancer care has evolved on many levels, from inpatient single-agent chemotherapy administered by an oncologist to multimodality treatment delivered in various settings using various routes using various modes of delivery. Since surgical resection plays a major role in treating cancer, a comprehensive preoperative evaluation is warranted, especially in those patients with numerous medical problems.[1]
- The goals of preoperative assessment are to identify the risk associated with the patient-specific type of surgery, identify patient comorbidities, document prior cancer treatments and side effects that affect the perioperative period, order appropriate diagnostic testing, assess the patient's medical and cardiovascular risks for the surgery, recommend perioperative medical strategies to optimize and reduce risk,[2] and weigh the risks and benefits of delaying surgery for medical optimization and/or further diagnostic workup.[3]

24.2 Surgery-Specific Risks

- A patient with cancer may undergo surgery for a variety of reasons, including[4]:
  - Preventive: to prevent cancer by removing tissue and/or organs
  - Diagnostic: to establish a diagnosis
  - Staging: to establish the stage of disease and the prognosis
  - Curative: to provide a cure

S.K. Sahai (✉)
Department of General Internal Medicine, The University of Texas
MD Anderson Cancer Center, 1515 Holcombe Blvd, Houston, TX, USA
e-mail: ssahai@mdanderson.org

S.L. Cohn (ed.), *Perioperative Medicine*,
DOI: 10.1007/978-0-85729-498-2_24, © Springer-Verlag London Limited 2011

- Cytoreductive: to partially remove (debulk) a tumor
- Palliative: to relieve pain or organ dysfunction
- Supportive to install a central line or feeding tube
- Unrelated: to undergo surgery unrelated to cancer treatment or surgery in a cancer survivor

- Understanding the type of, reasons for, and risks of surgery is essential in providing an appropriate perioperative risk assessment. Various procedures are associated with different levels of surgical stress. For example, while it may not be necessary to obtain an echocardiogram to assess systolic function prior to placement of a permanent venous catheter, an echocardiogram may be indicated prior to a Whipple procedure.
- In general, adherence to the American College of Cardiology (ACC)/American Heart Association (AHA) guidelines is recommended to determine surgical risk.[5] However, it must be noted that while the guidelines place most intra-abdominal procedures in the moderate-risk category, there is a notable difference in risk, even though both are "moderate risk," between a hysterectomy and a cystoprostatectomy.

24.3 Patient-Specific Risk Factors

- Proper identification of comorbid conditions is essential for accurate assessment of patient-specific risk factors. In general, it is important to determine whether the patient has any of the revised cardiac risk index (RCRI) conditions: diabetes, ischemic heart disease (coronary artery disease, prior myocardial infarction, angina), congestive heart failure, renal insufficiency, or stroke.
- Cancer patients set to undergo surgery may have other comorbidities associated with malignancy in general (e.g., anemia or venous thromboembolism) or specific conditions more likely to be found in conjunction with specific cancers (e.g., chronic obstructive pulmonary disease, hepatitis or cirrhosis, or seizures). For each condition, a thorough documentation of its onset, present treatment, and stability is needed.

24.4 Preoperative Evaluation and Management

- Cancer is, for all practical purposes, a derangement of cellular regulation. As such, cancer treatments are designed to eliminate the cells that are out of control (i.e., the cancer cells). In the absence of therapies targeted to the cancer, chemotherapy or radiation therapy can have a toxic effect on healthy tissue. When evaluating a patient with cancer for surgery, it is important to know the details of prior cancer treatments and how those treatments may affect perioperative care.
- In general, chemotherapy agents from the same class have similar side effects. Table 24.1 lists representative chemotherapy agents and their perioperative concerns. It is important

Table 24.1 Chemotherapy agents and perioperative concerns

Class	Agent	Common perioperative concern
Alkylating agent		
Nitrosourea	Carmustine Lomustine	Pulmonary fibrosis
Methylating agent	Procarbazine	Edema, tachycardia
	Dacarbazine	Hepatic necrosis and occlusion Hepatic vein thrombosis
	Temozolomide	Seizure and gait abnormality Peripheral edema
Platinum	Cisplatin	Acute renal tubular necrosis Magnesium wasting
	Carboplatin	Peripheral sensory neuropathy
	Oxaliplatin	Paresthesia Ototoxicity
Nitrogen mustard	Cyclophosphamide Ifosfamide	Pericarditis Pericardial effusions Pulmonary fibrosis Hemorrhagic cystitis Water retention Anemia
	Melphalan	SIADH
	Chlorambucil	SIADH Seizures
Antimetabolite		
Anthracycline/ Anthraquinolone	Doxorubicin Daunorubicin Epirubicin Idarubicin Mitoxantrone Valrubicin	Cardiomyopathy Electrocardiogram changes
Antitumor antibiotic: natural product	Bleomycin Mitomycin C	Pulmonary fibrosis Pneumonitis Pulmonary hypertension
Pyrimidine analogue	Capecitabine	Myocardial ischemia/ infarction
	Cytarabine (Ara-C)	Coronary vasospasm Edema
	Fluorouracil	
	Gemcitabine	Proteinuria

(continued)

Table 24.1 (continued)

Class	Agent	Common perioperative concern
Purine analogue	Thioguanine	Hepatotoxicity
	Pentostatin	Pulmonary toxicity Deep vein thrombophlebitis Chest pain Edema Atrioventricular block Arrhythmia Hypo- or hypertension
	Cladribine	Thrombosis Tachycardia Acute renal failure Tumor lysis syndrome
	Fludarabine	Cerebrovascular accident/ transient ischemic attack Angina Thrombosis Arrhythmia Congestive heart failure Acute renal failure Tumor lysis syndrome
	Mercaptopurine	Intrahepatic cholestasis and focal centrilobular necrosis
Folate antagonist	Methotrexate	Elevated liver enzymes Pulmonary edema Pleural effusions Encephalopathy Meningismus Myelosuppression
Substituted urea	Hydroxyurea	Seizure Edema
Microtubule Assembly Inhibitor		
Taxane	Paclitaxel	Peripheral neuropathy
	Docetaxel	Bradycardia Autonomic dysfunction
Alkaloid	Vinblastine	Hypertension Angina Cerebrovascular accident Coronary ischemia Electrocardiogram abnormalities Raynaud phenomenon SIADH Gastrointestinal bleed

Table 24.1 (continued)

Class	Agent	Common perioperative concern
	Vincristine	Paresthesia Recurrent laryngeal nerve palsy Autonomic dysfunction Orthostasis Hypo- and hypertension SIADH
Biologic Agent		
Monoclonal antibody	Alemtuzumab	Dysrhythmia/tachycardia/supraventricular tachycardia Hypo- or Hypertension
	Bevacizumab	Pulmonary bleeding Hypertension Thromboembolic events
	Cetuximab	Cardiopulmonary arrest
	Rituximab	Tumor lysis syndrome Electrolyte abnormality
	Trastuzumab	Cardiomyopathy Thrombus formation Pulmonary toxicity Tachycardia Hypertension
	Daclizumab	Chest pain Hyper- and hypotension Thrombosis
	Ibritumomab	Peripheral edema
	Palivizumab	Arrhythmia
	Muromonab-CD3	Tachycardia Hyper- and hypotension
Biological Response Modulator		
Interleukin	Aldesleukin Denileukin Diftitox	Capillary leak syndrome Peripheral edema Hypotension Electrocardiogram changes
Interferon	Interferon Alfa-2b Interferon Alfacon-1	Arrhythmia Chest pain Pulmonary pneumonitis Ischemic disorders Hyperthyroidism Hypothyroidism

(continued)

Table 24.1 (continued)

Class	Agent	Common perioperative concern
	Peginterferon Alfa-2a Peginterferon Alfa-2b	Pulmonary infiltrates Ischemic disorders Hyperthyroidism Hypothyroidism
Vascular Endothelial Growth Factor Inhibitor		
Tyrosine kinase inhibitor	Imatinib	Edema Left ventricular dysfunction
	Sorafenib	Cardiac ischemia and infarction Hypertension Thromboembolism
	Sunitinib	Cardiac ischemia and infarction Thromboembolism Adrenal insufficiency Pulmonary hemorrhage Hypertension Hypothyroidism Cardiomyopathy QT prolongation Torsade de pointes
	Dasatinib	Fluid retention Cardiomyopathy QT prolongation Pulmonary hemorrhage Platelet dysfunction
	Nilotinib	QT prolongation Hypertension Peripheral edema
Epidermal Growth Factor Receptor Inhibitor		
	Erlotinib	Deep venous thrombosis arrhythmia Pulmonary toxicity Cerebrovascular accidents Myocardial ischemia Syncope Edema
	Lapatinib	Cardiomyopathy Pulmonary toxicity QT prolongation
	Panitumumab	Pulmonary fibrosis Peripheral edema

Table 24.1 (continued)

Class	Agent	Common perioperative concern
Angiogenesis Inhibitor		
Immunomodulator	Thalidomide Lenalidomide	Thromboembolism Edema Bradycardia
Enzyme		
	Asparaginase	Thrombosis Glucose intolerance Coagulopathy
Miscellaneous		
Topoisomerase I inhibitor	Irinotecan Topotecan Rubitecan	Neutropenia Diarrhea Cholinergic syndrome
Epipodophyllotoxin topoisomerase II inhibitor	Etoposide	Neutropenia Stevens-Johnson syndrome Toxic epidermal necrolysis Myocardial infarction Congestive heart failure

Adapted from Sahai et al.[6], with permission from Elsevier
SIADH syndrome of inappropriate antidiuretic hormone

to note that chemotherapy side effects may manifest during the treatment cycle and may persist for months after treatment ends; it is usually the late effects that concern the perioperative evaluation. Also of importance is that many cancer medications and treatments are known by their brand names and/or acronyms. For the purposes of this chapter, we elected to use the generic names wherever possible.

24.4.1 Cardiovascular

- Various chemotherapy agents directly affect the cardiovascular system (Table 24.1), usually in a dose-dependent fashion. The most well-known side effect is cardiomyopathy, followed by ischemia. A small number of agents can affect the electrophysiology of the heart, inducing arrhythmia.
- Radiation therapy may accelerate coronary/carotid/aortic atherosclerosis, induce pericarditis, and induce or exacerbate valvular disease.
- Combinations of chemotherapy and radiation therapy may have a synergistic effect and worsen cardiomyopathy.

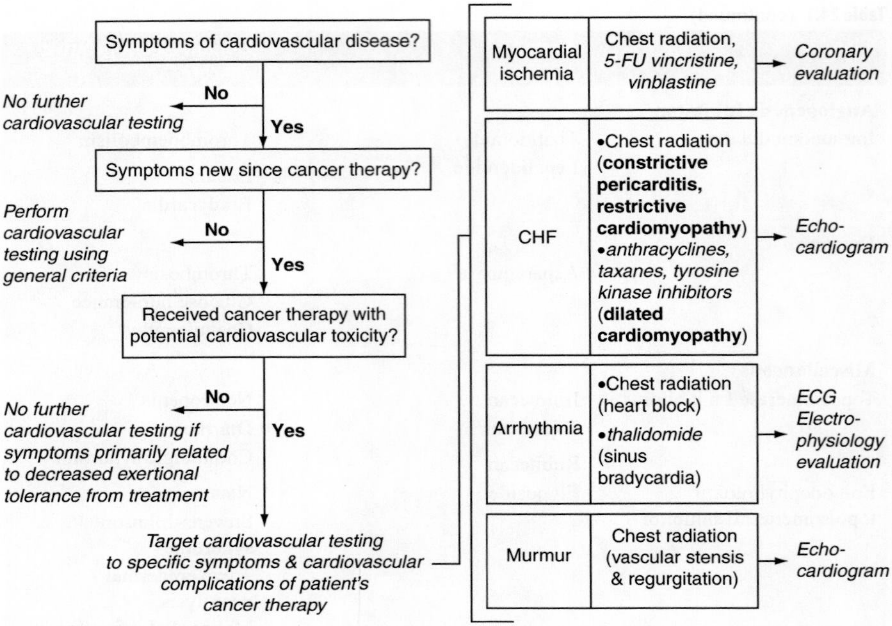

Fig. 24.1 Preoperative cardiac risk evaluation of the patient with cancer. (*5-FU* 5-fluorouracil, *CHF* congestive heart failure, *ECG* electrocardiogram) (Reprinted with permission from Sahai[7])

- In general, we recommend that cancer patients be evaluated using the ACC/AHA guidelines for preoperative evaluation.[5] The challenge for the perioperative practitioner is to determine whether a patient's cardiovascular symptoms are due to natural disease progression or to the side effects of chemotherapy.
  - A previously asymptomatic patient who does not achieve a value of 4 in metabolic equivalent testing may have preexisting, undiagnosed cardiac disease that has been exacerbated by chemotherapy, or the patient may be fatigued from the cancer treatment itself. Recognition of the former may affect perioperative outcomes, whereas a focus on the latter may lead to unneeded testing. Therefore, it is important to determine risk based on the following pathway (Fig. 24.1):

1. Does the patient have any of the revised cardiac risk index risk factors?
   (a) NO: Proceed to step 2.
   (b) YES: Proceed to targeted, noninvasive cardiovascular testing per the ACC/AHA guidelines.
2. Are symptoms of cardiovascular disease present?
   (a) NO: No need for further cardiovascular testing.
   (b) YES: Proceed to step 3.

3. Did the symptoms start during or after cancer therapy?
   (a) NO: Proceed with targeted, noninvasive cardiovascular testing per the ACC/AHA guidelines.
   (b) YES: Proceed to step 4.

4. Did the patient receive potentially cardiotoxic chemotherapy?
   (a) NO: No need for further evaluation if the symptoms can be explained by common chemotherapy side effects.
   (b) YES: Proceed with targeted, noninvasive cardiovascular testing.

Targeted testing should evaluate the patient for the following cardiovascular conditions using the tests noted for each:

- Ischemia: electrocardiogram and stress testing
- Cardiomyopathy: echocardiogram
- Arrhythmia: electrocardiogram and consider Holter monitor
- Valvular/Atherosclerotic disease: echocardiogram or carotid Doppler

24.4.2 Pulmonary

- As listed in Table 24.1, several chemotherapy agents can cause pulmonary symptoms, ranging from mild bronchospasm to pulmonary fibrosis.
- In the preoperative evaluation of a cancer patient with shortness of breath, a detailed history is needed, particularly regarding the nature of the onset of symptoms.
- As with cardiovascular disease, preexisting stable pulmonary disease is not usually an issue, but sudden onset accompanied by tachycardia may be consistent with a pulmonary embolism. Additionally, progressive shortness of breath may be consistent with acute or chronic pulmonary embolism and/or pulmonary hypertension.
  - Echocardiographic findings of unexpected pulmonary hypertension should prompt the physician to consider a pulmonary embolism in the differential diagnosis.
- Need for perioperative pulmonary screening is limited except in patients set to undergo lung resection. Also, during cancer treatment a patient may develop a pleural effusion that necessitates a therapeutic thoracentesis prior to surgery to relieve symptoms and improve ventilation.

24.4.3 Gastrointestinal and Hepatobiliary

- The diagnosis of cancer is frequently preceded by a period of weight loss. As such, nutritional issues may be at the forefront of optimizing care during cancer therapy. Patients with gastrointestinal malignancies are especially prone to nutritional compromise.

- Radiation therapy may exacerbate malabsorption secondary to radiation enteritis. Early and aggressive nutrition counseling and therapy may reduce perioperative complications with regard to wound healing and overall physical deconditioning. Nutrition therapy includes the placement of an enteral feeding tube or supplementation via parenteral nutrition.
- Chemotherapy agents can be toxic to the liver, and elevations of liver enzymes can be a marker of liver toxicity or reactivation of hepatitis B.[8] Frequently, oncologists will discontinue statins during chemotherapy to avoid further hepatotoxicity[9]; however, this practice remains controversial, as statins may have a cardioprotective effect during surgery.[10]

24.4.4 Genitourinary and Renal

- Renal side effects occur via two basic mechanisms:
  1. Direct nephrotoxicity from the chemotherapy, and
  2. Intrinsic or extrinsic renal dysfunction resulting from the tumor mass.
- Additionally, the patient with renal insufficiency may also need to be evaluated for perioperative dialysis if an acute kidney injury from surgery exacerbates a chronic condition.
- In patients undergoing chemotherapy, renal function may vary widely owing to individual treatment regimens and resultant dehydration issues. Medications that may have been dosed appropriately prior to treatment may need the dose adjusted based on the changing renal function to avoid an overdose.
- Patients with primary renal or bladder cancers may also pose a challenge from an anticoagulation perspective. These patients, along with patients who have central nervous system or gastrointestinal malignancies, may require either antiplatelet or anticoagulation treatment because of cardiovascular disease or venous thrombosis; however, ongoing bleeding from the cancer may prevent optimal treatment.

24.4.5 Hematology

- Cancer is associated with an inflammatory and hypercoagulable state,[11,12] and as a result, venous thrombosis is a prevalent complication throughout the entire treatment cycle.
- Prophylaxis for venous thromboembolism should follow accepted guidelines unless contraindicated.[13,14]
  - In general, low-molecular-weight heparin is recommended for both prophylaxis and treatment. Additionally, the high-risk cancer patient should receive extended venous thromboembolism prophylaxis after release from the hospital for up to 1 month from the date of surgery (see Chap. 5).

24.4.6 Neurology

- Many patients with central nervous system tumors are receiving corticosteroids to reduce inflammation. Steroids may induce several complications, particularly elevated serum glucose levels and poor wound healing. Steroid-induced diabetes should be treated just like any other case of type II diabetes; however, close follow-up is indicated as discontinuation of steroid therapy can precipitate hypoglycemia.
- Two paraneoplastic syndromes are prevalent in patients with cancer. Myasthenia gravis may be present in 30% of patients with thymomas.[15] Additionally, Eaton-Lambert syndrome may be present in patients with small cell lung cancer.[16]
- Patients with central nervous system malignancies and hematologic issues pose a challenge in the perioperative period. For those at risk of cerebellar hemorrhage or of postoperative venous thromboembolism, an inferior vena cava filter may be indicated.

24.4.7 Endocrinology

- Management of diabetes in cancer patients is similar to management of diabetes in non-cancer patients (see Chap. 22).
- Cushing syndrome may be present as a paraneoplastic disorder, especially in patients with small cell lung cancer, pancreatic cancer, and carcinoid tumors. Another paraneoplastic finding common in cancer patients is the syndrome of inappropriate secretion of antidiuretic hormone. This tends to be a chronic condition of slow onset, and asymptomatic mild hyponatremia is not a contraindication to surgery.
- As steroids are a major component of chemotherapy regimens, both steroid-induced hyperglycemia and adrenal insufficiency are common conditions in cancer patients.
- The patient who has received radiation therapy to the head and neck area may be at risk for hypothyroidism.
- An elevated calcium level is common in cancer patients. While many practitioners may relate this to a paraneoplastic process, primary hyperparathyroidism should be suspected as a potential concurrent diagnosis.

24.5 Preoperative Testing

- As shown in the literature, preoperative testing remains controversial. For the cancer patient with multiple homeostatic disruptions from inadequate nutrition, therapy, dehydration, etc., it is tempting to use the "shotgun" approach to preoperative laboratory tests. However, in the absence of significant suspicion of metabolic derangement, the need for testing is limited.

For example, many patients get a chest X-ray for cancer staging purposes. In the absence of symptoms or findings on physical examination, there is rarely a need to repeat radiography before surgery. Additionally, cancer patients usually have a wealth of laboratory data available. Therefore, repeat testing of routine blood work is not necessary unless suspicion exists.

24.6 Conclusion

- The perioperative care of a cancer patient can be challenging for many reasons. The clinician must take into consideration several factors, such as the patient's cancer history, the cancer treatment received, and the presence of other comorbid conditions. With the use of a systematic approach, however, the cancer patient's risk going into surgery can be assessed and the patient's condition optimized as much as possible for the desired procedure.

References

1. Geraci JM, Escalante CP, Freeman JL, Goodwin JS. Comorbid disease and cancer: the need for more relevant conceptual models in health services research. *J Clin Oncol*. 2005;23(30): 7399-7404.
2. Sahai SK, Zalpour A, Rozner MA. Preoperative evaluation of the oncology patient. *Med Clin North Am*. 2010;94(2):403-419.
3. Ewer MS. Specialists must communicate in complex cases. *Intern Med World Rep*. 2001;16(5):17.
4. Surgery. Web Page. 2010; http://www.cancer.org/docroot/ETO/content/ETO_1_2X_Surgery.asp. Accessed 09/19, 2010.
5. Fleisher LA, Beckman JA, Brown KA, et al. ACC/AHA 2007 guidelines on perioperative cardiovascular evaluation and care for noncardiac surgery: A report of the American College of Cardiology/American Heart Association Task Force on practice guidelines (writing committee to revise the 2002 guidelines on perioperative cardiovascular evaluation for noncardiac surgery). 2007; http://circ.ahajournals.org/cgi/content/short/116/17/e418 file://C:\A_journals\Guidelines\Fleisher_Circ2007_.pdf.
6. Sahai SK, Zalpour A, Rozner MA. Preoperative evaluation of the oncology patient. *Med Clin North Am*. 2010;94(2):403-419.
7. Sahai SK. Perioperative care of the patient with cancer. Johns Hopkins Consultative Medicine Essentials for Hospitalists Web site. Available at: http://www.jhcape.com/images/mod-10Feb10/fig2_large.jpg. Published: March 1, 2010. Accessed: August 13, 2010.
8. Borentain P, Colson P, Coso D, et al. Clinical and virological factors associated with hepatitis B virus reactivation in HBsAg-negative and anti-HBc antibodies-positive patients undergoing chemotherapy and/or autologous stem cell transplantation for cancer. *J Viral Hepat*. 2010;17(11):807-815.
9. Jakobisiak M, Golab J. Statins can modulate effectiveness of antitumor therapeutic modalities. *Med Res Rev*. 2010;30(1):102-135.

10. Feldman LS, Brotman DJ. Perioperative statins: more than lipid-lowering? *Cleve Clin J Med.* 2008;75(9):654-662.
11. Adcock DM, Fink LM, Marlar RA, Cavallo F, Zangari M. The hemostatic system and malignancy. *Clin Lymphoma Myeloma.* 2008;8(4):230-236.
12. Gouin-Thibault I, Achkar A, Samama MM. The thrombophilic state in cancer patients. *Acta Haematol.* 2001;106(1–2):33-42.
13. Lyman GH, Khorana AA, Falanga A, et al. American Society of Clinical Oncology guideline: recommendations for venous thromboembolism prophylaxis and treatment in patients with cancer. *J Clin Oncol.* 2007;25(34):5490-5505.
14. Wagman LD, Baird MF, Bennett CL, et al. Venous thromboembolic disease NCCN. Clinical practice guidelines in oncology. *J Natl Compr Canc Netw.* 2008;6(8):716-753.
15. Maggi L, Andreetta F, Antozzi C, et al. Thymoma-associated myasthenia gravis: outcome, clinical and pathological correlations in 197 patients on a 20-year experience. *J Neuroimmunol.* 2008;201–202:237–244.
16. O'Neill GN. Acquired disorders of the neuromuscular junction. *Int Anesthesiol Clin.* 2006; 44(2):107-121.

HIV

25

Richard B. Brooks

25.1 Introduction

- In the past, HIV was often detected late in the disease course and management consisted primarily of treating associated opportunistic infections. With better surveillance and the development of more effective antiretroviral medications with fewer toxic side effects, HIV is in many ways now viewed as a chronic illness requiring long-term management. Despite these advances, an estimated 21% of HIV-infected individuals are unaware of their infection.[1] More attention has therefore been focused on identifying these individuals through screening and targeted testing.
- Many data suggest that people with HIV may be susceptible to an accelerated aging process and the chronic medical conditions associated with aging. If present, these comorbid conditions may confer additional perioperative risk for HIV+ persons.[2]
- Prospective studies have estimated the risk of HIV transmission to healthcare personnel via a percutaneous exposure to be approximately 0.3%. Mucous membrane exposures carry a significantly lower risk, approximately 0.09%. Risk of transmission is increased for procedures using hollow-bore needles, deeper injuries, when blood is visible on the device, when a needle is placed directly into the patient's vein or artery, and for exposures to blood from patients with terminal illnesses, likely reflecting exposure to a greater number of infectious particles. The risk of HIV transmission from healthcare personnel to patients is exceedingly low. As of 2009, only four instances involving nine patients had been documented in the literature. Healthcare workers should use universal precautions for all patients, regardless of HIV infection status. This should include wearing gloves and masks with face shields when handling blood, semen, or vaginal secretions.[3]

R.B. Brooks
Department of Medicine, University of California,
San Francisco General Hospital,
San Francisco, CA, USA
e-mail: richard.brooks@ucsf.edu

S.L. Cohn (ed.), *Perioperative Medicine*,
DOI: 10.1007/978-0-85729-498-2_25,

25.2 Patient-Specific Risk-Factors

- An individual's CD4 count determines his/her immune status and risk for opportunistic infections (see Table 25.1).
- An individual's HIV viral load is directly proportional to the rate of disease progression and the risk of infecting others. The viral load is also used to determine a person's response to antiviral therapy.
- Potential perioperative problems associated with HIV infection or antiretroviral treatment include the following:
  - Cytopenias, including anemia, leukopenia, and thrombocytopenia may increase risk of infection and bleeding
  - Coagulopathy
    - Lupus anticoagulant and elevated PTT (generally a lab artifact with no true elevated risk for bleeding or thrombosis)
    - Particularly if co-infected with HCV or HBV causing advanced liver disease
  - Adrenal insufficiency (conflicting data about whether this is truly more common among the general HIV+ population) can be caused by the interaction of ritonavir and corticosteroids – may increase risk of hypotension.
  - Drug-induced hepatotoxicity
  - Drug-induced nephrotoxicity
  - HIV-associated nephropathy

Table 25.1 Common opportunistic infections in HIV+ persons and recommended prophylactic regimens

Opportunistic infection	CD4 count at which pt. is at risk	First-line prophylaxis	Second-line prophylaxis
***Pneumocystis* Pneumonia (PCP)**	CD4 <200 cells/mm^3 or history of thrush	Trimethoprim/ sulfamethoxazole 160/800 mg PO daily	Dapsone 100 mg PO daily
Mucocutaneous Candidasis (thrush)	CD4 <200 cells/mm^3	None for primary prophylaxis	
***Toxoplasma gondii* encephalitis**	CD4 <100 cells/mm^3 and positive IgG serology	Trimethoprim/ sulfamethoxazole 160/800 mg PO daily	Dapsone 50 mg daily + pyrimethamine 50 mg PO qweek + leucovorin 25 mg PO qweek
Disseminated *Mycobacterium avium* complex (MAC)	CD4 <50 cells/mm^3	Azithromycin 1,200 mg PO weekly or clarithromycin 500 mg PO BID	Rifabutin 300 mg PO daily

– Metabolic disturbances, e.g., insulin resistance, dyslipidemia, lipodystrophy, leading to premature atherosclerosis
– Malnutrition and wasting, which may inhibit optimal wound healing
– Hyperbilirubinemia from atazanavir – This is harmless but may be confused with other causes of hyperbilirubinemia (see Chap. 42- postoperative jaundice)
– Drug–drug interactions
– Increased risk for drug reactions and hypersensitivity reactions

25.3 Surgery-Specific Risk Factors

- Overall, most surgical procedures can be safely performed in HIV+ patients who generally tolerate surgery very well.
- Based on the findings of a retrospective case–control study, HIV+ patients may have an increased risk for postoperative pneumonia compared to their HIV- counterparts. This study included patients undergoing a wide variety of surgeries. Importantly, rates of other complications did not differ between HIV+ and HIV- patients. Patients in this study had relatively well-preserved CD4 counts and suppressed viral loads. Having a viral load of >30K copies/mL conferred higher risk for complications.[4]
- A retrospective study of trauma patients showed that HIV+ patients had higher risks for certain infectious postoperative complications, such as pneumonia, bacteremia, and wound infections. Mortality, however, did not differ compared to HIV- patients.[5]
- In a retrospective study of HIV+ patients undergoing total knee and hip replacements, complication rates did not differ between HIV+ and HIV- patients.[6]
- A retrospective study comparing HIV+ women to HIV- women undergoing cesarean section revealed higher postoperative complication rates, including endometritis, need for transfusion, pneumonia, maternal sepsis, ICU admission, and maternal death even after adjustment for confounding factors. Of note, however, data on CD4 count and viral load were not collected, and two of three deaths in the HIV+ group were in women who met diagnostic criteria for AIDS.[7]
- HIV is no longer a criterion for exclusion for organ transplants. Outcomes for HIV+ patients vary depending on the organ being transplanted and the underlying disease necessitating the need for transplant. For optimal outcomes, transplant patients' HIV should be well-controlled with a suppressed viral load on a stable antiretroviral regimen prior to transplant.[8]

25.4 Preoperative Evaluation

- The preoperative evaluation should begin with taking a thorough history, including assessing the patient's risk factors for HIV infection, such as intravenous drug use, history of transfusions, sexual history, history of trading sex for money or drugs, and number of sexual partners.

- If the patient is already known to be infected with HIV, obtain additional history including length of infection, current and nadir CD4 count, current HIV RNA level, history of opportunistic infections, and the presence of any comorbidities, especially cardiac, renal, liver disease, and diabetes.
- If the patient is at increased risk for HIV or has never been tested before, they should be offered an HIV test. The Centers for Disease Control and Prevention (CDC) now recommends routine screening HIV tests for all persons aged 13–64 although it is unlikely to change management in the perioperative setting. HIV testing is now considered part of routine medical care by the CDC and thus in many states no longer requires separate, written consent.[9]
- Be sure to thoroughly review the patient's current medications, with particular attention paid to antiretroviral medications and opportunistic infection prophylaxis. Do not forget to ask about over-the-counter and herbal medication use. Also ask about allergies, as HIV+ patients have higher rates of allergic reactions to many medications.[10]
- Ask about current and past tobacco use, as it is more common in HIV+ individuals, and encourage smoking cessation (see Chap. 21 on pulmonary complications). Ascertain history about abuse of other substances as well, and watch patients with a history of alcohol dependence for signs and symptoms of alcohol withdrawal.
- Perform a complete review of symptoms to elicit any symptoms of underlying disease that the patient may not have volunteered.
- Perform a thorough physical exam focusing on the cardiopulmonary system and looking for oropharyngeal thrush, lymphadenopathy, or other signs of infection.
- While physicians may be tempted to do an extensive laboratory workup for HIV+ patients prior to surgery, there is little data to support the clinical benefit or cost-effectiveness of doing so. A reasonable approach would be to check a CBC and basic metabolic panel. If the patient has a known history of or risk factors for liver disease, one could check a liver panel. If not checked in the last 3–6 months, a CD4 and HIV viral load should be ordered. Unless indicated by history or abnormalities found on physical exam, there is no proven utility in ordering a PT/PTT, electrocardiogram, or chest X-ray (see Chap. 2 on Preoperative Testing).
- If information on co-infections such as HBV, HCV, syphilis, other sexually transmitted diseases and TB is not available by chart review or history, one should use clinical judgment to determine whether to send the appropriate tests to evaluate for these. For example, there would be little utility with regard to perioperative risk reduction in testing a patient for TB who has no prior history of TB and no history of cough, fever, hemoptysis, weight loss, or TB exposures.
- As with all patients, discuss and document preferences for a health care proxy and advanced directives.

25.5 Perioperative Management

- Direct, ongoing communication with the patient's primary care provider and/or HIV provider can be extremely useful to ensure continuation of the correct medication regimen and for confirmation of past medical history.

Table 25.2 2009 Department of Health and Human Services revised guidelines on when to start antiretroviral therapy in HIV+ persons

CD4 count at which to start treatment*	Level of recommendation** and evidence***
<350 or AIDS-defining illness	AI
350–500	AII (55% of panel), BII (45% of panel)
>500	BIII (50% of panel), CIII (50% of panel)

*Regardless of CD4 count, all pregnant patients, those with HIV-associated nephropathy, and those co-infected with HBV requiring treatment should receive antiretroviral therapy
**Level of recommendation: *A*=strong, *B*=moderate, *C*=Optional
***Level of evidence: *I*=data from RCTs, *II*=data from well-designed non-randomized trials or observational cohort studies with long-term clinical outcomes, *III*=expert opinion

- New guidelines released by the DHHS in December 2009 have expanded treatment recommendations to include more people (see Table 25.2). Given that studies have found higher post-operative complication rates for people with elevated viral loads, it would be reasonable to delay elective procedures until a patient is on a fully suppressive antiviral regimen, assuming s/he meets criteria for treatment. Ensure the patient is on appropriate prophylaxis for opportunistic infections (OIs) based on CD4 count and history of previous OIs (see Table 25.1).[11]
- With each missed dose of antiretroviral medications, risk for development of resistant virus increases. Therefore, continuation of a patient's antiretroviral medications, even while NPO, is preferred. In the case the patient is unable to tolerate pills, some antiretroviral medications come in liquid forms or in tablets that can be dissolved and given via feeding tube. Discuss options with an HIV specialist or an experienced pharmacist. Because of more complicated pharmacokinetics, NNRTI-containing antiretroviral regimens have a lower threshold for fostering resistance; therefore, if there is a need to stop a patient's NNRTI-based regimen for any length of time, it should only be done with expert guidance.
- Be aware that certain drugs (e.g., statins, PPIs) often used prophylactically for surgical or hospitalized patients may have drug interactions or contraindications for use with certain antiretroviral drugs.
- Given the increased rates of malnutrition and wasting among HIV+ patients, especially those with advanced disease, it would be reasonable to encourage increased caloric and protein intake for these patients prior to surgery. However, data showing improved outcomes with use of appetite stimulants or specific nutritional supplements in this setting are lacking.
- HIV+ patients require standard antibiotic prophylaxis for surgical wound infections based on the type of surgery and other underlying medical conditions. HIV in and of itself does not necessitate additional or broader coverage.
- To prevent perinatal HIV transmission, scheduled cesarean section at 38 weeks of gestation is recommended for pregnant women with an HIV viral load >1,000 copies/mL near the time of delivery or who have unknown HIV viral load levels.[12]
- Indications for prevention of postoperative venous thromboembolic disease are no different for HIV+ patients than for the HIV- population.

- The workup for postoperative fever in HIV+ patients should be largely the same as for HIV- patients (see Chap. 33). Given that several studies have found increased rates of pneumonia and wound infections in this population, particular attention may be given to ruling out these infections. In patients with low CD4 counts, opportunistic infections can be the cause of postoperative fever but are significantly less common.
- In critically ill patients who have hypotension of unclear etiology, consider testing and treating for adrenal insufficiency, as some studies have suggested an increased risk for adrenal insufficiency in HIV+ patients.
- HIV+ patients are at increased risk of neutropenia; however, treating neutropenia with granulocyte-colony stimulating factor (G-CSF) in this population is controversial. No prospective trials have demonstrated any mortality benefit to doing so. On the other hand, one open-label, randomized, controlled trial in HIV+ patients with a CD4 count <200 cells/mm^3 and absolute neutrophil count <1,000 cells/mm^3 demonstrated reduced rates of bacterial infections, shorter length of hospitalization, and shorter duration of treatment with intravenous antibiotics when the neutropenia was treated w/ recombinant G-CSF.[13]
- In the event that a healthcare provider may have had an occupational exposure to HIV, their local occupational health office should be contacted immediately. Postexposure prophylaxis is effective at preventing infection with HIV but must be instituted as soon as possible. A national telephone hotline with advice regarding postexposure prophylaxis is available at 1-888-448-4911.

References

1. CDC. HIV prevalence estimates–United States, 2006. MMWR. 2008;57[No. 39]:1073–1076.
2. Desquilbet L, Jacobson L, Fried LP, et al. Multicenter AIDS cohort study. HIV-1 infection is associated with an earlier occurrence of a phenotype related to frailty. *J Gerontol Biol Sci Med Sci*. 2007;62A:1279-86.
3. CDC. Updated U.S. Public Health Service guidelines for the management of occupational exposures to HIV and recommendations for postexposure prophylaxis. MMWR. 2005;54[No. RR-09]: 1–17.
4. Horberg MA, Hurley LB, Klein DB, et al. Surgical outcomes in human immunodeficiency virus-infected patients in the era of highly active antiretroviral therapy. *Arch Surg*. 2006; 141:1238-45.
5. Morrison CA, Wyatt WM, Carrick MM. Effects of human immunodeficiency virus status on trauma outcomes: a review of the national trauma database. *Surg Infect*. 2010;11:41-7.
6. Habermann B, Eberhardt C, Kurth AA. Total joint replacements in HIV positive patients. *J Infect*. 2008;57:41-6.
7. Louis J, Landon MB, Gersnoviez RJ, et al. Perioperative morbidity and mortality among human immunodeficiency virus infected women undergoing cesarean delivery. *Obstet Gynecol*. 2007;110:385-90.
8. Blumberg EA, Stock P. The AST Infectious Diseases Community of Practice. Solid organ transplantation in the HIV-infected patient. *Am J Transplant*. 2009;9:S131-S135.

9. CDC. Revised recommendations for HIV testing of adults, adolescents, and pregnant women in health-care settings. MMWR. 2006;55[No. RR-14]:1–17.
10. Coopman SA, Johnson RA, Platt R, Stern RS. Cutaneous disease and drug reactions in HIV infection. *N Engl J Med*. 1993;328:1670-1674.
11. Panel on Antiretroviral Guidelines for Adults and Adolescents. Guidelines for the use of antiretroviral agents in HIV-1-infected adults and adolescents. Department of Health and Human Services. January 10, 2011; 1–161. Available at http://www.aidsinfo.nih.gov/ContentFiles/AdultandAdolescentGL.pdf. Accessed 5/7/10.
12. Perinatal HIV Guidelines Working Group. Public Health Service Task Force. Recommendations for Use of Antiretroviral Drugs in Pregnant HIV-Infected. Women for Maternal Health and Interventions to Reduce Perinatal HIV Transmission in the United States. May 24, 2010; pp 1–90. Available at http://aidsinfo.nih.gov/ContentFiles/PerinatalGL.pdf. Accessed 3/3/10.
13. Kuritzkes DR, Parenti D, Ward DJ, et al. Filgrastim prevents severe neutropenia and reduces infective morbidity in patients with advanced HIV infection: results of a randomized, multicenter, controlled trial. G-CSF 930101 Study Group. *AIDS*. 1998;12:65-74.

Chronic Kidney Disease 26

Mihaela S. Stefan and Adam C. Schaffer

26.1 Introduction

- The estimated prevalence of chronic kidney disease (CKD) (Table 26.1) is 23.2 million or 11.5% of the U.S. adult population[1] and millions of patients with renal dysfunction have surgery each year.
- Patients with CKD have a two- to fivefold higher risk of death and cardiovascular complications after elective, noncardiac surgery than those with normal renal function. The level of baseline renal function prior to surgery influences the risk of both postoperative acute kidney injury (AKI) (see AKI definition in Table 26.2) and postoperative mortality.[2]
- Patients who develop postoperative AKI have an increased length of stay and higher mortality.
- Although patients with CKD usually have multiple comorbidities and risk factors for postoperative complications, CKD per se is an independent predictor for postoperative death and complications.
- Patients on dialysis have the highest risk of postoperative death and complications and they pose specific challenges in the pre and postoperative period.
- Most death are caused by cardiovascular events, myocardial infarction, congestive heart failure (CHF), pulmonary edema, cardiac arrest, and arrhythmia followed by sepsis.
- Patients with CKD are at higher risk for developing postoperative sepsis, fluid overload, acid–base and electrolyte disturbances (especially hyperkalemia), acute kidney injury and bleeding.
- A comprehensive preoperative evaluation with particular attention to cardiac function and volume status optimization is essential for minimizing postoperative complications.
- As for other patients, the risk of postoperative complications in patients with CKD is dependent on the type of surgical procedure, whether the surgery is emergent or elective, patient-specific risk factors, and the degree of renal dysfunction.
- Postoperative renal failure (Chap. 40), fluid and electrolyte disorders (Chap. 39), and anesthesia (Chap. 8) are discussed separately.

M.S. Stefan (✉)
Department of Medicine, Baystate Medical Center/Tufts University School of Medicine,
759 Chestnut Street, Springfield, MA 01199, USA
e-mail: mihaela.stefan@bhs.org

S.L. Cohn (ed.), *Perioperative Medicine*,
DOI: 10.1007/978-0-85729-498-2_26,

Table 26.1 Stages of chronic kidney disease

Stage	Description	GFR (mL/min/1.73 m²)
1	Kidney damage with normal or increased GFR	>90
2	Kidney damage with mild decrease in GFR	60–89
3	Moderate decrease in GFR	30–59
4	Severe decrease in GFR	15–29
5	Kidney failure	<15 (or dialysis)

Chronic kidney disease (CKD) is defined as either kidney damage or GFR <60 mL/min/1.73 m² for≥3 months. Kidney damage is defined as pathologic abnormalities or markers of damage, including abnormalities in blood or urine tests or imaging studies

Table 26.2 Classification/staging system for acute kidney injury[15]

Stage serum creatinine criteria	Urine output criteria
1 Increase in serum creatinine ≥0.3 mg/dL (≥26.4 mol/L) or increase to more than or equal to 150–200% (1.5- to 2-fold) from baseline	Less than 0.5 mL/kg/h for more than 6 h
2 Increase in serum creatinine to more than 200–300% (>2- to 3-fold) from baseline	Less than 0.5 mL/kg/h for more than 12 h
3[a] Increase in serum creatinine to more than 300% (>3-fold) from baseline or serum creatinine ≥4.0 mg/dL [≥354 mol/L] with an acute increase of at least 0.5 mg/dL [44 mol/L]	Less than 0.3 mL/kg/h for 24 h or anuria for 12 h

Modified from RIFLE (Risk, Injury, Failure, Loss, and End-stage kidney disease) criteria. The staging system proposed is a highly sensitive, interim staging system and is based on data indicating that a small change in serum creatinine influences outcome. Only one criterion (creatinine or urine output) has to be fulfilled to qualify for a stage

[a]Given wide variation in indications and timing of initiation of renal replacement therapy (RRT), individuals who receive RRT are considered to have met the criteria for stage 3 irrespective of the stage they are in at the time of RRT

26.2 Patient-Specific Risk Factors (Table 26.3)

- Preoperative renal dysfunction is the strongest predictor for postoperative renal failure.
  - Patients with a mild decrease in glomerular filtration rate (GFR > 60 mL/min) undergoing noncardiac surgery do not have a higher risk of major postoperative complications or death compared with patients with normal renal function. The management of such patients in the perioperative period should include the standard precautions for renal protection taken for any other patients.

Table 26.3 Risk factors for postoperative acute kidney injury (AKI) or acute renal failure (ARF) after noncardiac surgery

Patient risk factors	Surgical risk factors
Preexisting CKD	High-risk surgery – intraperitoneal or vascular
Advanced age	Emergency surgery
CHF	
HTN	
DM	
COPD	
Liver disease	
Ascites	
Gender (men)	

- A recent study[3] of patients undergoing general surgery found mild and moderate renal insufficiency (serum creatinine 1.2–2 mg/dL) to be major predictors for postoperative acute kidney injury (hazard ratio 3.2). Other independent predictors were intraperitoneal surgery, active heart failure, ascites, emergency surgery, diabetes mellitus (DM), hypertension (HTN), male gender, and age >56.
- There is a graded relationship between the serum creatinine (and estimated glomerular filtration rate) and postoperative morbidity and mortality. Patients with creatinine between 1.5 and 3 mg/dL undergoing general surgery have a significant higher rate of 30-day mortality and morbidity (10.1% and 21.6%, respectively) than patients with creatinine less than 1.5 mg/dL (3.5% and 12%, respectively). The mortality and morbidity rates increase to 20% and 31%, respectively, for patients with a creatinine >3 mg/dL.[4] The risk of postoperative complications, such as sepsis, cardiac arrest, bleeding, and respiratory complications, is also higher in patients with a creatinine >3 mg/dL.

• Patients with end-stage renal disease (ESRD) on dialysis have an even higher risk of death and postoperative complications.

- Advanced renal dysfunction is an immunocompromised state (with reduced chemotaxis of neutrophils and decreased antibody response) predisposing patients to impaired wound healing and postoperative infections.
- Overall reported postoperative complication rate for patients on hemodialysis (HD) is 54–64%. The most common complication is hyperkalemia.[5] Other frequent complications are infections, hemodynamic instability, fluid overload, and operative site hematoma.
- Patients on peritoneal dialysis pose an increased challenge when undergoing abdominal surgeries. They have a high risk of developing peritonitis, incisional hernia, and protracted wound healing.
- Autonomic neuropathy is frequent in patients with end-stage renal disease and may result in delayed gastric emptying, variable blood pressure, and cardiac arrhythmias.

26.3 Surgery-Specific Risk Factors

- The most common procedure for patients with advanced CKD is access for dialysis, followed by procedures for peripheral vascular disease, coronary artery disease (CAD), and kidney transplantation.[6]
- Overall postoperative in-hospital mortality of patients with ESRD on dialysis undergoing general surgery is 4–10% and postoperative morbidity is between 46% and 54%.[7]
- Emergent surgery is associated with an increased risk for morbidity and mortality in CKD patients. For example, emergent abdominal surgery in patients on dialysis has a mortality rate of 24–40% and complications rate of 54–62%. There is an unusually high prevalence of nonocclusive mesenteric ischemia, and bowel infarction seems to be a common cause of acute abdomen in HD patients.[8]
- Abdominal laparoscopic surgical techniques may decrease renal perfusion as intra-abdominal pressure increases. To lessen the effects of elevated intra-abdominal pressure, preoperative euvolemia or fluid loading is advocated.[9]

26.3.1 Aortic and Vascular Surgery

- After abdominal aortic aneurysm repair, the postoperative mortality is 3.2% in patients with preoperative normal renal function and 9.2% in patients with chronic kidney disease.[2]
- Outcome is also poor after infrainguinal bypass procedures in patients on maintenance dialysis: 9% mortality and 39% morbidity. Complications include wound breakdown, graft thrombosis, and limb amputation, and only half of the patients survive 2 years.[10]
- Perioperative mortality is also much higher after carotid endarterectomy in patients with CKD compared with those with normal renal function (3.9% vs. 1%).[11] Mortality is as high as 17% in patients with creatinine > 3 mg/dL and stroke rate is 4.3%, raising the question if selection criteria should be different for patients with CKD.

26.3.2 Obstructive Jaundice

- The association between obstructive jaundice and perioperative renal failure is well known, but the etiology of renal dysfunction is less clear. Patients with obstructive jaundice have a significant decrease in the effective plasma volume with volume depletion of 3–4% of body weight (1.8–2 L) and may have systemic endotoxemia. Serum bilirubin, patient's age, degree of volume depletion, and urinary sodium excretion are important predictors of the renal dysfunction in patients with obstructive jaundice.[12]

26.3.3 Anesthesia

- The anesthesia team needs to be aware of the degree of patient's renal dysfunction to be able to choose the appropriate anesthetic and method of anesthesia. Dosing may need to be reduced, and long-acting muscle relaxants should be avoided.
- The presence of platelet dysfunction and bleeding tendency in patients with advanced CKD raises concerns regarding possible increased risk of epidural hematoma with the use of epidural anesthesia.

26.4 Preoperative Evaluation

26.4.1 General Issues

- Patients with CKD may have overlapping comorbidities such as diabetes mellitus, cardiovascular disease, hypertension, anemia, neuropathy, poor nutritional status, bone disease, and dyslipidemia. The goal of the preoperative evaluation is to optimize any of the above modifiable factors before surgery (Table 26.4).
- The preoperative evaluation should include a detailed review of systems with particular attention to renal-related comorbidities, a careful physical exam, electrocardiogram, and screening laboratory tests including a blood count, metabolic panel, serum magnesium, and phosphorus levels, as well as a coagulation profile.[13]

Table 26.4 Factors that increase postoperative morbidity in patients with chronic kidney disease

Renal factors	Nonrenal factors
Decrease ability to dilute urine	Anemia
Impaired sodium excretion	Bleeding tendency
Limited ability to excrete acid	Immunocompromised state
Decreased capacity to excrete drugs	Autonomic neuropathy
	Malnutrition
	Arrhythmia
	Multiple comorbidities (DM, HTN, CAD, CHF)

26.4.1.1
Assessing GFR

- Traditionally, plasma creatinine has been used for preoperative assessment of renal function. Although creatinine level is a specific marker of renal impairment, it has a low sensitivity for mild and moderate degrees of renal dysfunction because it depends on many extra renal factors such as muscle mass, gender, and age. GFR may be reduced by as much as 50% with serum creatinine still in the normal range.
- Creatinine clearance (CrCl) can be calculated by Cockcroft–Gault formula or by Modification of Diet in Renal Disease Study Group (MDRD) formula.

Cockcroft–Gault equation:
Men: 140 − age (years) × weight (kg)/serum creatinine (mg/dL) × 72
Women: 140 − age (years) × weight (kg) × 0.85/serum creatinine (mg/dL) × 72
MDRD equation: GFR (mL/min/1.73 m^2) = 175 × (serum creatinine)$^{-1.154}$ × (Age)$^{-0.203}$ × (0.742 if female) × (1.212 if African American)

- As already demonstrated by multiple studies, estimated GFR is a much more powerful predictor of perioperative mortality risk as serum creatinine alone and a graded relationship exists between the severity of preoperative renal impairment and the incidence of postoperative adverse events.
- If AKI is identified in a patient with preexisting CKD, a thorough evaluation of the precipitating factors should be performed. If the procedure is urgent (for example, surgery for hip fracture), the goal is to manage precipitating factors and optimize patient's status before the underlying condition deteriorates further. Elective surgery should be postponed if new, significant AKI is identified preoperatively and a workup to determine the cause of the renal dysfunction should be undertaken. See Chap. 40 regarding the workup of postoperative AKI.

26.4.1.2
Cardiovascular Risk Stratification

- Cardiovascular disease remains the main factor for death in patients with ESRD. A preoperative creatinine of more than 2 mg/dL was found to be associated with major cardiac complications in 9% of cases,[14] was included in the Lee Revised Cardiac Risk Index (RCRI), and as one of the prognostic variables in the American College of Cardiology/American Heart Association (ACC/AHA) guidelines on perioperative cardiovascular evaluation. (See Chap. 20 regarding the cardiac risk assessments).
  - The prevalence of coronary artery disease (CAD) in patients with ESRD on dialysis is approximately 40% and of left ventricular hypertrophy is approximately 75%.[7]
  - In patients with advanced CKD, assessing functional capacity, (which is an essential part of the ACC/AHA preoperative algorithm), may be difficult because patients with ESRD may have anemia, bone disease, neuropathy, claudication, and weakness secondary to dialysis.

 - Clinical manifestations of CAD and CHF may be atypical in patients with ESRD. If preoperative stress testing is indicated, pharmacologic testing with dipyridamole-thallium imaging or dobutamine stress echocardiography is often necessary in ESRD and renal transplant patients. If the patient has history of CHF, a resting echocardiogram can be obtained to evaluate the left ventricular ejection fraction.

- Prospective recipients for renal transplant at risk for cardiovascular complications (diabetics, long duration of dialysis, vascular disease, and any history of CAD or CHF) often have cardiac workup prior to transplantation even when they are asymptomatic. The goal is to optimize long-term survival since the number of donor kidneys is limited. If significant coronary artery stenosis is found, revascularization is most likely recommended.

26.4.1.3 Renal Transplant Patients

- To avoid deterioration of the renal function, consultation with patient's nephrologist is strongly recommended.
  - Patients with a renal transplant are maintained on immunosuppressive therapy and glucocorticoids and some might have secondary adrenal insufficiency caused by chronic glucocorticoid therapy. Depending on the type of surgery, stress-dose steroid might be indicated in the perioperative period. If the patient develops unexplained findings consistent with adrenocortical insufficiency, such as hypotension, hyponatremia, hyperkalemia, stress-dose steroids should be considered.
  - In hospitalized renal transplant patients on calcineurin inhibitors, such as tacrolimus or cyclosporine, levels of the calcineurin inhibitors should be monitored.

26.5 Preoperative Management (Risk Reduction Strategies)

- Patients with underlying preoperative renal dysfunction have a lower renal reserve and are more susceptible to perioperative insults and to development of new renal injury.
- The major goals of preoperative management are to ensure euvolemia, adequately control blood pressure, correct hyperkalemia and acidosis, minimize bleeding tendency in uremic patients, and avoid nephrotoxic agents (Table 26.5).

26.5.1 Fluid Management

- Volume status needs to be optimized before surgery to assure an adequate kidney perfusion and avoid renal ischemic insult. For those patients not on dialysis, judicious use of diuretics and hydration as appropriate can achieve euvolemia.

Table 26.5 Common postoperative complications in patients with chronic kidney disease

Acute kidney injury
Arrhythmia
Hyperkalemia
Fluid and electrolytes imbalance
Metabolic acidosis
Pericarditis
Postoperative infections
Hypo/hypertension
Bleeding
Acute congestive heart failure
Perioperative myocardial infarction
Worsening anemia

- Maintenance of euvolemia is the goal in the perioperative period and for fluid management, crystalloids are used. It is commonly recommended to titrate crystalloid infusion to maintain mean arterial pressure >65–70 mmHg, urine output>0.5 cc/kg/h, and central venous pressure 10–15 mmHg.
- Patients with CHF and advanced CKD not on dialysis represent a challenge, and very careful assessment of daily weights, amount of fluid infused, and urinary output is necessary. For these patients, a multidisciplinary approach, including a renal consultation is recommended. In the postoperative period, careful recording of the daily weights, intake and output of fluids, clinical assessment of the fluid status, and daily electrolytes and creatinine must be performed until the patient is stable.

26.5.2 Hyper- and Hypotension Management

- Intraoperative hypotension is considered a risk factor for AKI after surgery, and hypotension or hypertension during surgery is correlated with perioperative cardiac events.
- Approximately 5% of patients on HD have chronic hypotension. During the postoperative period, hypotension might be exacerbated by bleeding, arrhythmia, or low intravascular volume. If a patient is on midodrine (a selective alpha-1 adrenergic agonist), this should be continued without interruption during the perioperative period.
- Difficult-to-control hypertension is frequent in patients with advanced CKD. Antihypertensive medications need to be continued through the perioperative period. If the patient is NPO or the blood pressure does not respond to the oral medications, intravenous labetalol or hydralazine can be used.

26.5.3 Electrolyte Management

- Hyperkalemia is the most frequent electrolyte abnormality in the postoperative period. The management of hyperkalemia in patients with CKD is not different from other patients. An electrocardiogram should be obtained, and if there are signs of hyperkalemia, such as peaked T waves or QRS prolongation, aggressive medical management to reduce the potassium level is needed.
  - Calcium gluconate (1 ampule of 1,000 mg) helps stabilize the cardiac membranes.
  - Insulin (10 units intravenous) and dextrose (1/2 or 1 ampule of Dextrose 50%) reduces the serum potassium level by shifting the potassium from the serum compartment to the intracellular compartment.
  - Sodium polystyrene sulfonate (a cation exchange resin) given orally 15–30 g is useful in removing potassium via stool.
  - Patients on dialysis should undergo emergent dialysis to remove potassium if medical management is not successful.

26.5.4 Metabolic Acidosis

- Patients with CKD and metabolic acidosis have a reduced ability to compensate for respiratory acidosis. In the perioperative period, hypercapnia can be worsened by sedatives and analgesics.
  - Patients who already use positive pressure devices should bring their CPAP/BIPAP in the hospital and use them after surgery.

26.5.5 Anemia

- Anemia is frequent in patients with CKD and may necessitate preoperative transfusion or treatment with iron or erythropoietin, especially for surgeries with expected significant blood loss. Patients with concomitant CAD and CHF should have their hematocrit optimized and for intermediate and high-risk surgeries, a hematocrit>28% is recommended.
- Desmopressin (dDAVP, L-desamino-8-D-arginine vasopressin) can be used in case of bleeding in uremic patients.

26.5.6 Medications

- Medications should be adjusted for the GFR level, and all potential nephrotoxic medications should be avoided. Dose adjustment is generally not necessary until the GFR is less than 60 mL/min/1.73 m^2.

- Perioperative antibiotics may require dosage adjustment based on GFR.
- When selecting an analgesic, anesthetic, or neuromuscular agent, consideration should be given to the impact of the altered renal function on the elimination of the drug, potential for accumulation and active metabolites.
- Nonsteroidal anti-inflammatory agents (NSAIDs), including Ketorolac (a parenteral compound), have multiple side effects in patients with CKD and should not be used in the perioperative period. NSAIDS are nephrotoxic and can precipitate an acute decrease in GFR and also increase the risk of gastrointestinal bleeding.
- Angiotensin-converting enzyme inhibitors (ACEI) and angiotensin II antagonists (ARA) are commonly used by patients with CKD and might be associated with intraoperative hypotension with induction of general anesthesia. It is advisable to discontinue these agents on the morning of surgery requiring general anesthesia, particularly in a patient whose blood pressure is on the low side.
- Antiplatelet therapy (aspirin and/or clopidogrel) is commonly used in this population. The decision to continue or stop them depends on the surgical bleeding risk, the risk assessment of the underlying condition, and the choice of anesthetic technique. Dual antiplatelet therapy should be continued for at least 1 month after placement of a bare metal stent and for at least 12 months after placement of a drug-eluting stent to minimize the risk of stent thrombosis (see Chap. 20).
- Narcotics
  - Morphine is metabolized in the liver but its active metabolite, morphine-3-glucoronide is renal eliminated, and its half-life is significantly prolonged in renal failure. Morphine is eliminated with HD.
  - Fentanyl is extensively metabolized in the liver, and <10% is eliminated unchanged in the urine.
  - Oxycodone is metabolized in the liver to oxymorphone, half-life of which is significantly prolonged in renal failure.
  - The dosage of the opioids should be reduced and the interval of administration increased in patients with renal failure.
  - Meperidine is contraindicated in patients with renal failure; its active metabolite normeperidine is associated with seizures, myoclonus, and altered mental status in patients with CKD.

26.5.7 Patients on Dialysis

- To minimize the risk of fluid overload, electrolyte imbalance, and hemodynamic instability, patients on HD should have dialysis within 24 h of surgery and be at or close to their "dry weight." Postoperatively, patients should undergo heparin-free dialysis if the anticipated bleeding risk of surgery is high. Close collaboration with a nephrologist is essential.
- Intravenous access can be more difficult in this population and some patients may require central venous access if postoperative intravenous therapy is needed.

- Patients on chronic peritoneal dialysis should have the abdomen drained before any abdominal surgery. Draining the peritoneal fluid decreases the intra-abdominal pressure, making ventilation easier and decreasing the risk of aspiration. For nonabdominal surgery, peritoneal dialysis can be restarted immediately after the procedure. Following abdominal surgery the patient should be maintained on hemodialysis until the surgical site is healed, to decrease the risk of anastomotic leak, wound dehiscence and infection, and incisional hernia.

26.5.8 Use of Intravenous Contrast Agents

- Patients who already have renal insufficiency are at high risk of developing contrast-induced nephropathy.
- Pre and postinfusion of the contrast agent hydration with normal saline or sodium bicarbonate and N-acetylcysteine are the main prophylactic strategies to decrease the risk of contrast-induced nephropathy.

26.5.9 Obstructive Jaundice Surgery

- Preoperative lactulose and bile salts to prevent postoperative endotoxemia and adequate hydration are paramount in the prevention of postoperative renal failure in patients with obstructive jaundice (Table 26.5).

26.6 Summary

Patients with chronic kidney disease undergoing surgery have a high risk of perioperative death and complications. For those with advanced kidney disease, a comprehensive approach achieved by a multidisciplinary team comprised of the surgeon, anesthesiologist, nephrologist, and medical consultant is necessary to minimize morbidity and mortality.

References

1. Levey AS, Stevens LA, Schmid CH, et al. A new equation to estimate glomerular filtration rate. *Ann Intern Med.* 2009;50(9):604-612.
2. Mathew A, Devereaux PJ, O'Hare A, et al. Chronic kidney disease and postoperative mortality: a systematic review and meta-analysis. *Kidney Int.* 2008;73(9):1069-1081.

3. Kheterpal S, Tremper KK, Englesbe MJ, et al. Predictors of postoperative acute renal failure after noncardiac surgery in patients with previously normal renal function. *Anesthesiology*. 2007;107(6):892-902.
4. O'Brien MM, Gonzales R, Shroyer AL, et al. Modest serum creatinine elevation affects adverse outcome after general surgery. *Kidney Int*. 2002;62(2):585-592.
5. Schreiber S, Korzets A, Powsner E, Wolloch Y. Surgery in chronic dialysis patients. *Isr J Med Sci*. 1995;31(8):479-483.
6. Krishnan M. Preoperative care of patients with kidney disease. *Am Fam Physician*. 2002;66(8):1471-1476.
7. Kellerman PS. Perioperative care of the renal patient. *Arch Intern Med*. 1994;154(15): 1674-1688.
8. Wind P, Douard R, Rouzier R, Berger A, Bony C, Cugnenc PH. Abdominal surgery in chronic hemodialysis patients. *Am Surg*. 1999;65(4):347-351.
9. Demyttenaere S, Feldman LS, Fried GM. Effect of pneumoperitoneum on renal perfusion and function: a systematic review. *Surg Endosc*. 2007;21(2):152-160.
10. Baele HR, Piotrowski JJ, Yuhas J, Anderson C, Alexander JJ. Infrainguinal bypass in patients with end-stage renal disease. *Surgery*. 1995;117(3):319-324.
11. Debing E, Van den Brande P. Chronic renal insufficiency and risk of early mortality in patients undergoing carotid endarterectomy. *Ann Vasc Surg*. 2006;20(5):609-613.
12. Padillo FJ, Cruz A, Briceno J, Martin-Malo A, Pera-Madrazo C, Sitges-Serra A. Multivariate analysis of factors associated with renal dysfunction in patients with obstructive jaundice. *Br J Surg*. 2005;92(11):1388-1392.
13. Joseph AJ, Cohn SL. Perioperative care of the patient with renal failure. *Med Clin North Am*. 2003;87(1):193-210.
14. Lee TH, Marcantonio ER, Mangione CM, et al. Derivation and prospective validation of a simple index for prediction of cardiac risk of major noncardiac surgery. *Circulation*. 1999;100(10):1043-1049.
15. Bellomo R, Ronco C, Kellum JA, Mehta RL, Palevsky P. Acute renal failure – definition, outcome measures, animal models, fluid therapy and information technology needs: the Second International Consensus Conference of the Acute Dialysis Quality Initiative (ADQI) Group. *Crit Care*. 2004;8(4):R204-R212.

GI Disease 27

Nomi L. Traub and Richard B. Brooks

This chapter will discuss three distinct areas of gastrointestinal disease – acid peptic disorders, inflammatory bowel disease, and liver disease.

27.1 Acid-Peptic Disorders and Stress-Related Mucosal Disease

27.1.1 Introduction

Common acid-peptic disorders include gastroesophageal reflux (GERD), gastric and duodenal ulcers (DU), and gastritis.

- The incidence of peptic ulcer disease (PUD) has decreased over the past 2 decades, in association with the development of potent acid suppressants, and the discovery of *Helicobacter pylori* (*H. pylori*). The vast majority of ulcers stem from *H. pylori* infection or the use of nonsteroidal anti-inflammatory drugs (NSAIDs). Despite advances in medical therapy, data suggest that hospitalization rates for complications of PUD remain stable. Surgical procedures to address these complications seem to be on the wane due to advances in endoscopic therapy and pharmacologic regimens to eradicate *H. pylori*. While formerly aimed at curing PUD, currently, surgical intervention is frequently an emergency procedure to control hemorrhage in high-risk patients.
- Stress-related mucosal disease (SRMD) may be considered a form of *H. pylori* – negative and NSAID-negative ulcer, occurring in critically ill patients. The pathogenesis is not well defined. In a small percentage of patients, stress ulcers cause clinically significant hemorrhage, and less commonly, lead to perforation. Hemorrhage and perforation are associated with high mortality rates.

Few data exist on patients with established PUD and nonulcer surgical procedures.

N.L. Traub (✉)
Department of Graduate Medical Education, Atlanta Medical Center, Atlanta, Georgia, USA and Department of Medicine, Medical College of Georgia, Augusta, Georgia, USA
e-mail: nomi.traub@emory.edu

S.L. Cohn (ed.), *Perioperative Medicine*,
DOI: 10.1007/978-0-85729-498-2_27,

27.1.2
Patient-Specific Risk Factors

27.1.2.1
Age

- Esophageal sphincter pressure and peristalsis decrease with age, increasing risk of GERD.
- The prevalence of *H. pylori* infection increases with age, and in the United States, 50% of the population is seropositive by age 60.
- Peptic ulcer bleeding occurs predominantly in the elderly (68% are over the age of 60) in whom it is associated with a high mortality rate.[1]

27.1.2.2
Medications and Substance Use

- NSAIDS and aspirin use increase risk of PUD and bleeding.
- Corticosteroids and anticoagulants increase risk of ulcer bleeding when used with NSAIDs.
- Cigarette smoking may contribute to ulcer risk in patients infected with *H. pylori*.[2]
- History of ulcer complications predicts future ulcer complications associated with NSAID use.

27.1.2.3
Critical Care Issues

- Risk factors for mortality in perforated ulcers include preoperative shock, major medical illnesses, perforation $>$24 h,[3] and age over 70 years, which is associated with use of NSAIDs.[4]
- Mechanical ventilation $>$48 h and coagulopathy (defined as platelet count $<$50,000/μL, INR $>$1.5, or PTT $>$2 times the control value) are risks for SRMD which may lead to erosive gastritis.[5]
- Postoperative ileus, abdominal distention, and nasogastric tube use may worsen GERD and increase risk of aspiration.

27.1.3
Surgery-Specific Risk Factors

The choice of surgical procedure for a particular patient hinges on numerous factors – ulcer location, the indication for surgery, the condition of the patient, prior procedures, and the need for future NSAID therapy. In general, resective procedures have lower ulcer recurrence rates, but higher morbidity and mortality.

- For DU bleeding – first priority is control of bleeding, and a definitive acid-reduction procedure is often performed. There is still controversy in the literature over the need for a definitive acid-reducing operation.

For gastric ulcer (GU) bleeding – the risk of malignancy in this setting necessitates biopsy. Resection, often accompanied by a Billroth I or II reconstruction is the preferred procedure, but patient morbidity may preclude it. Patients with bleeding GU tend to be older and medically complicated.

For perforated DU: simple closure ± omental patch, PPI, and *H. pylori* eradication if needed, yields a <5% recurrence rate at 1 year.[6]

- For perforated GU, associated with a 10–30% risk of gastric cancer and a 10–40% mortality rate – resection of GU with an adequate margin + frozen section is performed. Simple closure of benign lesions with omental patch + PPI ± *H. pylori* eradication if indicated, is associated with a high risk of GU recurrence and reperforation.
- For SRMD: Although the largest study of ICU patients did not identify surgery-related risk factors for patients with SRMD, smaller studies found that neurosurgical patients (head and spinal trauma), trauma patients, patients with severe burns, and organ transplant patients were at greatest risk for postoperative bleeding.

27.1.4 Preoperative Evaluation

- Evaluate for coagulopathy, with platelet count, PT/INR, PTT, and correct abnormalities.
- Stop NSAIDs to prevent gastropathy and for their antiplatelet effect. If NSAIDs cannot be stopped, use concomitant proton pump inhibitor (PPI) or misoprostol. Cyclo-oxygenase 2 (COX-2) inhibitors reduce but do not eliminate the risk of PUD and complications. In patients with a history of previous PUD bleeding, and a need for an anti-inflammatory agent, use a COX-2 inhibitor with PPI or misoprostol.[7]
- Stop aspirin 1 week prior to surgery if possible, but only if the benefit of aspirin cessation outweighs the risk of continuation (see Chap. 3).
- Counsel patient about smoking cessation as smoking may be associated with poorer ulcer healing.
- Evaluate and treat *H. pylori* in patients with known PUD or past history of documented PUD.
- Consider postponing elective surgery in patients with active ulcer disease.
- Consider prophylaxis for SRMD in high-risk patients, with PPI or histamine 2 receptor antagonists.

27.2 Inflammatory Bowel Disease

27.2.1 Introduction

- Though medical treatment currently predominates in the management of inflammatory bowel disease, surgery continues to play an important role. Clinicians seek surgical solutions when complications occur, or aggressive medical management fails, whether due to the severity of illness, adverse effects of medications, or nonadherence.

- Historically, the majority of patients with Crohn's disease (CD) have undergone a surgical procedure at some point during the course of their illness, but the rate of surgical intervention may be decreasing due to the advent of newer biological therapies.
- Surgery, less frequently performed in patients with ulcerative colitis (UC), often cures the disease. Elective surgery may be done for strictures, fistulas, malignancy or prevention of malignancy, malnutrition, or poorly controlled disease. Emergent surgery is required for fulminant colitis, toxic megacolon, bowel obstruction, abscess, perforations, or severe hemorrhage.

27.2.2 Patient-Specific Risk Factors

- Smoking increases the risk of recurrence in CD[8]; smoking protects against UC.[9]
- Medications:
- Corticosteroids may increase the risk of perioperative infections.[10]
- Azathioprine and 6-mercaptopurine (6-MP) are not associated with an increased risk of infection in studies of elective surgery.[10]
- Data on infliximab and postoperative complications are inconsistent.[11] NSAIDs may lead to disease flares.[12]

27.2.3 Surgery-Specific Risk Factors

- No significant data are published on patients with IBD and nonrelated surgical procedures.
- Choice of surgical procedure for IBD and expected outcomes hinge on a correct diagnosis.
  - CD is panenteric and therefore not curable. Surgery for small bowel disease may lead to short bowel syndrome, with diarrhea, malnutrition, and electrolyte imbalance.
  - For UC, multiple procedures exist for elective colectomy. Proctocolectomy with permanent ileostomy cures UC, but many patients prefer a continence preserving procedure.
- Emergency surgery is inherently of higher risk compared to elective surgery, but many patients with IBD are young, and mortality is low, unless a perforation occurs (mortality rate of 27–57%).[13]

27.2.4 Preoperative Evaluation

- History should focus on accuracy of diagnosis of IBD, and differentiating CD from UC, as this distinction affects surgical options.
- Evaluate the adequacy of past medical treatment, current disease severity, complications, extraintestinal manifestations.

- Assess the patients's psychological status and treat depression or anxiety.
- Seek multidisciplinary input from a gastroenterologist, surgeon, and primary care physician to facilitate smooth management of complex medications in the perioperative period.
- Counsel patients and families about surgical options, realistic expectations for postoperative outcomes, and risks of disease recurrences and complications.
- Assess for malnutrition, which occurs frequently due to poor oral intake and malabsorption. Check weight, complete blood count, albumin, calcium, phosphorus, magnesium, vitamin levels, prothrombin time, folate, and iron.
- Assess the patient for coagulopathy due to vitamin K-dependent factor deficiencies (from malabsorption and broad spectrum antibiotics).
- Evaluate anemia, which is often multifactorial due to blood loss, chronic inflammation, and malabsorption.
- Medications used for treatment of bowel inflammation, such as 5' aminosalicylate (ASA) drugs, may be able to be discontinued preoperatively if the diseased bowel segment will be resected.
- Many authors recommend preoperative discontinuation of drugs causing leukopenia, such as azathioprine or methotrexate, but no clear evidence is cited (see Chaps. 3 and 28).
- Consider empiric stress dose steroids or evaluation of the hypothalamic-pituitary-adrenal (HPA) axis for patients on chronic intermediate- to high-dose steroids (see Chaps. 3 and 22).

27.2.5 Perioperative Management

- Treat any identified infection aggressively preoperatively; prophylactic antibiotics should be given prior to surgery and for up to 24 h. Bowel preparation should be pursued if possible.
- Total parenteral nutrition for 7–14 days preoperatively is only recommended for severely malnourished patients.[14]
- In severe or fulminant colitis, aggressive treatment should be attempted with corticosteroids and possibly cyclosporine. If no improvement ensues within 96 h, surgery should proceed, in an effort to avoid perforation.
- Prophylaxis for venous thromboembolism should be used as patients with IBD are considered at increased risk for thrombotic events.[15]
- Consider stress dose steroids as previously mentioned. The dose depends on the complexity of the surgical procedure.
- Correct coagulopathy, common due to malabsorption and use of antibiotics, with vitamin K or fresh frozen plasma
- Closely monitor patients with CD for development of the short bowel syndrome post small bowel resection and maintain hydration, electrolyte balance, and nutrition.
- Adjust preoperative medications, with input from gastroenterologist and surgeon, based on risk of infection, recurrence, and knowledge of the patient's postoperative anatomy. Oral 5'-ASA compounds will not come in contact with a blind-ending pouch and may

need to be changed to topical treatment or immunosuppressives, if there is still active inflammation. For patients with CD, recurrence is common, and data support using 5'-ASA drugs, metronidazole, and azathioprine/6-MP to prevent recurrence.
- Smoking cessation helps maintain remission in CD[8] and should be strongly promoted preoperatively and postoperatively.

27.3 Liver Disease

27.3.1 Introduction

- The liver plays several important roles in regard to perioperative health:
  - Production of coagulation factors necessary for hemostasis.
  - Production of proteins needed for wound healing and maintenance of intravascular volume.
  - Storage of glycogen and release of glucose into the bloodstream via gluconeogenesis.
  - Metabolism of many anesthetic and narcotic agents used during and after surgery for sedation and to help control pain.
  - Portal hypertension may result in splenic sequestration of platelets and thrombocytopenia, further worsening bleeding risks.
- Underlying liver disease at the time of surgery may negatively impact any of the above processes, resulting in poor hemostasis, ineffective wound healing, postoperative hypoglycemia, and prolonged effects of anesthesia and narcotic pain medications. Additionally, poor albumin production by the liver may result in reduced oncotic pressure and therefore increased ascites and interstitial edema.
- Advanced liver disease may be associated with other end-organ pathology, such as the hepatorenal and hepatopulmonary syndromes.

27.3.2 Patient-Specific Risk Factors

- Individual patients' risks are largely determined by the degree of underlying liver disease. Patients with lower Child-Pugh or MELD scores have consistently been shown to have better outcomes than those with higher scores (see Tables 27.1 and 27.3). Risk factors in these scores include ascites, encephalopathy, albumin, bilirubin, INR, and creatinine.[16]
- Patients with other comorbidities in addition to their liver disease are at higher risk for complications. These comorbidities include heart failure, coronary artery disease, chronic obstructive pulmonary disease, pneumonia, diabetes mellitus, renal insufficiency, malnutrition, and preoperative infection.

Table 27.1 Child-Pugh Turcotte score and classification

	Total bilirubin (mg/dL)	Serum albumin (g/dL)	INR	Ascites	Encephalopathy
1 point	<2	>3.5	<1.7	None	None
2 points	2–3	2.8–3.5	1.7–2.2	Medically controlled	Grade I–II
3 points	>3	<2.8	>2.2	Poorly controlled	Grade III–IV
Total points		**Classification**		**30-day mortality**	
<7		Class A		10%	
7–9		Class B		30%	
>9		Class C		>70%	

- Patients with abdominal ascites undergoing intraabdominal surgery may have particular difficulty with wound healing and abdominal infection.
- Patients with alcoholic liver disease who are still drinking carry the additional risks associated with alcohol withdrawal, including alcohol withdrawal delirium and seizures. Abstinence for 1 month prior to surgery has been shown to reduce postoperative morbidity in alcohol abusers.[17]
- Acute hepatitis (alcoholic or viral) significantly increases postoperative morbidity and mortality.
- Patients with liver disease caused by hepatitis B may have acute exacerbations or flares surrounding surgical interventions.
- Patients with autoimmune liver or biliary disease on chronic steroid therapy may need to receive perioperative stress-dose steroids.
- Patients with hereditary hemochromatosis undergoing liver transplant have lower 1- and 5-year survival rates than other patients receiving transplants.[18]

27.3.3 Surgery-Specific Risk Factors

Surgical factors associated with increased risk in patients with liver disease include:

- Urgent and emergency surgery.
- Duration of surgery.
- Intraoperative hypotension and hypercarbia-induced splanchnic vasoconstriction resulting in ischemic liver injury.[19]
- Abdominal surgery and general anesthesia often result in minor elevations in LFTs. These typically resolve in several days in patients with normal hepatic function but may be more pronounced and prolonged in patients with underlying liver disease.
  - Open procedures carry greater risk than laparoscopic procedures.
  - In particular, laparoscopic cholecystectomy in cirrhotic patients results in less intraoperative blood loss, shorter operative time, and shorter length of hospital stay.[20]

- Cardiac surgery can be safely performed in some patients with mild cirrhosis (Child-Pugh score ≤ 7 in one series), but it carries a high risk for morbidity and mortality in patients with more advanced disease. In addition, the use of cardiopulmonary bypass appears to further increase the risk for perioperative complications and death.[21]
- Several studies of orthopedic surgeries in cirrhotic patients have demonstrated increased perioperative complication rates compared to noncirrhotic patients; however, elective total hip and total knee arthroplasties are generally well tolerated by people with Child's class A or B cirrhosis.[22]
- Endovascular abdominal aortic aneurysm (AAA) repair has been successfully used in patients with liver disease and other comorbidities conferring higher risk for open surgery. In contrast, even mild liver disease has been shown to increase risk for postoperative mortality in patients undergoing open AAA repair.[23,24]
- After hepatectomy, liver dysfunction is the most common cause of death. Additionally, age, cirrhosis, and postoperative sepsis have been shown to be independent predictors of death after hepatectomy.[25]

27.3.4 Preoperative Evaluation (Fig. 27.1)

- The most important aspects of the preoperative evaluation are based on a clinical assessment of the patient and his lab values rather than on pathological staging of the individual's liver disease.

27.3.4.1 History

- Ask about risk factors for liver disease, including intravenous drug use, birth in a country with endemic hepatitis B (or to a mother born there), amount and frequency of alcohol use, and exposure to herbal medications, mushrooms, or other medications that may cause liver injury.
- Determine the time of the patient's last alcohol intake to help predict the time of onset of any impending alcohol withdrawal.
- Take a family history with particular attention to any family members with liver disease.

27.3.4.2 Physical Exam

- Pay particular attention to signs that may indicate underlying cirrhosis, such as caput medusa, spider angiomata, palmar erythema, and gynecomastia. Assess the patient's mental status and look for asterixis to evaluate for encephalopathy. Look for jaundice and bruising of the skin.
- Hepatomegaly may indicate congestion from cardiac disease or an infiltrative liver disease.

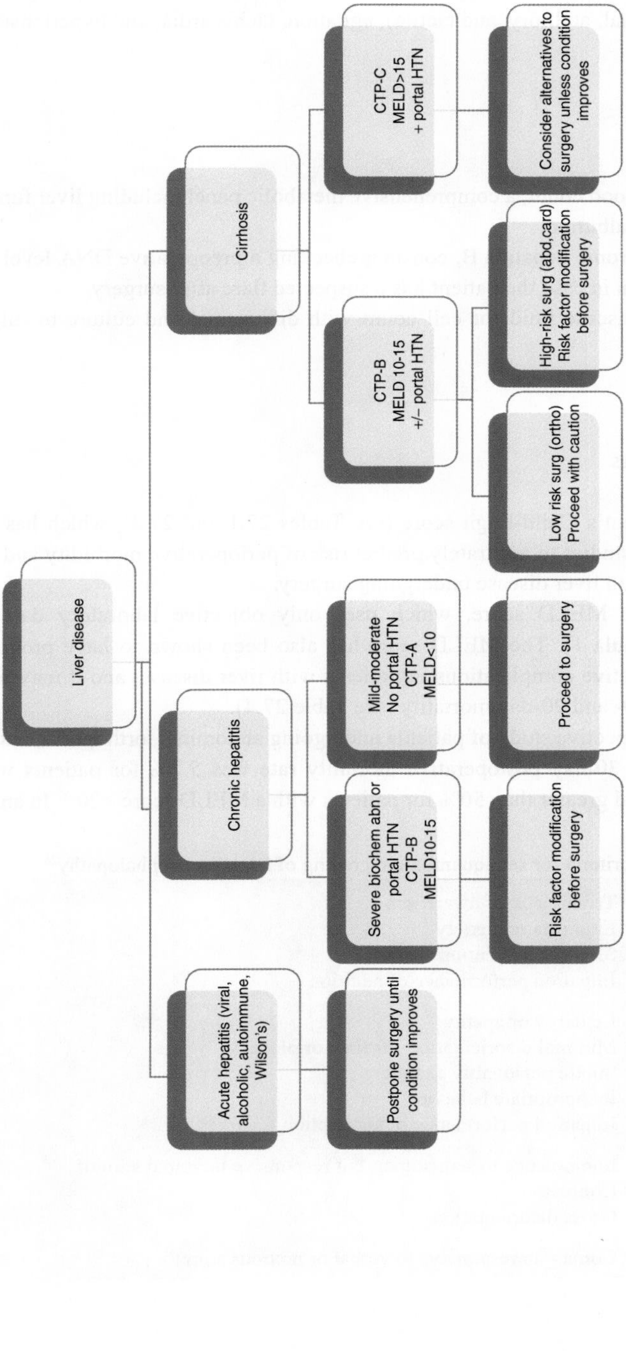

Fig. 27.1 Algorithm for preoperative assessment for elective surgery in patients with known liver disease. Contraindications to surgery include: acute hepatitis (viral, alcoholic), fulminant hepatic failure, Child C cirrhosis, severe coagulopathy (despite treatment), severe extrahepatic complications (acute renal failure, cardiomyopathy, hypoxemia) (Adapted from Friedman[30], Malik and Abmad[31], Milwala et al.[32])

- Assess the patient for any signs of concomitant infection that may need to be treated prior to surgery. In particular, the diagnosis of spontaneous bacterial peritonitis (SBP) can be challenging, and patients can be relatively asymptomatic.
- Look for signs of alcohol withdrawal, such as tremulousness, delirium, diaphoresis, hallucinations (visual, auditory, and tactile), agitation, tachycardia, and hypertension.

27.3.4.3 Laboratory Examination

- Send a complete blood count, a comprehensive metabolic panel including liver function tests, PT/PTT, and albumin.
- In patients with chronic hepatitis B, consider checking a preoperative DNA level for a point of comparison in case the patient has a suspected flare after surgery.
- Consider sending ascitic fluid for cell count with differential and culture to rule out infection.

27.3.4.4 Risk Stratification Schemes

- Calculate the patient's Child-Pugh score (see Tables 27.1 and 27.2), which has been shown in multiple studies to accurately predict risk of perioperative morbidity and mortality in patients with liver disease undergoing surgery.
- Also calculate the MELD score, which uses only objective laboratory data (see Table 27.3 – Formula 1). The MELD score has also been shown to have prognostic utility for perioperative complications in patients with liver disease, and it may be the best predictor of 30- and 90-day mortality (see Table 27.4).
- In one large, retrospective study of patients undergoing abdominal, orthopedic, and cardiac surgeries, the 30-day postoperative mortality rate was 5.7% for patients with a MELD score <8 and greater than 50% for patients with a MELD score >20.[27] In another

Table 27.2 West Haven criteria for semiquantitative grading of hepatic encephalopathy[26]

Grade 1	Trivial lack of awareness Euphoria or anxiety Shortened attention span Impaired performance of addition
Grade 2	Lethargy or apathy Minimal disorientation for time or place Subtle personality change Inappropriate behavior Impaired performance of subtraction
Grade 3	Somnolence to semistupor, but responsive to verbal stimuli Confusion Gross disorientation
Grade 4	Coma – unresponsive to verbal or noxious stimuli

Table 27.3 MELD scores

Formula 1
MELD = 3.8[Ln serum bilirubin (mg/dL)] + 11.2[Ln INR] + 9.6[Ln serum creatinine (mg/dL)] + 6.4
Formula 2
iMELD = MELD + (0.3 × age) − (0.7 × serum sodium [mEq/L]) + 100

Table 27.4 Relationship between MELD score and postoperative mortality in a cohort of 772 patients undergoing major digestive, orthopedic, and cardiovascular surgeries[27]

MELD score	Mortality, %					
	7 days	30 days	90 days	1 year	5 years	10 years
0–7	1.9	5.7	9.7	19.2	50.7	72.6
8–11	3.3	10.3	17.7	28.9	58.5	78.1
12–15	7.7	25.4	32.3	45.0	69.5	87.3
16–20	14.6	44.0	55.8	70.5	94.1	94.1
21–25	23.0	53.8	66.7	84.6	92.3	100
≥26	30.0	90.0	90.0	100	100	100

Adapted from Teh et al.[27], with permission from Elsevier

Table 27.5 Relationship between iMELD score and postoperative mortality in a cohort of 191 patients undergoing a variety of digestive, hepatic, and extradigestive surgeries[28]

iMELD score	Mortality within 30 days of surgery or during hospitalization
<35	4%
35–45	16%
>45	50%

retrospective study, the "integrated MELD" score (iMELD), which adds age and sodium level to the traditional factors calculated in the score (see Table 27.3 – Formula 2), was shown to have superior predictive capacity when compared to both traditional MELD and Child-Pugh scores. An iMELD score <35 carried a risk of perioperative death of 4%, a score of 35–45 a risk of 16%, and a score of >45 a risk of 50% (see Table 27.5).[28]

27.3.5 Perioperative Management (Risk-Reduction Strategies)

- Advise patients who abuse alcohol to abstain for at least the month prior to surgery.
- Control ascites with diuretics or paracentesis prior to going to surgery.
- Do not overdiurese given the risk of inducing or worsening hepatorenal syndrome.
- Correct coagulopathy with vitamin K supplementation, FFP, and/or cryoprecipitate. Transfuse platelets to keep >50,000 cells/mm^3, though particular surgeries may require higher thresholds.
- Control hepatic encephalopathy with lactulose or rifaximin.

- Treat any underlying infections, including SBP, prior to surgery.
- Use hepatically metabolized agents such as benzodiazepines and opiates judiciously. Remember that they may not be cleared as quickly in patients with hepatic disease.
- Avoid emergency surgery if possible, as it clearly confers a higher risk of postoperative morbidity and mortality.
- Opt for laparoscopic or other less-invasive surgeries over open surgeries.
- Patients with more advanced liver disease (e.g., Child-Pugh class C), who are therefore poor surgical candidates, may benefit from less invasive procedures, such as radiofrequency ablation (RFA), transarterial chemoembolization (TACE), or transjugular intrahepatic portosystemic shunt (TIPS) in place of partial hepatectomies or surgical shunt placement.
- Avoid intraoperative hypotension and the resulting risk for hepatocellular damage.
- Optimize preoperative nutritional status with supplements and appetite stimulants. Consider referral to a nutritional expert. Include thiamine in the medication regimen for patients with a history of alcoholic liver disease.
- Start secondary prevention of esophageal variceal bleeding in patients with documented varices using beta-blockers (propranolol) to reduce portal pressures. The data to support use of TIPS preoperatively to decompress portal pressures with a goal of reducing perioperative complications in operations other than liver transplants come from small retrospective studies. TIPS is not currently used routinely for this indication.[29]

References

1. Ohmann C, Imhof M, Ruppert C, et al. Time–trends in the epidemiology of peptic ulcer bleeding. *Scand J Gastroenterol*. 2005;40:914-920.
2. Kurata JH, Nogawa AN. Meta-analysis of risk factors for peptic ulcers. Nonsteroidal anti-inflammatory drugs, *Helicobacter pylori*, and smoking. *J Clin Gastroenterol*. 1997;24:2-12.
3. Boey J, Choi SKY, Alagaratnam TT, Poon A. Risk stratification in perforated duodenal ulcers: a prospective validation of predictive factors. *Ann Surg*. 1987;205:22-26.
4. Irvin TT. Mortality and perforated peptic ulcer: a case for risk stratification in elderly patients. *Br J Surg*. 1989;76:215-218.
5. Cook DJ, Fuller HD, Guyatt GH, et al. Risk factors for gastrointestinal bleeding in critically ill patients. *N Engl J Med*. 1994;330:377-381.
6. Ng EKW, Lam YH, Sung JJY. Eradication of *Helicobacter pylori* prevents recurrence of ulcer after simple closure of duodenal ulcer perforation. *Ann Surg*. 2000;231:153-158.
7. Malfertheiner P, Chan FKL, McColl KEL. Peptic ulcer disease. *Lancet*. 2009;374: 1449-1461.
8. Cosnes J, Beaugerie L, Carbonnel F, Gendre JP. Smoking cessation and the course of Crohn's disease: an intervention study. *Gastroenterology*. 2001;120:1093-1099.
9. Lindberg E, Tysk C, Andersson K, Jarnerot G. Smoking and inflammatory bowel disease. A case control study. *Gut*. 1988;29:352-357.
10. Aberra FN, Lewis JD, Hass D, Rombeau JL, Osborne B, Lichtenstein GR. Corticosteroids and immunomodulators: postoperative infectious complication risk in inflammatory bowel disease patients. *Gastroenterology*. 2003;125:320-327.
11. Sewell JL, Mahadevan U. Infliximab and surgical complications: truth or perception? *Gastroenterology*. 2009;136:354-355.

12. Evans JMM, McMahon AD, Murray FE, McDevitt DG, MacDonald TM. Non-steroidal anti-inflammatory drugs are associated with emergency admission to hospital for colitis due to inflammatory bowel disease. *Gut*. 1997;40:619-622.
13. Metcalf AM. Elective and emergent operative management of ulcerative colitis. *Surg Clin North Am*. 2007;87:633-641.
14. The Veterans Affairs Total Parenteral Nutrition Cooperative Study Group. Perioperative total parenteral nutrition in surgical patients. *N Engl J Med*. 1991;325:525-532.
15. Miehsler W, Reinisch W, Valic E, et al. Is inflammatory bowel disease an independent and disease specific risk factor for thromboembolism? *Gut*. 2004;53:542-548.
16. Suman A, Barnes DS, Zein NN, Levinthal GN, Connor JT, Carey WD. Predicting outcome after cardiac surgery in patients with cirrhosis: a comparison of Child-Pugh and MELD scores. *Clin Gastroenterol Hepatol*. 2004;2:719-723.
17. Tonnesen H, Rosenberg J, Nielsen HJ, et al. Effect of preoperative abstinence on poor postoperative outcome in alcohol misusers: randomized controlled trial. *BMJ*. 1999;318: 1311-1316.
18. Kowdley KV, Brandhagen DJ, Gish RG, et al. Survival after liver transplantation in patients with hepatic iron overload: the national hemochromatosis transplant registry. *Gastroenterology*. 2005;129:494-503.
19. Murray JF, Dawson AM, Sherlock S. Circulatory changes in chronic liver disease. *Am J Med*. 1958;24:358-367.
20. Puggioni A, Wong LL. A metaanalysis of laparoscopic cholecystectomy in patients with cirrhosis. *J Am Coll Surg*. 2003;197:921-926.
21. Filsoufi F, Salzberg SP, Rahmanian PB, et al. Early and late outcome of cardiac surgery in patients with liver cirrhosis. *Liver Transpl*. 2007;13:990-995.
22. Cohen SM, Te HS, Levitsky J. Operative risk of total hip and knee arthroplasty in cirrhotic patients. *J Arthroplasty*. 2005;20:460-466.
23. Bush RL, Johnson ML, Hedayati N, Henderson WG, Lin PH, Lumsden AB. Performance of endovascular aortic aneurysm repair in high-risk patients: results from the Veterans Affairs National Surgical Quality Improvement Program. *J Vasc Surg*. 2007;45:227-233.
24. Pronovost P, Dorman T, Sadovnikoff N, Garrett E, Breslow M, Rosenfeld B. The association between preoperative patient characteristics and both clinical and economic outcomes after abdominal aortic surgery. *J Cardiothorac Vasc Anesth*. 1999;13:549-554.
25. Capussotti L, Viganò L, Giuliante F, Ferrero A, Giovannini I, Nuzzo G. Liver dysfunction and sepsis determine operative mortality after liver resection. *Br J Surg*. 2009;96:88-94.
26. Ferenci P, Lockwood A, Mullen K, Tarter R, Weissenborn K, Blei AT. Hepatic encephalopathy – definition, nomenclature, diagnosis, and quantification: final report of the working party at the 11th World Congresses of Gastroenterology, Vienna, 1998. *Hepatology*. 2002;35:716-721.
27. Teh SH, Nagorney DM, Stevens SR, et al. Risk factors for mortality after surgery in patients with cirrhosis. *Gastroenterology*. 2007;132:1261-1269.
28. Costa BP, Sousa FC, Serôdio M, Carvalho C. Value of MELD and MELD-based indices in surgical risk evaluation of cirrhotic patients: retrospective analysis of 190 cases. *World J Surg*. 2009;33:1711-1719.
29. Schlenker C, Johnson S, Trotter JF. Preoperative transjugular intrahepatic portosystemic shunt (TIPS) for cirrhotic patients undergoing abdominal and pelvic surgeries. *Surg Endosc*. 2009;23:1594-1598.
30. Friedman LS. The risk of surgery in patients with liver disease. *Hepatology*. 1999;29:1617-1623.
31. Malik SM, Ahmad J. Preoperative risk assessment for patients with liver disease. *Med Clin N Am*. 2009;93:917-929.
32. Millwala F, Nguyen GC, Thuluvath PJ. Outcomes of patients with cirrhosis undergoing non-hepatic surgery: risk assessment and management. *World J Gastroenterol*. 2007;13:4056-4063.

Suggested Reading

Acid-Peptic Disorders and Stress-Related Mucosal Disease

ASHP. Therapeutic guidelines on stress ulcer prophylaxis. *Am J Health Syst Pharm.* 1999;56: 347-379.

Dellinger RP, Levy MM, Carlet JM, et al. Surviving sepsis campaign: international guidelines for management of severe sepsis and septic shock. *Crit Care Med.* 2008;36:296-327.

Gralnek IM, Barkun AN, Bardou M. Management of acute bleeding from a peptic ulcer. *N Engl J Med.* 2008;359:928-937.

Sung JJY, Barkun A, Kuipers EJ, Mössner J, Jensen DM, et al. Intravenous esomeprazole for prevention of recurrent peptic ulcer bleeding. *Ann Intern Med.* 2009;150:455-464.

Sung JJY, Lau JYW, Ching JYL, Wu JCY, Lee YT, et al. Continuation of low-dose aspirin therapy in peptic ulcer bleeding. *Ann Intern Med.* 2010;152:1-9.

Inflammatory Bowel Disease

Cohen JL, Strong SA, Hyman NH, et al. Practice parameters for the surgical treatment of ulcerative colitis. *Dis Colon Rectum.* 2005;48:1997-2009.

Colombel JF, Sandborn WJ, Reinisch W, Mantzaris GJ, Kornbluth A, et al. Infliximab, azathioprine, or combination therapy for Crohn's disease. *N Engl J Med.* 2010;362:1383-1395.

Cullen JJ, Martin RF. *Surgical Clinics of North America: Current Management of Inflammatory Bowel Disease*. Philadelphia: W.B. Saunders; 2007:87.

Marrero F, Qadeer MA, Lashner BA. Severe complications of inflammatory bowel disease. *Med Clin N Am.* 2008;92:671-686.

Podolsky DK. Inflammatory bowel disease. *N Engl J Med.* 2002;347:417-429.

Liver Disease

Garrison RN, Cryer HM, Howard DA, Polk HC Jr. Clarification of risk factors for abdominal operations in patients with hepatic cirrhosis. *Ann Surg.* 1984;199:648-655.

Kim JJ, Dasika NL, Yu E, Fontana RJ. Cirrhotic patients with a transjugular intrahepatic portosystemic shunt undergoing major extrahepatic surgery. *J Clin Gastroenterol.* 2009;43:574-579.

Mansour A, Watson W, Shayani V, Pickleman J. Abdominal operations in patients with cirrhosis: still a major surgical challenge. *Surgery.* 1997;122:730-735; discussion 735–736.

Rice HE, O'Keefe GE, Helton WS, Johansen K. Morbid prognostic features in patients with chronic liver failure undergoing nonhepatic surgery. *Arch Surg.* 1997;132:880-885.

28 Rheumatic Disease

Brian F. Mandell

28.1 Introduction

- The consultant should not assume baseline laboratory tests will be normal.
- The medical consultant should try to confirm the rheumatologic diagnosis by discussion with the patient, the patient's rheumatologist, and review of records in order to assess the disease-specific risks of surgery.
- Assess disease activity and the degree of end organ damage that may influence the perioperative course. In general, elective surgery is deferred during times of active disease.
- Patients frequently utilize many prescribed and "alternative" medications. These must be carefully reviewed, e.g., fish oil is used as an anti-inflammatory agent and causes platelet dysfunction.
- Consider postoperative rehabilitation: recommendations regarding pain and restarting anti-inflammatory medications may impact postoperative recovery, particularly important in patients with inflammatory arthritis undergoing arthroplasty.

28.2 Patient with Inflammatory Arthritis (Rheumatoid Arthritis (RA), Psoriasis, Spondylopathies)

28.2.1 Patient/Disease-Specific Risk Factors

- Involvement of the cervical spine and jaw movement may influence the ease and safety of endotracheal intubation.[1]

B.F. Mandell
Center for Vasculitis Care and Research, The Cleveland Clinic, Cleveland Clinic Lerner College of Medicine, Cleveland, OH, USA
e-mail: mandelb@ccf.org

S.L. Cohn (ed.), *Perioperative Medicine*,
DOI: 10.1007/978-0-85729-498-2_28, © Springer-Verlag London Limited 2011

- Sixty percent of patients with longstanding RA have radiographic cervical instability that may predispose to cervical cord injury.[2]
- Greater than 80% of patients with radiographic instability are asymptomatic. Peripheral joint destruction or compressive neuropathies may complicate interpretation of the exam.
- C1-2 is the most common site of laxity and instability, followed by subaxial disease and then cranial settling. Pannus from synovial proliferation may also narrow the canal and put the cord at risk of injury, without visualization on radiographs.
- Patients with recent onset disease are unlikely to have significant cervical spine instability, which occurs due to ligamentous laxity following years of inflammatory disease.

- Cardiovascular risk is increased with RA and psoriasis.
  - Patients may be unable to exert themselves to permit historical assessment of significant coronary artery disease. Patients with severe articular involvement are also likely to be deconditioned.
  - Patients with spondylitis or the HLAB27 gene are at risk for aortitis that may be accompanied by aortic valve insufficiency, conduction disease, or atrial fibrillation.

- Patients with RA may have unrecognized interstitial lung disease or pleural effusions.
- Patients with RA have a greater risk of infected arthroplasties than patients with osteoarthritis.

28.2.2 Surgery-Specific Risk Factors

- The RA does not generally involve the lumbar spine, thus epidural procedures may not be affected. However, the possibility for need to convert from spinal to general anesthesia must be considered.
- Patients with polyarticular joint inflammation or deformity may be uncomfortable during positioning in the OR and thus regional anesthesia may be difficult.
- Simultaneous bilateral knee arthroplasty carries an increased of cardiac complications (compared to staged procedures).

28.2.3 Preoperative Evaluation

- **Rheumatoid arthritis**
  - Hoarseness can be a sign of cricoarytenoid joint dysfunction, and its presence should prompt ENT preoperative evaluation in order to avoid a potential postextubation airway catastrophe due to vocal cord closure from joint dysfunction.[3] The joints can be injected with corticosteroids preoperatively if necessary.
  - Hyperreflexia may indicate asymptomatic cervical myelopathy. Document the neurologic exam.

– Preoperatively, obtain cervical spine radiographs in the neutral position as well as with flexion and extension views looking for radiographic instability.
– If there are signs or symptoms suggestive of cord compression, obtain a neurosurgical evaluation and an MRI in flexion and extension to evaluate bone or soft tissue compression of the cord prior to elective surgery.
– Communicate with the anesthesiologist and surgeon regarding any concerns.
– Cervical stabilization procedures are associated with morbidity and mortality and are not routinely considered prior to other surgery.
– [3]Evaluate cardiovascular risk using the ACC/AHA guidelines (Chap. 20), recognizing the increased incidence of CAD and the potential difficulty of assessing symptoms in these patients who may have limited physical activity.
– Sjogren's syndrome is common in patients with RA. Prior to long surgical procedures, lubricating eye ointment (not drops) should be applied.

- **Spondylitis (e.g., ankylosing spondylitis {AS})**

– AS may involve all levels of the spine and the peripheral joints.
– Spine involvement is characterized more by fusion and reduced mobility than by instability potentially compromising the ability to easily intubate or position the patient.
– Heterotopic ossification may develop around arthroplasties, adversely affecting outcomes. This is especially true in patients who had prior heterotopic ossification. Ossification may be prevented (limited data) with the preoperative use of radiation, nonsteroidal anti-inflammatory drugs, or bisphosphonate therapy.[4]

28.2.4
Perioperative Medication Management (also see Table 28.1)

- **Nonsteroidal Anti-inflammatory Drugs (NSAIDs)**

– Nonselective NSAIDs depress platelet function and are associated with surgical bleeding, but provide insufficient prophylaxis against thrombosis. They are generally discontinued 1–3 days prior to surgery; drugs with longer half-life (piroxicam) should be stopped even earlier. Aspirin, unlike other NSAIDs, is an irreversible inhibitor of platelet cyclooxygenase, platelet function may take up to a week following discontinuation to fully return to normal. Nonacetylated salicylates do not affect platelet function.
– The cyclooxygenase 2 (COX-2) selective NSAIDs (e.g., celecoxib) do not affect platelet function. In short term, small trials they have not adversely affected bleeding. They may provide sufficient analgesia when given preoperatively to reduce the need for postoperative narcotics. There are controversial concerns regarding their association with increased cardiovascular morbidity.
– All NSAIDs are associated with (usually reversible) renal insufficiency, particularly in the setting of decreased renal blood flow.
– Parenteral administration offers no gastric safety advantage over orally administered NSAID.

Table 28.1 Rheumatic disease medications in the perioperative period

Drug	Preoperative recommendations	Comments
NSAID (nonselective)	Stop 2–3 half lives prior to surgery	Reversibly inhibit platelet function, demonstrated increased postoperative bleeding Can effective analgesia may decrease narcotic requirement, decrease renal function, decrease drug excretion
Aspirin	Unless used as antithrombotic drug, stop ASA ~1 week pre-op	Irreversible platelet inhibition Increased postoperative bleeding
COX 2 selective	Can continue through surgery unless renal concerns	No antiplatelet effects. May be prothrombotic Can decrease renal function Effective as analgesic: narcotic sparing
Prednisone	Continue Consider short-term hydrocortisone 50–100 IV q 8 h	Concern with wound healing and infection with chronic use Cause leukocytosis, hyperglycemia No need for protracted tapering if "stress doses" are Rx Study shows baseline dosing is sufficient to avoid hypotension
Hydroxychloroquine	Can continue	Some antithrombotic effect (has been used as prophylactic antithrombotic in orthopedic surgery)
Methotrexate	Can continue	Avoid administration within 24–48 h of possible acute renal insufficiency. Pre-op discontinuation associated with flares in RA
Azathioprine	Can continue	
Leflunomide	Can continue	Limited data
Cyclophosphamide	Can continue	Acute renal failure could cause buildup of metabolites
Sulfasalazine	Can continue	
IVIg	Can continue	Avoid within few days of potential acute renal injury (i.e., hypoperfusion)
Colchicine	Can continue in baseline chronic dose	Watch for drug interactions, discontinue if acute renal failure occurs. Can cause diarrhea
Allopurinol, febuxostat	Can continue	Resume as soon as possible post-op. Do not initiate therapy in the acute perioperative period

- **Methotrexate (MTX)**
  - MTX is generally taken once weekly, along with daily folic acid (1 mg) to reduce side effects. Since the kidney excretes MTX, it should not be given immediately prior to any procedure likely to be complicated by renal insufficiency. The drug is normally cleared rapidly from the circulation following each administration.
  - Several small controlled studies have demonstrated the safety of providing MTX the week before surgery. Withdrawal of the drug can be associated with postoperative flare in the underlying disease, adversely affecting rehabilitation. MTX is generally not withheld for ≥ 1 week prior to a procedure.[5]
- **Leflunomide**
  - Leflunomide is a pyrimidine antagonist used in the treatment of RA and other inflammatory disorders. It has an extremely long tissue half-life. Withdrawal preoperatively is not likely to affect tissue or plasma levels. Studies have provided mixed results regarding risk for postoperative infections in patients taking leflunomide.
- **Corticosteroids**
  - Daily low dose (<10 mg/day) or intermittent prednisone as therapy for inflammatory arthritis is common. Patients taking supraphysiologic (>7.5 mg/day) doses of prednisone for greater than 2 weeks in the past year have a submaximal cortisol release response to challenge with ACTH. However, it has not been demonstrated that this blunting of the "stress response" has any clinically significant effect on the outcome to surgery.[6]
  - It has become routine practice to administer 50–100 mg of IV hydrocortisone prior to general anesthesia, and 25–50 mg every 8 h until the patient is stable. Nonetheless, several small studies have shown that patients who receive only their baseline corticosteroid dose do not suffer adverse effects (see Chap. 22).
  - If perioperative corticosteroid supplementation is provided, baseline corticosteroid dose should be resumed as soon as the patient is stable. There is no need for prolonged tapering regimens.
  - Chronic corticosteroid therapy may adversely affect wound healing, although there are limited supportive data from controlled studies in humans.
  - Corticosteroids elicit neutrophilia, hyperglycemia, and may blunt postoperative fever.
- **Antitumor Necrosis Therapies**
  - Limited data exist on the perioperative effects of these drugs (i.e., adalimumab, etanercept, infliximab, golimumab) on postoperative infection. Retrospective studies in patients with inflammatory bowel disease did not suggest an increased wound infection rate. However, some studies in RA patients with orthopedic procedures indicated an increased infection rate.[7]
  - Many rheumatologists now suggest holding anti-TNF therapy for 3–5 estimated half-lives of the drug prior to surgery, restarting it when the patient is stable postoperatively without evidence for infection.
  - This may cause some perioperative flares in arthritis which will require short courses of corticosteroid therapy.

28.2.5 Postoperative Complications

- Postoperative neurological complications are commonly due to compressive neuropathies but rarely from myelopathy.
- Flares in disease are usually due to withholding medications. Reinstitute anti-inflammatory medications as soon as possible. Low-dose corticosteroids (≤7.5 mg prednisone daily) may be helpful, as may NSAIDs.
- Postoperative fever is not likely due to a flare in these diseases.
- A monoarticular "flare" should be assumed to be an infection until proven otherwise with arthrocentesis.

28.3 Crystalline Arthritis

28.3.1 Preoperative Evaluation and Management

- Most patients with postsurgical gout have a history of prior attacks, although this history is infrequently recorded in preoperative assessment.
- Try to determine the validity of the prior diagnosis of gout or pseudogout. The finding of hyperuricemia alone is often (unreliably) the basis for the diagnosis of gout.
- Ascertain the frequency of attacks and the need for aggressive prophylaxis from the patient and records.
  - For patients with frequent attacks, consider adding once daily 0.6 mg colchicine pre and postprocedure if there are no contraindications (i.e., CKD, biliary disease, drug interactions, known intolerance). Even low-dose colchicine can, however, cause diarrhea.
- Hyperuricemia is strongly associated with coronary artery disease and the metabolic syndrome.

28.3.2 Medications

- Continue hypouricemic therapy up to the time of surgery and restart it immediately thereafter.
- Postoperative flares are common and may prolong hospitalization.[8]
  - Fluctuation in the serum urate level, up or down, can elicit an attack.

- If the patient has been using low-dose colchicine prophylaxis (0.6 mg qd to bid), continue it up to the time of surgery and reinstitute it as soon as possible following surgery. Given orally, side effects include diarrhea or nausea, but it is not ulcerogenic. Drug interactions (i.e., clarithromycin) or renal insufficiency can increase colchicine levels and cause serious toxicity including myopathy.
- NSAIDs theoretically can be used as prophylactic therapy, but due to side effects in the postoperative setting, they are generally utilized only if an attack occurs.

28.3.3 Postoperative Complications

- Flares (attacks) are common and are frequently associated with fever.
  - Mean time of occurrence ~4 days post-op
- Acute arthritis in the postoperative setting warrants arthrocentesis to exclude infection. Indirect evaluation (presence or absence of fever, leukocytosis, ESR elevation) cannot distinguish infection from crystalline arthritis.
- Similarly, radiographs or nuclear imaging studies are of no diagnostic value since they cannot distinguish between septic and crystalline arthritis.
  - The serum urate level is not a reliable diagnostic test for gout, especially at the time of an attack, and will not distinguish between infection, pseudogout, or gout.
- Treatment options include:
  - Corticosteroids in moderate to high doses (i.e., approximately 40 mg daily) are effective, continue until attack completely resolves.
  - NSAIDs – selective vs. nonselective based on the clinical concern for suppression of platelet function and induction of gastric injury.

    All NSAIDs can adversely affect renal function.
    High doses are generally needed to resolve a gout attack
  - Oral colchicine can be used to treat acute attacks, but the dose required to totally alleviate the attack is likely to cause GI symptoms in many patients, and thus not ideal in the post-op setting.
  - IL1 antagonists (i.e., anakinra) are very effective, and avoid systemic complications of the other medications, but are very expensive.
  - Do not initiate or significantly alter hypouricemic therapy in the setting of an acute flare of gout.
  - Intra-articular steroid injections can be used in some joints, but infection should have been excluded.

28.4 Myositis

28.4.1 Preoperative Evaluation and Management

28.4.1.1 Patient/Disease Associated

- These patients are at increased risk for cardiac, pulmonary, and gastrointestinal abnormalities.
  - Patients with active disease or muscle fibrosis may be difficult to wean from a ventilator. Respiratory muscle weakness by objective testing should prompt consideration to delay major elective procedures.
  - Weaning may be facilitated in a partially seated position to enhance diaphragm function.
  - Polymyositis and dermatomyositis can cause cardiomyopathy, cardiac conduction abnormalities, interstitial lung disease, dysphagia, and respiratory muscle dysfunction.
- Obtain baseline enzyme measurements. Transaminases, CPK MB, and troponin may be elevated in patients with peripheral myositis (without cardiac involvement).
- Initiation of swallowing may be compromised and can increase risk for aspiration. Inquire about the previous ability to swallow pills.

28.4.2 Perioperative Medications

- Steroids, methotrexate, calcineurin antagonists, and azathioprine are frequently utilized in relatively high doses to induce or maintain remission.
  - Although myositis is not likely to flare with short-term holding of (noncorticosteroid) medications, there is no evidence that continuing them up until surgery compromises outcome.
  - Resume meds postoperatively as soon as the patient is stable and renal function is known (MTX).
- IVIg
  - Some patients with myositis receive this in high doses on a monthly basis to induce or preserve remission.
  - Avoid administration in temporal proximity to potential renal insult as it can cause intrarenal hypoperfusion and renal failure.

28.4.3
Postoperative Complications

- Diagnosis of MI may be difficult due to baseline elevation of troponin T or more frequently, the baseline increase of the MB fraction of CPK (from regenerating skeletal muscle).
- Weaning from a ventilator may be difficult. Placing the patient in a seated position and noninvasive ventilatory support may be helpful.

28.5
Systemic Lupus Erythematosus

28.5.1
Patient-/Disease-Specific Risk

- Lupus can affect multiple organ systems increasing the risk of perioperative complications.
  - Cardiac: increased risk for coronary artery disease, beyond that explained by traditional risk factors, and valve disease.
  - Pulmonary: risk for pulmonary hypertension (may be asymptomatic), pulmonary embolism, and less commonly interstitial lung disease.
  - Hematologic: may be at increased risk for bleeding (secondary to thrombocytopenia) or thrombosis (lupus anticoagulant, antiphospholipid antibodies).
  - Renal: function may be abnormal despite a normal creatinine. Glomerulonephritis (GN) may be misinterpreted as a urinary tract infection
  - Patients with SLE may also have myositis.
  - Central nervous system: may cognitive dysfunction and deficient memory.

28.5.2
Preoperative Evaluation and Management

- Obtain a baseline CBC, basic metabolic panel, PT/PTT, and urinalysis. Cytopenias are common.
  - Thrombocytopenia should prompt questioning regarding bruising, bleeding, miscarriage, or thrombosis (antiphospholipid syndrome).
  - Do not assume that a newly discovered prolonged PTT reflects a lupus anticoagulant (LAC) without a full coagulation evaluation (rare patients have antifactor antibodies which can cause significant bleeding).
  - Glomerulonephritis (GN) is usually asymptomatic. The urine in GN may have significant pyuria, although red cells should be present as well. Microscopic evaluation is mandatory in the evaluation of possible GN. An abnormal preoperative urine dipstick (blood, leukocytes) should not be assumed to be due to urinary infection.

28.5.3
Perioperative Management of Medications

- Drugs, other than corticosteroids, used to maintain remission may be held during the immediate perioperative period as noted above and in Table 28.1, but they generally do not need to be discontinued in advance of surgery.
  - Hydroxychloroquine has some antithrombotic effect, but is unlikely to cause bleeding, and it can be continued perioperatively.
  - Continue corticosteroids during the perioperative period. Some clinicians recommend a slight elevation in corticosteroid dose to prevent a flare in SLE induced by the stress of surgery.

28.5.4
Postoperative Complications

- Fever may be a manifestation of disease activity, thrombosis, infection, or drug reaction.
- Disease flares may occur perioperatively and be difficult to distinguish from infection, corticosteroid withdrawal syndromes, thromboembolism, drug reactions, or a surgical complication.
- Antiphospholipid antibodies (APLA) or lupus anticoagulant (LAC) may be present in >30% of patients with SLE and may predispose some of these patients to thrombosis.
  - They may also have thrombocytopenia or hemolysis.
  - In the absence of thrombocytopenia <50,000, routine prophylactic anticoagulation should be prescribed.
  - Patients with APLA/LAC and prior thrombosis should receive aggressive prophylactic anticoagulation (similar to high-risk patients with prosthetic valves).

28.6
Scleroderma

28.6.1
Patient-/Disease-Specific Risk

- Intubation may be difficult due to facial tightening with decreased ability to open the mouth wide enough. Dental health may be poor. Sjogens with dry mouth is common.
- Peripheral vascular access may be limited making central venous access necessary.
- Vasospasm is frequently severe. As a result, digital oximetry may not be reliable and the ulnar pulse may be absent (ulnar occlusion is frequent).

28.6.2 Preoperative Evaluation

- Carefully evaluate the need for arterial lines as digital circulation is often tenuous.
- Pulmonary hypertension may be severe, yet clinically unrecognized.[9] Modest hypovolemia or anesthetic-induced vasodilation may elicit hypotension.
- Baseline EKG may reveal conduction disease or a pseudoinfarction pattern.
- Interstitial lung disease is common.
- Myositis occurs (usually subclinical).

28.6.3 Perioperative Medication Management

- Continue drugs given for pulmonary hypertension and review these in advance with anesthesiologist.
- There are no specific drugs that are effective in the treatment of scleroderma. Continue drugs given as symptomatic therapy for Raynaud's if they are tolerated.
- Continue aggressive antireflux therapies, including positioning in bed.

28.6.4 Postoperative Complications

- Fever is not expected from scleroderma.
- Due to gut involvement, oral drug absorption may be slow and unreliable. Bacterial overgrowth is common. Postop ileus may be problematic.
- Reflux and esophageal dysmotility increase risk for aspiration.
- Hypothermia may cause peripheral, renal, or central vasoconstriction. Severe vasospastic ischemia may warrant vasodilator therapy. Prostaglandin E infusion is well tolerated, effective, and easily titrated.
- Do NOT interrupt continuous epoprostenol (Flolan®) infusion in patients being treated for pulmonary hypertension.

28.7 Antiphospholipid Syndrome (APLS)

- APLS includes venous and arterial thrombosis.
- Patients with a history of thrombotic events and persistent antiphospholipid antibodies (APLA) or the lupus anticoagulant are at extremely high risk for perioperative thrombosis[10] and should receive aggressive prophylaxis with combination therapy – pharmacologic and mechanical.

- Patients with APLA or LAC without any history of thrombosis may not be at significantly increased risk for thrombosis.
- Patients may be at particularly high risk for thrombosis at initiation of warfarin, especially if accompanied by the additional thrombotic risk of surgery.
- The presence of thrombocytopenia is not protective against thrombosis in the setting of APLS. Corticosteroid or IVIg therapy may be used to increase the platelet count if necessary to permit anticoagulation.
- Immunosuppressive therapy is unlikely to acutely prevent thrombosis.
- Women with a history of unexplained miscarriages and APLA may also be at increased risk for thrombosis.
- In the presence of a lupus anticoagulant, routine monitoring of the PTT may be unreliable. Dose LMW heparin by weight. Alternatively, monitor factor Xa activity or thrombin time.
- Patients with APLA are predisposed to cardiac valve disease. Monitoring of heparin effect during bypass may be unreliable if the ACT is used. Consider monitoring heparin levels.

28.8 Osteoarthritis and Osteoporosis

- Pain may limit activity, and thus exertional symptoms of CAD or PVD may be absent.
- Severe kyphoscoliosis may decrease lung volumes and affect positioning in the operating room.
- Attention should be devoted to the prescription and alternative medications that the patient is taking for pain relief (Table 28.1).

References

1. Grauer JN, Tingstad EM, Rand N, Christie MJ, et al. Predictors of paralysis in the rheumatoid cervical spine in patients undergoing total joint arthroplasty. *J Bone Joint Surg Am.* 2004;86-A:1420-1424.
2. Gurley JP, Gordon RB. The surgical management of patients with rheumatoid cervical spine disease. *Rheum Dis Clin North Am.* 1997;23:317-332.
3. Segebarth PB, Limbird TJ. Perioperative upper airway obstruction secondary to severe rheumatoid arthritis. *J Arthroplasty.* 2007;22:916-919.
4. Pakos EE, Ioannidis JP. Radiotherapy vs. nonsteroidal anti-inflammatory drugs for the prevention of heterotopic ossification after major hip procedures: a meta-analysis of randomized trials. *Int J Radiat Oncol Biol Phys.* 2004;60:888-895.
5. Pieringer H, Stuby U, Biesenbach G. The place of methotrexate perioperatively in elective orthopedic surgeries in patients with rheumatoid arthritis. *Clin Rheumatol.* 2008;27:1217-1220.
6. deLange DW, Kars M. Perioperative glucocorticosteroid supplementation is not supported by evidence. *Eur J Intern Med.* 2008;19:461-467.

7. Pappas DA, Giles JT. Do antitumor necrosis factor agents increase the risk of postoperative orthopedic infections? *Curr Opin Rheumatol.* 2008;20:450-456.
8. Kang EH, Lee EY, Lee YJ, Song YW, Lee EB. Clinical features and risk factors for postsurgical gout. *Ann Rheum Dis.* 2008;67:1271-1275.
9. MacKnight B, Martinez EA, Simon BA. Anesthetic management of patients with pulmonary hypertension. *Sem Cardiothorac Vasc Anesth.* 2008;12:91-96.
10. Kapural L, Sprung J. Perioperative anticoagulation and thrombolysis in congenital and acquired coagulopathies. *Anesthesiol Clin North Am.* 1999;17:923-958.

Neurological Disease

29

Lane K. Jacobs and Benjamin L. Sapers

29.1 Introduction

Patients with neurologic disease tend to be older or sicker than those without these conditions. Preexisting neurologic disease may influence preoperative evaluation and preparation for surgery, selection of anesthetic agents and technique, and perioperative management. Various neurologic conditions share common clinical physiology and have similar risk factors that need to be addressed. This chapter focuses on the evaluation and management of patients with cerebrovascular disease, neuromuscular, and movement disorders undergoing noncardiac surgery. Differences between cardiac and noncardiac surgery will be highlighted where appropriate.

29.2 General Considerations (Table 29.1)

Patients with disparate neurological diseases often have similar symptoms, take similar medications, and respond similarly to anesthetics and perioperative physiological changes. Given this, general comments and recommendations can be made for the neurological conditions discussed in this chapter.

29.2.1 Advanced Age

- The elderly patient with neurological disease will have less reserve and a higher likelihood of more severe complications from surgery.
  - General operative risk increases by six times if over 80 years of age.

L.K. Jacobs (✉)
Section of General Internal Medicine, Carolinas Medical Center,
1000 Blythe Blvd, 5th Floor MEB, 28203 Charlotte, NC, USA
e-mail: ljacobs@carolinas.org

S.L. Cohn (ed.), *Perioperative Medicine*,
DOI: 10.1007/978-0-85729-498-2_29,

Table 29.1 General considerations and risk factors for surgical patients with neurologic diseases

Patient-specific risk factors	Surgery-specific risk factors	Risk reduction strategies
Advanced age (>80)	Type of surgery	Optimize medical therapy
Maintenance medications	Anatomical area of surgery	Continue meds on AM of surgery and perioperatively
Volume depletion	Specific anesthetic agents	Early mobilization
Cardiac disease	Drug interactions	DVT prophylaxis
Autonomic dysfunction	NPO status	Lung expansion maneuvers
Pulmonary disease		Optimize respiratory status and monitor closely postop
Neurologic deficit		Volume expansion preop
Mobility/functional status		Delirium prophylaxis
Nutritional status		Monitor electrolytes
Bladder dysfunction		Accurate analgesia
Hyperglycemia		

- Volume depletion, hypotension, and hypercoagulable state related to age and neurological disease are compounded by those that are commonly associated with surgery alone.
- Postoperative delirium, especially with the use of anticholinergic medications, is frequent in this population.
- Clearance of anesthetics, analgesics, and sedatives is often impaired.

29.2.2 Volume Depletion

- Many patients with neurologic disease will be hypovolemic at a baseline which can exaggerate the tendency to have induction-related hypotension.
  - Hold diuretics perioperatively for at least 24 h where possible
  - Perioperative volume expansion will decrease the risk of anesthesia-induced hypotension.
- Diabetes insipidus and SIADH are conditions commonly associated with active neurological disease.
- Poor nutritional status and volume depletion are commonplace and can lead to hypokalemia, hypophosphatemia, and hypomagnesemia with resultant cardiac arrhythmia or rhabdomyolysis.

29.2.3 Medications

- Continue all maintenance medications including those to be given on the morning of surgery.
- High-dose opioids carry higher risk in neurologically impaired patients because of an increased frequency of delirium, impaired cough, reduced mobility, and constipation.
  - Meperidine is contraindicated in patients also receiving MAO-B inhibitors.
  - Aspirin decreases risk of perioperative stroke in carotid endarterectomy (CEA) surgery and in this setting should be continued. For intracranial and spinal surgery where bleeding could be catastrophic, it should be stopped 5–7 days before.
  - Clopidogrel should be held, when possible, seven days prior to surgical procedures.
- For patients on chronic glucocorticoid therapy, consider the need for stress-dose steroids.

29.2.4 Pulmonary Status

- Where appropriate, pulmonary parameters such as negative inspiratory force (NIF) or peak expiratory flow (PEF), and baseline functional vital capacities (FVC) may be useful for anticipating severity of complications, but not in predicting the likelihood of them.
- Incentive spirometry is useful in preventing postoperative pulmonary complications in high-risk patients.[7]
- Intraabdominal and intrathoracic procedures may increase risk of postoperative pulmonary complications.

29.2.5 Cardiovascular Status

- Assess functional capacity and look for symptoms and signs of heart disease.
- Look for evidence of autonomic dysfunction, including orthostatic hypotension, constipation, sialorrhea, and a neurogenic bladder.
  - Orthostatic hypotension may need to be addressed by increasing salt intake, or using fludrocortisone, and midodrine (The FDA (United States Food and Drug Administration) on 8/16/10 recommended the removal midodrine from market.)
  - Patients with autonomic, motor, or cognitive impairment are at increased risk of postoperative falls.
- Electrocardiograms are helpful in the perioperative period for detecting conduction abnormalities, such as QT prolongation, that may predict perioperative arrhythmia.

29.2.6
Nutritional Status

- Serum albumin inversely correlates with length of stay, wound infection rate, pneumonia risk, and mortality. However, aggressive short-term treatment of nutritional deficiency has not consistently been shown to improve outcome though it appears to be helpful in smaller studies.

29.2.7
Venous Thromboembolism (VTE) Risks

- VTE risk is increased due to advanced age and limited mobility.
- Patients with prior stroke are at an elevated risk for venous thrombosis and thromboembolism above the risk usually associated with surgical procedures.
- Early mobilization decreases the risk of DVT, minimizes deconditioning, improves respiratory function, and reduces the risk of pressure ulcers.

29.2.8
Anesthesia Type

- As a rule, there is no clear risk differential between regional or general anesthesia, and in any case this decision is best left to the anesthesiologist.

29.2.9
Surgical Procedure

- Upper abdominal and non-sternotomy thoracic procedures in patients with neuromuscular disorders result in impairment of movement and increased risk for atelectasis and pneumonia.
- Head and neck surgery leads to increased risk for aspiration in patients at risk for or suffering from impairment of swallowing function or airway protection.
- Intracranial surgery is associated with an increased risk for seizures and mental status changes.
- Cardiac, carotid, aortic, and major vascular surgery are associated with a higher risk for perioperative stroke.

29.2.10
Miscellaneous

- Limited mobility is a risk factor for decubitus ulcers.
- Assess for risk of delirium and provide prophylaxis where appropriate.
- Bladder dysfunction is common and will increase the risk for incomplete voiding and urinary tract infection. One must minimize duration of indwelling urinary catheters.

29.3 Cerebrovascular Disease

- Perioperative strokes result in prolonged hospital stays, disability, and death. Most perioperative strokes are embolic or ischemic – hemorrhagic strokes are rare.
- Most strokes occurring after cardiac surgery are embolic and approximately 45% occur within the first day after surgery and are related to manipulations of the heart and aorta or release of particulate matter from the cardiopulmonary bypass pump. Another 20% occur by the second day, 10% more on the third day, the majority occurring within 10 days. The late strokes are felt to be precipitated by atrial fibrillation, myocardial infarction, and coagulopathy. Delayed hypoperfusion strokes are often related to postoperative dehydration or blood loss.
- Perioperative strokes after general surgery are also mainly embolic or ischemic; however, they typically occur much later – on average, on the 7th day.

29.3.1 Patient-Related Risk Factors (Table 29.2)

- The risk of cerebrovascular accident (CVA) in the general population rises with age from about 2/1,000 individuals at age 55 to 10–24/1,000 after age 74. Over 80% of patients survive their first stroke.

Table 29.2 Risk factors for perioperative stroke

Patient-specific	Surgery-specific
Advanced age (>70)	Type of surgery (CABG, valve, carotid, aortic, other vascular > noncardiac)
Female gender	Duration of surgery (card-pulm bypass pump and aortic cross-clamp time)
Prior stroke/TIA (recent [<1 month] > remote)	Arrhythmias (AF)
Cardiovascular disease: AF, CHF, MI, CAD, HTN, valvular disease	Anesthesia? (general vs local)
Cardiovascular risk factors: DM, hyperlipidemia, smoking, PAD	Intraoperative hypotension +/– hypertension
Other comorbidities: COPD, CKD, underlying malignancy	Hyperglycemia/dehydration
Discontinuation of antiplatelet or anticoagulant therapy	Emergency surgery, perioperative MI

AF atrial fibrillation, *CABG* coronary artery bypass grafting, *CAD* coronary artery disease, *CHF* congestive heart failure, *CKD* chronic kidney disease, *COPD* chronic obstructive pulmonary disease, *DM* diabetes mellitus, *HTN* hypertension, *MI* myocardial infarction, *PAD* peripheral arterial disease, *TIA* transient ischemic attack

Table 29.3 Risk of perioperative Ischemic stroke for types of surgery and clinical conditions

Type of surgery	Stroke risk (%)
General surgery with or without carotid bruit	0.08–0.7
General surgery after prior stroke or symptomatic carotid stenosis/bruit	1.5–2.9
Head and neck	4.8
Surgery with symptomatic vertebrobasilar stenosis	6.0
Peripheral vascular surgery	0.8–3
CEA	5.5–6.1
CABG	1.4–3.8
CABG after prior stroke/TIA	8.5
CABG + valve surgery	4–13
CABG + carotid stenosis/occlusion	3–7

- Other risk factors for cerebrovascular disease (CVD) include hypertension, cigarette smoking, hyperlipidemia, atrial fibrillation, renal insufficiency, peripheral vascular disease (PVD), diabetes, coronary artery disease (CAD), and dementia.
- Perioperative strokes may also be precipitated by abrupt discontinuation of antiplatelet or anticoagulant therapy.
- In healthy patients undergoing noncardiovascular surgery, the stroke risk is extremely small (0.04–0.8%). Compared to this population, patients with a history of CVA are at increased risk of perioperative stroke, and this risk varies with contemplated surgery, age, recentness of event, and underlying carotid disease state (Table 29.3).
- A history of stroke but not risk factors for it increases the risk of perioperative CVA.
- Surgery after a recent stroke is associated with a higher risk of recurrence. After 1–3 months, the risk of recurrent stroke returns to that for patients with prior more distant strokes.
  - Recovery of cerebral autoregulation probably occurs after 1–2 weeks.
  - Post-infarction inflammatory changes in cerebral tissue lead to softening and may make the surrounding areas vulnerable to hemorrhagic transformation or ischemia. These changes probably resolve within 1 month after the acute event.
- Elective surgery should probably be postponed for at least 1 month after an ischemic stroke.

29.3.2 Surgery-Related Risk Factors (Tables 29.2 and 29.3)

- Surgery type affects the risk of perioperative stroke.
- Cardiac, carotid, and aortic surgery are associated with a greater risk of stroke than are general surgery procedures.

- The type of anesthesia may influence stroke risk but the data are controversial.
- Unplanned intraoperative hypotension, hyperglycemia, dehydration, and blood loss may be associated with an increased risk.

29.3.3 Preoperative Evaluation

- Obtain a thorough history, including the timing and details of the neurologic event.
- Question the patient about symptoms of cardiac disease since the risk factors are similar.
- Assess mobility and exercise capacity.
- Review the medication history, especially antiplatelet and anticoagulant medications, and ask about compliance with the regimen.
- Evaluate the patient's mental status and document any baseline neurologic deficits on physical examination.

29.3.4 Perioperative Management

- In general, asymptomatic carotid bruits or stenoses do not require invasive management prior to noncardiac surgery.
- Continue antihypertensive medications and control blood pressure preoperatively and perioperatively.
- Continue aspirin for carotid, cardiac, and vascular procedures. For all others, assess the risks and benefits on an individual basis.
- Consider "bridging therapy" for patients on chronic anticoagulation at high risk for thromboembolism.
- Consider statin therapy if a patient is not already on it.
- Prescribe appropriate VTE prophylaxis and encourage early ambulation.

29.4 Seizure Disorders

- Incidence of epilepsy is approximately 0.5–2% in the general population with a prevalence of 0.54/100.
- Up to one-third of these patients can have seizures monthly despite appropriate therapy.
- Perioperative seizures can result in aspiration, delayed awakening from anesthesia, and disruption of the surgical wound.

29.4.1 Patient-Specific Risk Factors

- Noncompliance with antiepileptic drugs (AED) can increase risk of perioperative seizures.
- Certain medications may decrease seizure threshold.
  - Some antibiotics, analgesics, immunosuppressants, psychotropics, and sedative-hypnotic drugs can increase the risk for seizures.
- Medication interactions can change the amount of free AED available leading to sedation, hypoventilation, and aspiration.
- Accelerated or impaired metabolism of perioperative medications can lead to insufficient or excessive/prolonged drug effects.
  - Only four AEDs are <u>not</u> metabolized primarily via hepatic mechanisms: gabapentin, pregabalin, levetiracetum, and partially topiramate. All other AEDs are hepatically metabolized and will have predictable effects when interacting with perioperative medications and anesthetics also metabolized by the liver.
  - All AEDs are cytochrome p450 inducers <u>except</u> ethosuximide, gabapentin, levetiracetam, pregabalin, tiagabine, valproate (inhibitor), and zonisamide.
  - Highly protein-bound AEDs include carbamazepine, clonazepam, phenytoin, tiagabine, and valproate.

29.4.2 Surgery-Specific Risk Factors

- Prolonged NPO status may decrease AED drug level necessitating a change to parenteral administration or drug substitution.
- Anesthetics and certain opiates have variable degrees of seizure enhancing or suppressing effects, but the literature is varied and conflicting regarding the effects of specific agents.
  - Halothane and dihydrophenytoin may interact and have previously been implicated in contributing to post-halothane hepatitis.
- Excess sedation may predispose the patient to aspiration or respiratory problems.
- Intracranial surgery increases seizure risk.

29.4.3 Preoperative Evaluation

- Obtain a detailed history documenting the type and frequency of seizures, and when the last seizure occurred.
- Note any comorbid medical or neurologic conditions.

- Document medication history including AEDs and compliance.
  - Obtain drug levels if there is a question of compliance or toxicity.
- Inquire about illicit drug or alcohol use.
- Document any preexisting neurologic deficits.

29.4.4 Perioperative Management

- Preoperatively continue all medications at previous dosages, including on the morning of surgery.
- Postoperatively, if the patient has ileus or will be NPO for a prolonged period, the usual maintenance AED therapy will need to be changed.
  - It is important to know which AEDs are available in rectal and intravenous formulations (Table 29.4).
  - Resume the patient's usual AEDs as soon as the patient can resume oral intake.

29.5 Movement Disorders: Parkinson's Disease, Huntington's Disease, Spine Injury and Paralysis

- Reaction to anesthesia is generally normal.
- Early extubation to noninvasive ventilation seems to be of benefit over prolonged invasive ventilation.
- Many maintenance medications may prolong the patient's QT interval, increasing the risk for lethal arrhythmia in the setting of surgery.
- Obtain preoperative electrocardiogram, and baseline negative inspiratory flow or peak expiratory flows are needed.

29.5.1 Parkinson's Disease (PD)

- PD is one of the most common neurological diseases in the preoperative arena, second only to stroke. The prevalence is 1–2/100 population with an incidence of 1–2/10,000.
- Resting tremor, bradykinesia, rigidity, and postural instability are the primary symptoms of PD.
- Effective drugs include levodopa, anticholinergic agents, dopamine receptor agonists, and selective monoamine oxidase B (MAO-B) inhibitors. Levodopa is usually administered with carbidopa – a dopa-decarboxylase inhibitor – to minimize side effects due to systemic conversion to dopamine (see Table 29.5).

Table 29.4 Anti-epileptic drugs available for parenteral or rectal* administration

Medication	Route	Dose (mg/kg/dose)	Comments	ECG monitoring	Treatment type	Kinetics-peak concentration
Carbamazepine	PR[a]	20	Cathartic	No	Maint	80% Absorbed peak 4–8 h
Clonazepam	PR	0.02–0.10	Slow onset	No	Acute	10–120 min
Diazepam	IV[b]	0.04–0.03	Hypotension	No	Acute/maint	Rapid
Diazepam	Rectal	0.2–0.5 mg	Hypotension	No		Peak 2–30 min
Fosphenytoin	IM	15–20 load		No	Acute/maint	3 h
Fosphenytoin	IV	4–6 mg maint		Yes		Rapid
Lorazepam	PR[c]	0.05–0.1 mg	Hypotension	No	Acute	20–120 min
Lorazepam	IV[b]		Hypotension	No	Acute	Rapid
Midazolam	IV	0.15 load then 0.15–10 mcg/kg/min	Hypotension Resp failure	No	Acute	Rapid
Paraldehyde	Rectal[d]	0.3 ml/kg, max 5 ml (1 g/ml)	Dilute 2:1 with equal vol. olive/ cottonseed oil dissolves plastics	No	Acute	20–90 min
Pentobarbital	IV	5 load then 1–3 mg/kg/h	Hypotension resp. failure	Yes	Acute/maint	Rapid
Phenobarbital	IV[b]	10–20	Hypotension, arrhythmia	Yes	Acute/maint	Rapid
Phenobarbital	PR[c]	10–20	Hypotension Too slow onset for usual acute use	Yes	Acute	4–5 h, 90% absorbed
Phenytoin	IV[b]	10–20	Hypotension, arrhythmia	Yes	Acute/maint	0.5–1 h
Propofol	IV	1 mg/kg load then 2–4 mg/ kg/h max 15	Hypotension resp. failure	Yes	Acute/maint	Rapid

Valproate	IV		Minimal	No	Acute/maint	1
Valproic acid	PR[d]	5–20 mg 10–15 q 8 h Maint	Dilute syrup 1:1 with water Cathartic	No		80% Absorbed peak 2–4 h

[a]Suspension, [b]Contains propylene glycol, [c]Use parenteral solution, [d]Oral solution
*AEDs used rectally most often are carbamazepine, diazepam, phenobarbital, and valproate

Table 29.5 Common medications for patients with Parkinson's disease[6]

Medication class	Medication	Route	Adverse effects
Dopaminergic drugs	Carbidopa/levodopa	Oral	Nausea (*N*), vomiting (*V*), orthostatic hypotension (*OH*), hypertension, dyskinesias (*D*), confusion (*C*), hallucinations (*H*), cardiac arrhythmias
Dopamine agonists	First generation (rarely used)-Bromocriptine, Pergolide second generation – Pramipexole, Ropinirole	Oral	N/V/OH/C/H/D and edema First-generation medications are rarely associated with pulmonary and/or retroperitoneal fibrosis, while sleep attacks occur more frequently with second generation agents
Monoamine oxidase type B inhibitors	Selegiline, Rasagiline	Oral	N/OH/H, cardiac arrhythmias, drug interactions, serotonin syndrome reported with concurrent meperidine use
Indirect agonists	Amantadine	Oral	OH/H, dry mouth, livido reticularis, edema
Anticholinergic drugs	Trihexyphenidyl Benztropine Diphenhydramine	Oral Oral, IM, IV Oral, IM, IV	Somnolence, delirium, glaucoma, blurred vision, dry mouth, constipation, urinary retention
Catechol-*O*-methyltransferase inhibitors	Entacapone	Oral	N/OH/D/H, diarrhea, insomnia
Neuroleptics	Clozapine, Quetiapine	Oral	OH, somnolence, weight gain, tachycardia, hyperglycemia, fatal neutropenia (with clozapine)

29.5.2
Patient-Related Risk Factors

- Respiratory disorders are frequently present.
  - Both obstructive and restrictive patterns may be seen on pulmonary function tests.
  - Reduced respiratory muscle strength, impaired cough, and sleep apnea are common.[8]
- Asymptomatic cardiac disease may be present and undiagnosed due to the patient's limited mobility and dementia.
  - Levodopa increases heart rate, cardiac contractility, and is associated with both hypertension and hypotension.
- Oropharyngeal dysphagia and esophageal dysmotility may predispose to aspiration and may impair nutrition.
- Autonomic dysfunction is present in 15–20% of patients and may predispose patients to orthostatic hypotension, constipation and ileus, and voiding dysfunction associated with urinary tract infections.
- Dementia is seen in one-third of patients.
- Psychosis, including hallucinations, is common and is related to dopaminergic and anticholinergic therapies.[5]
- Fall risk is increased due to autonomic, motor, and cognitive impairment.
- Older age and immobility increase risk for venous thromboembolism and decubitus ulcers.

29.5.3
Surgery-Related Risk Factors

- Surgeries associated with prolonged NPO status may increase risk due to difficulty administering anti-Parkinsonian medications orally.
- Aspiration pneumonia, urinary tract infections, and longer hospital stays are more common in PD patients undergoing gastrointestinal and prostate surgery than in patients without this disease.
- Delirium may also be more frequent after these surgeries.[8]

29.5.4
Perioperative Management to Reduce Risk

- Optimize anti-Parkinsonian therapy to maximize mobility and minimize side effects.
  - Associated dysautonomias may not always respond to anti-PD therapy.[4]
- Absence of PD medications can exacerbate rigidity and other symptoms of PD.
  - Avoid postoperative withdrawal of anti-Parkinsonian medications, if possible.[2] A levodopa/carbidopa solution can be given via a feeding tube, if necessary.[3]

- Acute symptom exacerbation, including upper airway obstruction and respiratory failure, can occur with the short-term discontinuation of medication.[3]
- The severe complication of Parkinsonism-hyperpyrexia syndrome (PHS), which is similar to the neuroleptic malignant syndrome, can be triggered by withdrawal of PD medications.
- Some taper dopaminergic drugs to the lowest dose possible starting 2–3 weeks prior to surgery to minimize PHS risk.
- Orally disintegrating carbidopa–levodopa may be helpful in patients with dysphagia.
- Parenteral anticholinergic medications such as benztropine or diphenhydramine can be substituted for oral agents. In select cases, subcutaneous apomorphine may be cautiously administered to prevent or treat postoperative symptoms in patients unable to take oral medications. To minimize side effects pre-treat with trimethobenzamide hydrochloride for 3 days, if possible. Use of these drugs increases the risk of delirium due to anticholinergic effects.

- Optimize treatment of dementia and delirium.
  - Central cholinesterase inhibitors (rivastigmine, donepezil) may be moderately effective for dementia and psychosis but are associated with higher rates of nausea, vomiting, and tremor.[1]
  - Clozapine or quetiapine may be useful treatments for hallucinations and delirium. Clozapine requires monitoring for agranulocytosis with complete blood counts. Other antipsychotics – haloperidol, risperidone, and olanzapine – can worsen PD.[6]
- Early mobilization can decrease risk of VTE, pressure ulcers, and deconditioning.
- Incentive spirometry can help reduce postoperative pulmonary complications.

29.6 Neuromuscular Diseases

Patients with a history of neuromuscular disease, movement disorders, and central degenerative neurological processes have similar clinical manifestations including weakness, decreased mobility, muscle fatigability, and spasticity. Many patients are maintained on immunosuppressive agents, are subject to worsening with physical stressors, and are nutritionally compromised.

29.6.1 Multiple Sclerosis (MS)

- MS is an autoimmune neurodegenerative disease with sensory, motor, and cognitive manifestations.
- Prevalence is approximately 90/100,000 individuals.

29.6.1.1
Patient-Specific Risk Factors

- Medications used to treat MS patients may increase surgical risk.
  - Immune-suppressive agents can increase the risk of perioperative infection.
  - High-dose glucocorticoids can suppress the normal adrenal responses to the stress of surgery leading to secondary adrenal insufficiency.
- Bulbar or respiratory involvement may increase risk for postoperative pulmonary complications.
- MS patients are at increased risk for urinary tract infections related to urinary retention or incontinence.
- Immobility may increase risk of VTE and pressure ulcers.

29.6.1.2
Surgery-Specific Risk Factors

- Both spinal and general anesthesia can exacerbate underlying MS.
- Neuraxial anesthesia may cause hypotension.

29.6.1.3
Perioperative Management

- Preoperatively, document medications and neurologic status. Provide stress dose steroids if indicated. Prescribe VTE prophylaxis and incentive spirometry.
- Postoperatively, monitor for new deficits and treat fever aggressively.

29.6.2
Muscular Dystrophy (MD)

- Prevalence is approximately 1.3–1.8/10,000 males (under 5/1,000,000 total) for Duchenne and Becker muscular dystrophies. Limb-girdle muscular dystrophy (LGMD) is the most common and has an approximate prevalence of 20–40/1,000,000.
- Involvement of respiratory muscles and axial skeletal and respiratory muscles is rare; specific perioperative risks of MD are those associated with limitations to mobility.
- Malignant hyperthermia (MH) is more common in patients with MD
  - Dantrolene may be used as pretreatment by the anesthesiologist, or the patient may be closely monitored for MH with dantrolene at the bedside in the OR.

29.6.3
Myasthenia Gravis (MG)

- MG is rare autoimmune disease with a prevalence 2/100,000.
- Its primary manifestation – muscle weakness and fatigability – is due to the loss of acetylcholine (ACh) receptor function at the motor endplates.
- Anti-cholinesterase medications are frequently employed to increase the half-life of ACH in the synaptic cleft, enhancing motor response to nerve discharge.

29.6.3.1
Patient-Specific Risk Factors

- Patients may have respiratory muscle weakness causing restrictive lung disease, hypoventilation, and atelectasis.
- Bulbar muscle involvement may increase risk for aspiration.
- Muscle weakness and decreased mobility may predispose to VTE and pressure ulcers.
- Certain medications (antibiotics, anticholinergics, antiarrhythmics) may exacerbate symptoms.
  - Anticholinergic medications perioperatively may have prolonged or atypical effects.
- Glucocorticoid and other immune suppressant therapy may increase the risk of infection.

29.6.3.2
Surgery-Specific Risk Factors

- Thoracic and abdominal procedures may increase postoperative pulmonary complications and require prolonged mechanical ventilation.
- Anesthetic agents may increase risk of cardiac arrest [succinylcholine (SCH) and some volatile anesthetics] as well as hyperkalemia and malignant hyperthermia.
  - Holding anticholinesterase drugs for one or two doses may help to avoid increased effect of SCH, but this is only appropriate in patients who are not completely dependent on anticholinesterase medications.
- Anticholinesterase agents may interfere with neuromuscular blocking agents.

29.6.3.3
Preoperative Evaluation

- Determine the patient's usual activity level and exercise capacity.
- Identify cardiopulmonary disease and other diseases that may coexist with MG, such as thyroid disease, lupus, and rheumatoid arthritis.
- Assess for signs of respiratory compromise or aspiration.
- Consider obtaining PFTs with maximal inspiratory and expiratory pressures.

29.6.3.4
Perioperative Management

- Continue the patient's usual medications.
  - Consider the need for stress dose steroids.
  - Minimize use of narcotics.
- Prescribe appropriate VTE prophylaxis.
- Avoid use of non-depolarizing neuromuscular blocking agents such as curare, ancuronium, vecuronium, atracruium, and rocuronium.
- Continue mechanical ventilation as needed, and observe the patient's respiratory status in a monitored setting for 24 h post-extubation.
- Continue incentive spirometry.

29.6.4
Motor Neuron Diseases (MND): Amyotrophic Lateral Sclerosis (ALS), Spinal Muscular Atrophy (SMA)

- These illnesses are characterized by denervation of muscles due to loss of upper and lower motor neurons.
- Prevalence is about 5–6/100,000.
- The clinical course is usually rapidly progressive. Compromised movement, spasticity, cognitive impairment, and respiratory compromise are hallmarks of these disease processes.
- Cardiac involvement may increase risk for perioperative arrhythmia and congestive heart failure.
- Swallowing impairments lead to an increased risk of aspiration and harm from noninvasive mechanical ventilation.
- The proliferation of extrajunctional acetylcholine receptors due to denervation in these conditions can potentiate an exaggerated potassium efflux after SCH exposure causing a hyperkalemia-induced rhabdomyolysis.
- Depressed baseline cognitive function, and interactions with commonly used maintenance medications can magnify the side effects of opiates, GABA-ergic agents, and other sedating medications.

Reference

1. Emre M, Aarsland D, Albanese A, et al. Rivastigmine for dementia associated with Parkinson's Disease. *N Engl J Med*. 2004;351:2509.
2. Frucht SJ. Movement disorder emergencies in the perioperative period. *Neurol Clin*. 2004;22:379.
3. Galvez-Jimenez N, Lang AE. The perioperative management of Parkinson's disease revisited. *Neurol Clin*. 2004;22:367.

4. Goetz CG, Lutge W, Tanner CM. Autonomic dysfunction in Parkinson's disease. *Neurology*. 1986;36:73-75.
5. LeWitt PA. Levodopa for the treatment of Parkinson's Disease. *N Engl J Med*. 2008;359: 2468-2476.
6. Miyasaki J, Shannon K, Voon V, et al. Practice parameter: evaluation and treatment of depression, psychosis, and dementia in Parkinson disease (an evidence-based review): report of the quality standards subcommittee of the American academy of neurology. *Neurology*. 2006;66:996.
7. Oliveira E, Michel A, Smolley L. The pulmonary consultation in the perioperative management of patients with neurologic diseases. *Neurol Clin*. 2004;22:277.
8. Pepper PV, Goldstein MK. Postoperative complications in Parkinson's disease. *J Am Geriatr Soc*. 1999;47(8):967-972.

Suggested Reading

Blacker DJ, Flemming KD, Link MJ, Brown RD. The Preoperative cerebrovascular consultation: common cerebrovascular questions before general or cardiac surgery. *Mayo Clin Proc*. 2004;79:223-229.

Gelb AW, Cowie DA. Perioperative stroke prevention. IARS Review Course Lectures. 2001; 46-53.

Halaszynski TM, Juda R, Silverman DG. Optimizing postoperative outcomes with efficient preoperative assessment and management. *Crit Care Med*. 2004;32(Suppl):S76-S86.

Kofke WA. Anesthetic management of the patient with epilepsy or prior seizures. *Curr Opin Anaesthesiol*. 2010;23:391-399.

Lieb K, Selim M. Preoperative evaluation of patients with neurological disease. *Semin Neurol*. 2008;28(5):603-610.

Larsen SF, Zaric D, Boysen G. Postoperative cerebrovascular accidents in general surgery. *Acta Anaesthesiol Scand*. 1988;32:698-701.

Wong GY, Warner DO, Schroeder DR, et al. Risk of surgery and anesthesia for ischemic stroke. *Anesthesiology*. 2000;92:425-432.

Selim M. Perioperative stroke. *N Engl J Med*. 2007;356:706-713.

Psychiatric Conditions

30

Joleen Elizabeth Fixley and Meghan Collen Tadel

30.1 Introduction

- Psychiatric illness is highly prevalent and increasing. It has been estimated that roughly one-third of the population has a diagnosable mental disorder, and of these, one-third were receiving treatment from 2001 to 2003, which was increased from 20% a decade earlier.[1]
- A survey of patients being evaluated before elective surgery found 43% were taking psychotropic drugs. Of these, approximately one-third were taking antidepressants, one-third were taking benzodiazepines, and the remaining one-third were distributed among taking lithium, antipsychotics, or psychoactive over the counter medications.[2]
- Psychiatric disease can be exacerbated by surgery and can affect patient outcome. Familiarity with the effects of psychiatric diagnoses and medications is essential for the medical consultant providing perioperative care to the surgical patient.

30.2 Risk Factors for Perioperative Morbidity

30.2.1 Patient-Specific Risk Factors

30.2.1.1 Anxiety

- Preoperative "anxiety" as a transient state has been measured by patients' self-reporting specific fears, and its incidence is high in patients without history of psychiatric illness or anxiolytic use.[3]

J.E. Fixley (✉)
Department of Internal Medicine, Creighton University School of Medicine, Nebraska – Western Iowa Veterans Affairs Medical Center, 4101 Woolworth Ave, 11AC, Omaha, NE 68105, USA
e-mail: joleen.fixley@va.gov

S.L. Cohn (ed.), *Perioperative Medicine*,
DOI: 10.1007/978-0-85729-498-2_30, © Springer-Verlag London Limited 2011

- In contrast, no randomized controlled trials have studied the effects of anxiety as a psychiatric diagnosis on postoperative outcome.

30.2.1.2
Depression

- Risk factors potentially associated with postoperative complications in depressed patients include decreased appetite leading to poor wound healing, decreased motivation for rehabilitation, and difficulty assessing pain.
- Preoperative active depressive symptoms have been correlated with an increased incidence of postoperative delirium after hip fracture, vascular, and cardiac surgery.
- Postoperative pain intensity and analgesic use were higher in chronically depressed patients. This correlated with the degree of depression and catastrophizing a negative mental attitude characterized by helplessness, rumination, and magnification.[4,5]

30.2.1.3
Somatization Disorder

- Somatizers are significantly more likely to undergo more operations, be dissatisfied with the outcome, and have more hospitalizations. Although the diagnosis of somatization has been known to lead to iatrogenic morbidity for over 50 years, not much improvement has occurred in avoiding unnecessary procedures in these patients.[6]
- Frequent follow up, education about their diagnosis, and establishment of rapport with this patient population by one primary care provider are essential to building trust and avoiding "doctor shopping." The preponderance of evidence should be in favor of a surgical procedure before undertaking one, and exploratory or diagnostic procedures should be avoided as they historically do not resolve symptoms in these patients.

30.2.1.4
Schizophrenia

- A systematic literature review found that patients with serious mental illness (including schizophrenia and major depressive disorder) were more likely to suffer severe postoperative morbidity and mortality due to poor baseline health status, later presentation for treatment, inability to fully cooperate with rehabilitation and increased risk of postoperative confusion and delirium if their chronic medications are discontinued preoperatively.[7]
- Institutionalized patients including schizophrenics were shown to be 3.5 times more likely (26.5% vs. 7.5%) to have postoperative complications, primarily pulmonary, than age- and sex-matched controls, and severe mental retardation had an even higher complication rate.[8]

  - More recent epidemiologic studies in community dwelling patients aged ≥ 65 years old have linked antipsychotic use and dose with the development of pneumonia.[9]

- Case reports have provided anecdotal evidence of schizophrenics' unusual absence of sensation or reaction to painful stimuli, and it has been hypothesized that delayed presentation with acute appendicitis accounts for an increased morbidity in this population.[10]

  - An advanced stage of appendicitis was noted in 25.6% of the general veteran population in NSQIP data and in 82% of veterans with schizophrenia or schizoaffective disorder in the VA database.[10,11] The overall complication and mortality rates were much higher for those with schizophrenia than the non-schizophrenic group. It is possible that symptoms are not perceived in the early stages by the schizophrenics and lead to delays in presentation to the hospital.
  - The schizophrenic veterans also had increased rates of smoking, alcohol abuse, and illicit drug abuse compared to the general VA (NSQIP) population.[10,11] While none of these factors were reported as having a higher risk of 30-day morbidity in the NSQIP data, "completely dependent" functional status predicted a high risk of 30-day mortality, and "partially dependent" functional status was associated with an increased risk of morbidity.[11]

- It is important to contrast that while depressed patients may have increased perception or reporting of pain, schizophrenics may have decreased perception or reporting of pain. A schizophrenics' history may largely be difficult to obtain and seemingly not reality based. Although it seems counterintuitive, we must pay more attention to complaints of pain in this population, not less.

30.2.2 Surgery-Specific Risk Factors

Certain types of surgery may increase psychological morbidity.

- After coronary artery bypass surgery, postoperative depression can occur and may result in increased readmission rates.[12]
- Similarly, transplant surgery has been associated with increased rates of depression, either new onset or exacerbations. Transplant patients also developed a post-traumatic stress disorder (PTSD) related to being notified of a need for, waiting for a donor organ, or events of the perioperative period.[13]

  - Additional risk factors for developing psychiatric disorders postoperatively were listed as: pre-morbid psychiatric illness, female gender, longer hospitalization, more impaired physical functional status, and lower social supports.

30.2.3
Preoperative Evaluation

30.2.3.1
History

- Inquire about any past psychiatric history
  - Ask about any prior hospitalizations or visits to a psychiatrist.
  - Ask about current status of the illness and historical severity of disease, which will give insight into current level of functioning and possible need for a psychiatric consult.[14]
- Ask about previous operations and outcomes to determine if there were any problems or postoperative deterioration of the patient's psychiatric symptoms.
- Obtain an accurate medication history including adherence to prescribed medications.
  - If the patient is not responsible for taking his/her own medications, but they are administered by a family member or nursing home staff, these caregivers will be essential in obtaining an accurate list. This may also be a clue to mild cognitive impairment.
  - Scheduled and prn use should also be confirmed. A patient may not ask for the "prn" anxiolytic in the hospital that she takes TID at home, resulting in a postoperative withdrawal syndrome. Conversely, a patient with TID "scheduled" benzodiazepine who actually takes it only once a week will certainly experience somnolence with increased risk of respiratory compromise if it is given as per the recorded order.
- Document substance use and abuse – tobacco, alcohol, and recreational drugs

30.2.3.2
Physical Exam

- Assessing mental status will help establish a basis for capacity to consent as well as a baseline for comparing to postoperative cognition.
  - Initial screening for mental status may be as simple as orientation to self, date, and place or expanded to include planned procedure, date and surgeon's name.
  - Repeating three objects and recalling after 5 min demonstrates memory. A detailed review of systems also reveals ability to remember remote and recent history.
  - If these reveal any suspicious paucity of information, a traditional Mini-Mental Status Examination should be carried out including documentation of which tasks were missed. Even mild impairment of cognition increases risk of postoperative delirium.

30.2.3.3
Preoperative Labs/Evaluation

- Risk of sudden cardiac death is increased in patients taking typical (haloperidol, thioridazine) and atypical (ziprasidone, clozapine, olanzapine, quetiapine, risperidone) antipsychotics and is increased further with high doses.[15]
- Sodium and potassium flux during ventricular depolarization and repolarization is altered which results in prolongation of the QRS complex and QT interval. These EKG changes are not the direct cause of the arrhythmias but are important markers for the underlying electrolyte channel alterations.[16]
  - A baseline EKG should be obtained in any patient taking an antipsychotic or other medication known to potentiate QTc or QRS prolongation. Abnormalities which may contribute to QTc prolongation include hypothyroidism, hypocalcemia, hypokalemia, and hypomagnesemia.
  - If a patient is found to have prolonged QTc intervals on baseline preoperative EKG (>440 ms), other medications that can further alter cardiac conduction should be avoided. A list of psychotropic medications that require assessment of QTc by EKG is listed in Table 30.1 along with medications commonly given in the perioperative period also known to prolong QTc. QTc prolongation beyond 500 m/s has been associated with substantially higher risk of sudden death.
- Other pertinent preoperative labs should include drug levels, especially if any signs of toxicity are noted on history and physical examination.

Table 30.1 QTc prolongation[15-17]

Psychotropic medications known to prolong QTc interval	Perioperative medications or conditions which can prolong QTc interval
Tricyclic antidepressants	Electrolyte abnormalities: hypokalemia, hypomagnesemia
Tetracyclic antidepressants	Hypocalcemia
Neuroleptics including typical and atypical antipsychotics:	Hypothyroidism
High risk: Thioridazine, Phenothiazines, Haloperidol	Ischemic heart disease
	Hypothermia
	Droperidol Chloral hydrate Methadone Antiarrhythmics (class IA & III) including: quinidine, procainamide, sotalol Amiodarone Macrolide antibiotics including erythromycin Fluoroquinolones including: gatifloxacin, levofloxacin, moxifloxacin

30.3 Perioperative Management to Reduce Risk

30.3.1 Preoperative

- Perioperative risk reduction strategies for patients with psychiatric disease center around obtaining a thorough preoperative assessment of their baseline psychiatric status and a complete medication history.
- Risks and benefits of continuing or holding psychotropic medications must be individually determined for each patient based on specific patient comorbidities including the underlying psychiatric diagnosis, extent of surgery, anesthetic requirements, and the potential harm to the patient from withdrawal syndromes or psychological relapse. Each of these elements as well as preoperative testing recommendations is addressed in Table 30.2.
- Over the past few decades, as use of psychotropic medications has increased, practice patterns have shifted from stopping all psychotropics prior to surgery (which decreased drug interactions but increased withdrawal symptoms and postoperative delirium) to continuing most chronic medications.[23] Since each patient's risks are unique and there are no consistent evidence-based guidelines, only very basic generic recommendations based on expert opinion are provided. If one is uncertain of the timing or need for cessation or risk of patient harm from withdrawal or relapse, we recommend consultation with the patient's primary treating psychiatrist or an available psychiatry consultant.[19,14,20,17]
- Psychiatric medication use predisposes patients to the reactions of serotonin syndrome and neuroleptic malignant syndrome. These may be clinically similar and difficult to distinguish from malignant hyperthermia.
  - Serotonin syndrome is usually incited by combining more than one serotonergic medication or drug, thus the medication history is crucial in elucidating the offending agents.
  - Medication and family history are also essential for increased index of suspicion of neuroleptic malignant syndrome and malignant hyperthermia, respectively. However, family history is often lacking in patients with malignant hyperthermia, and the patients themselves will more often than not have had prior exposure to halogenated inhalants without complication. See Table 30.3 for differential diagnosis of these disorders and Table 30.4 for a list of serotonergic medications/drugs.
- The following are recommendations and concerns about the various classes of medications used to treat psychiatric illnesses:

Table 30.2 Psychotropic medication profiles and perioperative considerations[14,18-22]

Category	Examples	Receptors or transmitters effected	Side effects relevant to perioperative period	Potential interactions with anesthetics and perioperative medications	Symptoms of withdrawal	Potential preoperative testing	Special considerations
MAOIs	Phenelzine tranylcypromine selegiline	Serotonin norepinephrine α-adrenergic, histaminergic	Orthostatic hypotension with reflex tachycardia	Hypertensive crisis with sympathomimetics potentially fatal interaction with meperidine or dextromethrophan serotonin syndrome	Severe psychological relapse including suicidal ideations and delusions		MAOIs require at least 2 week washout to prevent interactions. Patients need to be on tyramine free diet while on MAOIs.
TCAs	Amitriptyline nortriptyline desipramine doxepin, imipramine protriptyline trimipramine amoxapine maprotilie trazodone	Norepinephrine serotonin muscarinic, histaminergic, α1 and α2–adrenergic	Lower seizure threshold, QRS and QTc prolongation, AV block, S-T & T abnormalities, tachycardia, fatal arrhythmias in overdose, anticholinergic effects, sedation	AV and ventricular conduction delays with B-blockers and calcium channel blockers, hypertensive crisis with sympathomimetics, possible paradoxical hypotension with epinephrine increased INR w/ warfarin, increased phenytoin levels serotonin syndrome	Nausea, abdominal pain, diarrhea, dizziness, cardiac arrhythmias, manic symptoms, extrapyramidal signs	ECG	TCAs have been largely supplanted by SSRIs for treatment of depression. However, TCAs have seen renewed interest as adjuvant therapy for chronic pain. In this capacity they are generally prescribed at lower doses than for depression.

(continued)

Table 30.2 (continued)

Category	Examples	Receptors or transmitters effected	Side effects relevant to perioperative period	Potential interactions with anesthetics and perioperative medications	Symptoms of withdrawal	Potential preoperative testing	Special considerations
SSRIs	Fluoxetine paroxetine sertraline fluvoxamine citalopram escitalopram	Serotonin	SIADH, agitation, possibly decreased platelet aggregation	Warfarin, digoxin, phenytoin through p450 system, Altered pharmacokinetics with midazolam, lidocaine and fentanyl, serotonin syndrome	Anxiety, agitation, insomnia, nausea, vomiting, diarrhea, palpitations, paresthesias, ataxia	Consider sodium level if signs of SIADH, new SSRI prescription or elderly patient	
Antipsychotics/ neuroleptics	Typicals – chlorpromazine thioridazine fluphenazine mesoridazine perphenazine trifluoperazine loxapine haloperidol	D2 dopamine receptor α-adrenergic	QTc prolongation with progression to torsades de pointes, toxic cardiomyopathy, anticholinergic effects, sedation, orthostasis Extrapyramidal syndromes: parkinsonism, tardive dyskinesia, akathisia, dystonia, Neuroleptic malignant syndrome	Increased sedation with narcotics, possible paradoxical hypotension with epinephrine, hypotension with B-blockers	Anticholinergic effects and early psychological relapse	ECG	IM formulation of haloperidol is available and has extensive history of use in ICU patients

	Atypicals– olanzapine risperidone quetiapine ziprasidone aripiprazole	Multiple dopamine receptor	QTc prolongation but no evidence of progression to torsades to pointes, cardiomyopathy and myocarditis postural hypotension, neuroleptic malignant syndrome	Potentiation of sedative effects of anesthetics, hypotension with anesthetics and B-blockers		ECG, Glucose to assess for diabetes	Parenteral and orally dissolving Preparations available for some formulations
	Clozapine	Dopamine	Agranulocytosis, hyperthermia	Potentiation of sedative effects of anesthetics, hypotension with anesthetics and B-blockers	Psychiatric emergency – psychosis, delirium, dystonia, dyskinesia	CBC for white cell count	All patients on clozapine require close cooperation with psychiatric team for management
Mood stabilizers	Lithium	Ion-channels	Nephrogenic diabetes insidious, renal dysfunction, abnormalities of electrolytes including magnesium, calcium	NMB prolongation, lithium levels raised by diuretics (thiazide more than loop), NSAIDs, metronidazole, ACE inhibitors can greatly increase lithium levels	None	ECG, lithium level 12 h after dose, electrolytes, renal function, consider thyroid function tests	Toxicity at levels > 2 mEq/L associated with delirium, coma, seizures, ventricular arrhythmias, should obtain levels daily in patients with changing clinical picture

(continued)

Table 30.2 (continued)

Category	Examples	Receptors or transmitters effected	Side effects relevant to perioperative period	Potential interactions with anesthetics and perioperative medications	Symptoms of withdrawal	Potential preoperative testing	Special considerations
	Anticonvulsants – valproate carbamazepine oxcarbazepine	Ion-channels, membrane stabilizers		Decrease efficacy of NMB, macrolide antibiotics increase serum levels	Seizures	Drug level if appropriate	
Benzodiazepines	Alprazolam chlordiazepoxide clonazepam diazepam lorazepam	GABA receptors	Sedation, confusion	Additive sedation effect with anesthetics and opioid analgesics	Severe agitation, seizures, may be fatal		Use of flumazenil in patients on chronic benzodiazepines can lead to withdrawal symptoms including seizures. IM/IV formulations available for some benzodiazepines
Psychostimulants	Methylphenidate dextroamphet-amine amphetamine modafinil	Dopamine serotonin norepinephrine α and β-adrenorecep-tors	Hypertension, tachycardia	Potential for increased response to sympathomimetics	Excessive sleepiness, agitation		Used in treatment of narcolepsy and ADD/ADHD
Other psychotropics	Bupropion	Norepinephrine dopamine	Decreased seizure threshold		Mild		Exists in both time release and repeat dosing formulations.

	Venlafaxine	Serotonin, norepinephrine	Hypertension, insomnia, somnolence		Nausea, agitation, anxiety, insomnia, somnolence		
	Duloxetine	Serotonin, norepinephrine dopamine	Fatigue, hypertension		Similar to SSRIs		
	Nefazodone	Serotonin	Anticholinergic effects, bradycardia, orthostasis	Pharmacokinetic alteration of benzodiazepines, digoxin, haloperidol, carbamazepine		Consider liver function tests	
	Mirtazapine	Serotonin Norepinephrine	Sedation, rare neuropenia or abnormal liver function	Decreased action of clonidine	Mild	Consider liver function tests and CBC	
	Buspirone	Serotonin	Sedation				For use in generalized anxiety disorder
	Disulfiram			Severe reaction to metronidazole			For use in treating substance abuse disorders

Table 30.3 Differential diagnosis of serotonin syndrome, neuroleptic malignant syndrome, and malignant hyperthermia[24, 25]

	Serotonin syndrome	Neuroleptic malignant syndrome	Malignant hyperthermia
Incidence	Unknown	1.5% of those taking neuroleptics	Rare
Mortality	Unknown	20%	Up to 20%
Etiology	Serotonin excess: overdose vs. interaction of two or more medications	Idiosyncratic reaction to neuroleptics	Inherited autosomal dominant
Onset	Evolving within 24 h of addition of serotonergic medications	Onset evolves over days to weeks after initiation of neuroleptic	Onset 1–10 h after exposure to medication : halogenated inhalants or succinylcholine
Clinical signs	Autonomic dysfunction: (fever, HTN, tachycardia) clonus, ocular clonus (slow continuous horizontal eye movement), dilated pupils, tremor, akithesia, **hyperreflexia**, bilateral babinski sign, agitated delirium, seizure, diaphoresis, dry mucous membranes, hyperactive bowel sounds, vomiting, diarrhea, rhabdomyolysis, renal failure, DIC, ARDS	Autonomic dysfunction: (fever, HTN, tachycardia) Muscle rigidity, mental status changes, **bradyreflexia**, respiratory distress, rhabdomyolysis, renal failure, acidosis	Autonomic dysfunction: (high fever, HTN, tachycardia) Muscle rigidity (**especially masseters**), **Hypercapnia** (early sign), cyanosis mottling, rhabdomyolysis, renal failure respiratory acidosis, DIC
Treatment	1. D/C all serotonergic medications 2. Sedate with benzodiazepine 3. Supportive care in ICU if severe 4. If above not helpful: cyproheptadine, paralyze and intubate	1. D/C offending medication 2. Bromocriptine or dantrolene 3. Supportive care in ICU	1. D/C offending agent 2. Dantrolene 3. Supportive care in ICU
Resolution	Usually within 24 h	Usually within 1–2 weeks	Should respond to dantrolene rapidly, may need ongoing doses for 48 h after resolution to prevent relapse

Table 30.4 Medications/drugs implicated in serotonergic syndrome[24]

Serotonergic medications	Over the counter serotonergic medications/ drugs	Perioperatively used serotonergic medications
SSRI (Fluoxetine, Sertraline, Paroxetine, Trazodone, Duloxetine, venlafaxine)	Dextromethorphan	Dextromethorphan
Tricyclics (amytriptyline, imiprimine, nortriptyline)	L-Tryptophan	Methylene blue
Buspirone	St. John's Wort	Ondansetron
Buproprion	Cocaine	Granisetron
Lithium	Alcohol	Fentanyl
MAO-I	Ecstasy	Meperidine
Olanzapine Linezolid	Amphetamines	Sufentanil
Sumatriptan	Methamphetamines	Alfentanil
Tramadol	LSD	Remifentanil

30.3.1.1
Monoamine Oxidase Inhibitors (MAOIs)

- Ideally MAOIs should be stopped 2 weeks prior to elective surgery in conjunction with patient's treating psychiatrist to prevent withdrawal symptoms or severe psychological relapse.
- Because of their significant side effect profile and the advent of other effective antidepressants, MAOIs have largely gone out of use but patients who continue to take them may have been nonresponsive to alternate effective therapies. If a patient is unable to tolerate 2 weeks without therapy or presents emergently, MAOI-safe anesthetic should be used with no meperidine, no serotonergic medications, and only direct acting vasopressors (phenylephrine).

30.3.1.2
Tricyclic Antidepressants (TCAs)

- TCAs are usually continued in the perioperative period; however, if cardiac comorbidities or high surgical risk dictate cessation, TCAs should be tapered gradually over 2 weeks to avoid a withdrawal syndrome. TCAs should be restarted when the patient is tolerating PO and euvolemic. There are no parenteral forms of TCAs.
- If TCAs are continued, perioperative hypotension should be treated with indirect acting vasopressors like ephedrine as direct acting sympathomimetics can cause hypertensive crisis. If hypertensive crisis occurs, it should be treated with vasodilators

like nitroprusside or nitroglycerin. If anticoagulation is necessary, warfarin should be titrated starting at lower doses than normal and INR closely followed.

30.3.1.3
Selective Serotonin Reuptake Inhibitors (SSRIs)

- SSRIs are generally continued throughout the perioperative period. Withdrawal syndromes can occur within 24 h of a missed dose, especially for shorter acting agents like paroxetine. There are no parenteral formulations.
- If a patient has previously experienced significant withdrawal and is planned for a long perioperative NPO period, consider transitioning to a long acting formulation like fluoxetine which has less likelihood of withdrawal.
- Several studies showed in vitro and in vivo risks for bleeding in patients taking SSRIs.[26,27]
  - Platelets actively uptake serotonin and store it in granules which are released to stimulate aggregation.
  - Patients with depression have decreased serotonin in their platelets, and patients who are on SSRIs, which inhibit the uptake of serotonin by platelets, have even lower levels. These decreased platelet levels contribute to abnormal ADP-induced aggregation with preservation of thrombin-induced aggregation and may explain the increased risk of bleeding.[28]
  - Clinical data, however, have been conflicting regarding the actual risk of bleeding. It seems that SSRI may cause a statistically significant but only clinically mild increased risk of bleeding.[29]
  - This risk should be discussed with the patient and surgical team in specific instances where small volume bleeding may result in significant morbidity such as intracranial and spine surgery.
  - If SSRIs are to be stopped for bleeding risk or other concerns they should be tapered over a few weeks to avoid withdrawal symptoms. There may, however, be a rebound effect on platelet activity during the first 30 days after stopping SSRIs where patients with cardiovascular disease may be at increased risk of myocardial infarction.

30.3.1.4
Antipsychotics/Neuroleptics

- Both atypical and typical antipsychotics should be continued throughout perioperative period including morning of surgery.
- Because of the high incidence of QTc prolongation and an association with sudden cardiac death, a baseline EKG should be obtained and the patient monitored for possible synergistic comorbidities and medications (see Table 30.1).

- If psychotic patients require prolonged period of NPO, IM or oral dissolving formulations of antipsychotics should be used. Haloperidol has been widely used, and newer agents are available.
- Clozapine use is carefully monitored because of its unique side effects including agranulocytosis. Clozapine should be continued, including the day of surgery to prevent relapse, but it has been implicated in intraoperative hypotension, likely secondary to its alpha-blockade. The hypotension is responsive to vasopressors.
  - If the patient is NPO for a prolonged period (>2 days), clozapine should not be restarted at the prior dose but rather re-titrated from low doses to prior dose to prevent severe hypotension.[14]

30.3.1.5
Mood Stabilizers

- Due to risk of toxicity with perioperative fluid shifts and multiple organ system effects, and no withdrawal symptoms, lithium should be held 2–3 days prior to all but the most minor surgical procedures. Lithium can be restarted when patient fluid status is stable and tolerating PO. Resume home dosing while monitoring lithium levels for at least the first week.[14,25]
- Other mood stabilizers and anticonvulsants should be continued throughout perioperative period.

30.3.1.6
Benzodiazepines

- Benzodiazepines should be continued throughout the perioperative period to prevent withdrawal symptoms and for anxiolysis.
- Patients on chronic benzodiazepines may require higher doses of amnestics and anesthetics for equivalent effects. Additionally, these patients must be closely monitored for additive sedation and respiratory depressant effects of opioids.

30.3.1.7
Psychostimulants

- These medications are primarily used for treatment of ADD/ADHD or sedating side effects of other psychotropics.
- They are generally withheld on the morning of surgery to prevent potential increased reaction to sympathomimetics, but no evidence exists to forgo surgery if the medications are taken, and some evidence suggests that they may improve recovery of mental state postoperatively.

30.3.1.8 Other Psychotropic Medications

- These medications include antidepressants with unique serotonin, dopamine and norepinephrine receptor effects as well as buspirone, an anxiolytic, and disulfiram, a substance abuse deterrent.
- In general, these medications can be continued, but if specific concerns exist they can be stopped, often requiring a taper and possibly consultation with a psychiatrist.

30.3.1.9 Herbal Remedies for Psychologic Ailments

- There are several herbal remedies used for psychologic ailments. These herbals are not technically medications yet there is no guarantee that they are free from harmful side effects and interactions around the time of surgery.
- The American Society of Anesthesiologists (ASA) recommends stopping all herbal supplements 2 weeks prior to surgery because oftentimes specific elements are not known to patient or medical practitioner.
  - Some herbs used for sedative properties can have additive sedating effects with anesthesia including valerian root, kavakava and St. John's wort which is frequently used as a natural alternative to antidepressants and can cause serotonin syndrome.
  - *Ginkgo biloba* taken for improved memory can potentiate bleeding as can ginseng which also affects pharmacokinetics of other medications.[20]

30.4 Intraoperative

- Potential anesthetic, perioperative comorbidity, and medication interactions are listed in Table 30.1 (QTc) and Table 30.2 (Psychotropics). These interactions should be taken into account when formulating the anesthetic plan.
- Postoperatively, patients with serious mental illness have increased likelihood of confusion and delirium in the post-anesthetic period which significantly decreases when chronic medications are maintained throughout the perioperative period.[23]
- Additionally, anesthetics that incorporate low dose ketamine have been shown to decrease post-anesthetic delirium, confusion, and pain scores in patients with major depression or schizophrenia.[30,31]

30.5 Postoperative

- Patient perception of pain is altered by psychiatric diseases.
  - Patients with depression tend to have lower thresholds for pain with greater morbidity from pain.

- Patients with schizophrenia are less likely to complain of pain and may have greater underlying pathology by the time they do complain of pain.
- Regardless of the psychiatric disease, these patients require adequate pain medication to allow participation in rehabilitation.
  - Use of epidural postoperative analgesia with local anesthetics has been shown to be effective in schizophrenic patients at reducing postoperative ileus which could contribute to a decrease in the higher complication rates seen in these patients after abdominal surgery.[32]
- If psychoactive medications were withheld at the time of surgery they should be restarted as soon as the patient is hemodynamically stable and able to tolerate oral intake. If a lengthy delay to PO intake is anticipated, a parenteral or oral dissolving formulation should be substituted to prevent withdrawal or relapse of underlying disease.
- To maintain psychiatric stability, minimize environmental disturbances and maximize postoperative education and support. Family members and psychiatric liaison are helpful.

30.6 Conclusion

Psychotropic drugs are included in the medication regimen of a significant and increasing proportion of the surgical patient population. These medications have a multitude of possible side effects, withdrawal syndromes, and potential for drug–drug interactions with anesthetic agents. However, the evidence base underlying current recommendations for perioperative medication management is lacking. Although different psychiatric conditions are known to predispose patients to specific postoperative complications, the current status of the psychiatric illness and degree of functional dependence are more predictive of postsurgical morbidity than specific diagnoses. As such, it is critical to obtain a complete psychiatric and medication history from patients preoperatively and seek psychiatric consultation when necessary.

References

1. Kessler RC, Demler O, Frank RG, et al. Prevalence and treatment of mental disorders, 1990 to 2003. *N Engl J Med.* 2005;352(24):2515-2523.
2. Scher CS, Anwar M. The self-reporting of psychiatric medications in patients scheduled for elective surgery. *J Clin Anesth.* 1999;11(8):619-621.
3. Perks A, Chakravarti S, Manninen P. Preoperative anxiety in neurosurgical patients. *J Neurosurg Anesthesiol.* 2009;21(2):127-130.
4. Kudoh A, Katagai H, Takazawa T. Increased postoperative pain scores in chronic depression patients who take antidepressants. *J Clin Anesth.* 2002;14(6):421-425.
5. Papaioannou M, Skapinakis P, Damigos D, et al. The role of catastrophizing in the prediction of postoperative pain. *Pain Med.* 2009;10(8):1452-1459.
6. Zoccolillo MS, Cloninger CR. Excess medical care of women with somatization disorder. *South Med J.* 1986;79(5):532-535.

7. Copeland LA, Zeber JE, Pugh MJ, et al. Postoperative complications in the seriously mentally ill: a systematic review of the literature. *Ann Surg*. 2008;248(1):31-38.
8. Cutler BS, Fink MP. Postoperative complications in patients with disabling psychiatric illnesses or intellectual handicaps. A case-controlled, retrospective analysis. *Arch Surg*. 1990;125(11):1436-1440.
9. Trifiro G, Gambassi G, Sen EF, et al. Association of community-acquired pneumonia with antipsychotic drug use in elderly patients: a nested case-control study. *Ann Intern Med*. 2010;152(7):418-425. W139-40.
10. Cooke BK, Magas LT, Virgo KS, et al. Appendectomy for appendicitis in patients with schizophrenia. *Am J Surg*. 2007;193(1):41-48.
11. Margenthaler JA, Longo WE, Virgo KS, et al. Risk factors for adverse outcomes after the surgical treatment of appendicitis in adults. *Ann Surg*. 2003;238(1):59-66.
12. Tully PJ, Baker RA, Turnbull D, et al. The role of depression and anxiety symptoms in hospital readmissions after cardiac surgery. *J Behav Med*. 2008;31(4):281-290.
13. Dew MA, Kormos RL, DiMartini AF, et al. Prevalence and risk of depression and anxiety-related disorders during the first three years after heart transplantation. *Psychosomatics*. 2001;42(4):300-313.
14. Desan PH, Powsner S. Assessment and management of patients with psychiatric disorders. *Crit Care Med*. 2004;32(4 Suppl):S166-S173.
15. Ray WA, Chung CP, Murray KT, et al. Atypical antipsychotic drugs and the risk of sudden cardiac death. *N Engl J Med*. 2009;360(3):225-235.
16. Glassman AH, Bigger JT Jr. Antipsychotic drugs: prolonged QTc interval, torsade de pointes, and sudden death. *Am J Psychiatry*. 2001;158(11):1774-1782.
17. Naguib M, Koorn R. Interactions between psychotropics, anaesthetics and electroconvulsive therapy: implications for drug choice and patient management. *CNS Drugs*. 2002;16(4):229-247.
18. Haddad PM. Antidepressant discontinuation syndromes. *Drug Saf*. 2001;24(3):183-197.
19. Huyse FJ, Touw DJ, van Schijndel RS, de Lange JJ, Slaets JP. Psychotropic drugs and the perioperative period: a proposal for a guideline in elective surgery. *Psychosomatics*. 2006;47(1):8-22.
20. Baerdemaeker L, Audenaert K, Peremans K. Anaesthesia for patients with mood disorders. *Curr Opin Anaesthesiol*. 2005;18(3):333-338.
21. Looper KJ. Potential medical and surgical complications of serotonergic antidepressant medications. *Psychosomatics*. 2007;48(1):1-9.
22. Khawam EA, Laurencic G, Malone DA Jr. Side effects of antidepressants: an overview. *Cleve Clin J Med*. 2006;73(4):351-353. 356–61.
23. Kudoh A, Katagai H, Takazawa T. Antidepressant treatment for chronic depressed patients should not be discontinued prior to anesthesia. *Can J Anaesth*. 2002;49(2):132-136.
24. Altman CS, Jahangiri MF. Serotonin syndrome in the perioperative period. *Anesth Analg*. 2010;110(2):526-528.
25. Merli GJ, Weitz HH. *Medical Management of the Surgical Patient*. 3rd ed. Philadelphia: Saunders/Elsevier; 2008:840. xviii.
26. Movig KL, Janssen MW, de MJ Waal, et al. Relationship of serotonergic antidepressants and need for blood transfusion in orthopedic surgical patients. *Arch Intern Med*. 2003;163(19):2354-2358.
27. Gartner R, Cronin-Fenton D, Hundborg HH, et al. Use of selective serotonin reuptake inhibitors and risk of re-operation due to post-surgical bleeding in breast cancer patients: a Danish population-based cohort study. *BMC Surg*. 2010;10:3.
28. Maurer-Spurej E, Pittendreigh C, Solomons K. The influence of selective serotonin reuptake inhibitors on human platelet serotonin. *Thromb Haemost*. 2004;91(1):119-128.

29. van Haelst IM, Egberts TC, Doodeman HJ, et al. Use of serotonergic antidepressants and bleeding risk in orthopedic patients. *Anesthesiology*. 2010;112(3):631-636.
30. Ishihara H, Satoh Y, Kudo H, et al. No psychological emergence reactions in schizophrenic surgical patients immediately after propofol, fentanyl, and ketamine intravenous anesthesia. *J Anesth*. 1999;13(1):17-22.
31. Kudoh A, Takahira Y, Katagai H, et al. Small-dose ketamine improves the postoperative state of depressed patients. *Anesth Analg*. 2002;95(1):114-118, Table of contents.
32. Kudoh A, Katagai H, Takazawa T. Effect of epidural analgesia on postoperative paralytic ileus in chronic schizophrenia. *Reg Anesth Pain Med*. 2001;26(5):456-460.

Substance Abuse

31

Nadene C. Fair and Howard S. Smith

31.1 Introduction

- The following are consensus definitions recognized by the American Academy of Pain Medicine, American Pain Society, and American Society of Addiction Medicine:
  - **Addiction**: A primary, chronic, neurobiologic disease with genetic, psychosocial, and environmental factors influencing its development and manifestations. It is characterized by behaviors that include one or more of the following (The 5 C's) impaired **C**ontrol over drug use, **C**ompulsive use, **C**hronic use, **C**ontinued use despite harm, and **C**raving.
  - **Physical Dependence**: A state of adaptation made evident by a drug-class-specific withdrawal syndrome that can be produced by abrupt cessation, rapid dose reduction, decreasing blood level of the drug, and/or administration of an antagonist.
  - **Tolerance**: A state of adaptation in which exposure to a drug induces changes that result in diminution of one or more of the drug's effects over time.
- Though discussed separately, it is important to remember that most patients will abuse more than one substance. The use of these substances concurrently confers greater risk than if used alone.

31.2 Alcohol

- To help with the perioperative care of patients with alcohol use disorders (AUDs), it is important to understand how this is defined. There are three broad categories: alcohol misuse, at risk drinking, and alcohol abuse and dependence.[1]

N.C. Fair (✉)
Department of Internal Medicine, Morehouse School of Medicine, 720 Westview Dr. SW
Atlanta, 30310 Atlanta, GA, USA
e-mail: nfair@msm.edu

S.L. Cohn (ed.), *Perioperative Medicine*,
DOI: 10.1007/978-0-85729-498-2_31,

- The US National Institute on Alcohol Abuse and Alcoholism (NIAAA) encourages physicians to screen their patients for identification of alcohol use disorders (alcohol dependence and alcohol abuse) as well as for at-risk drinking [defined as alcohol consumption of ≥ 5 and ≥ 4 drinks (~14 g pure alcohol) in a single day for men and women, respectively, or ≥ 14 and ≥ 7 drinks/week for men and women, respectively]..[2]
  - Identification of at-risk drinking:
    1. "Do you sometimes drink alcoholic beverages?"
    2. "How many times in the past year have you had five or more drinks in a day (for men) or four or more drinks in a day (for women)?"
  - The Alcohol Use Disorders Identification Test (AUDIT) is particularly sensitive in identifying less severe drinking problems.[3] The test was developed by the World Health Organization and consists of ten questions regarding alcohol consumption, drinking behavior, adverse reactions, and alcohol-related problems. Each question is scored according to a 5-point scale (0–4). The selected cut-off scores used in the present study were equal to 8 and 4 in men and women, respectively. The AUDIT performs best with a cutoff of 4 points for alcohol misuse, ≥5 points as a positive result for at risk drinking and 6 points for alcohol dependence.[4]

31.2.1 Patient-Specific Risks

- Patients may not be forthcoming with the extent of their use of alcohol or may be unable to provide an adequate medical history.
- AUDs are often associated with cigarette smoking and drug abuse as well as psychiatric disorders.
- Alcoholic patients are at increased risk for various medical complications and comorbid conditions including hepatitis, cirrhosis, portal hypertension, gastritis, pancreatitis, varices, peptic ulcer disease, cardiomyopathy, arrhythmias, hypertension, stroke, neuropathy, anemia, thrombocytopenia, neutropenia, malnutrition, electrolyte abnormalities, cancer, and psychosis. These patients also have 2–3 times more postoperative complications than nonalcoholic patients.
- The physician also needs to anticipate the occurrence of these complications in the postoperative period, even if not identified previously. Alcohol withdrawal syndrome (AWS) is associated with increased morbidity, and complications may be related to older age, seizure history, or delay in diagnosis.

31.2.2 Surgery-Specific Risks

- AUDs are more prevalent in the surgical setting than the general population, particularly in patients admitted for trauma, otolaryngology procedures, and general surgery.

– Emergent surgery may be more frequent related to trauma.

- The stress of surgery may predispose patients to or exacerbate AWS.

31.2.3 Preoperative Evaluation

- A thorough history and physical examination along with pertinent laboratory work up will help in the identification and optimization of patients with AUDs prior to surgery. Elicit symptoms and signs of complications from alcohol use.
- There are several screening tests for alcoholism. The most commonly used and simplest one is the CAGE questionnaire (Table 31.1). Elicit a history of other substances that may be abused as well. Once an AUD has been identified then the physician must note duration of alcohol use, type and quantity of alcohol use, and timing of last alcohol intake..[5]
- Anticipate acute intoxication prior to surgery. This may be delayed in the postoperative period related to the effects of anesthesia and opioids. Determine if patient has history of alcohol withdrawal syndromes. Are there any features of AWS? (see Table 31.2)
- Anesthesiologists need to be aware of the presence of acute alcohol intoxication and chronic alcohol abuse as well as the use of any preoperative drug treatments or prophylaxis for AWS as these issues may affect the patients' response to anesthesia.
- Encourage abstinence or reduced alcohol intake prior to elective surgery in an effort to reduce perioperative risk in patients with AUDs.
- There are no specific laboratory tests for alcoholism; however, certain lab results are sensitive for alcoholism and will detect abnormalities related to alcohol use. Abnormal labs, when found, indicate a higher risk in these patients and may be correlated with the amount and the duration of alcohol used.
- Tests to be included in the perioperative work up of the alcoholic patient include complete blood count, comprehensive chemistry panel (including glucose, electrolytes, liver enzymes, and albumin), prothrombin time, blood alcohol level, and EKG. Consider a urinary drug screen for possible abuse of other substances. Depending on the results of these tests, additional testing may be warranted.
- Consider the MELD score in patients with cirrhosis undergoing surgery to estimate risk of postoperative mortality (see Chap. 27).

Table 31.1 CAGE questions

C	Have you tried to **Cut** down on your drinking?
A	Are you **Angry** or **Annoyed** when others criticize your drinking?
G	Do you ever feel **Guilty** about your drinking?
E	Do you ever take an **Eye opener**?

Source: Reproduced from John and Ewing[6], with permission. Copyright © (1984) American Medical Association. All rights reserved

Table 31.2 AWS, symptoms and time related to last drink

Withdrawal syndrome	Time from last drink	Symptoms
Autonomic Hyperactivity	6 h Peak 24–48 h	Mild to moderate symptoms: tremulous, irritability, nystagmus, nausea and vomiting, hyperreflexia, sleep disorders, tachycardia, diaphoresis and fever. Resolve within 24–36 h
Hallucinations	12–24 h	Usually visual, tactile and auditory hallucinations also Resolve within 24 h but may persist for up to 6 days
Seizures	12–48 h	Generalized tonic clonic, single and short in duration with short post-ictal period. May occur as early as 2 h after last alcohol use
Delirium Tremens	5 days	Confusion, autonomic symptoms-hypertension, tachycardia and febrile-T>101 F-visual and auditory hallucinations. Lasts several days. Mortality-15% in untreated patients. Patients with concurrent acute medical illnesses are 5× more likely to experience DTs

31.2.4 Perioperative Management

- Alcohol use may alter metabolism of various medications. Anesthesia and analgesia dosing may be affected.
- Monitor for arrhythmias, bleeding, surgical site infections, and AWS.
- Provide supportive care for patients with AUDs throughout the entire perioperative period. Hypoxia and hypotension may increase the risk of postoperative delirium.
- Be prepared to use pharmacologic agents to treat early withdrawal symptoms and to prevent progression to more serious withdrawal states.
- Benzodiazepines are the mainstay of therapy and are used to control sympathetic overactivity, hallucinations and to prevent seizures or subsequent seizures. Front loading or scheduled, fixed dosing of benzodiazepines is recommended to minimize seizures associated with AWS.
- Selected patients with AWS may benefit from the addition of a nonselective beta blocker, added to benzodiazepines and titrated to BP and heart rate to help minimize sympathetic overactivity and minimize cardiac complications.
- Clonidine may be useful in patients who cannot tolerate beta blockers and are in need of further control of sympathetic overactivity. Alternatively, dexmedetomidine may be useful as an intravenous infusion therapy in addition to benzodiazepines, for control of sympathetic overactivity.
- Carbamazepine can be used in patients who cannot take benzodiazepines.
- Haloperidol may be used for management of hallucinations that fail to respond to adequate doses of benzodiazepines.

- Supportive adjuncts include maintaining adequate hydration and nutrition and monitoring of blood glucose levels. Ensure thiamine, folate, and electrolyte replacement (including magnesium) as needed and psychosocial support as necessary.
- Postoperatively patients should be monitored closely for clinical and laboratory evidence of complications arising from alcohol use during the immediate postoperative period and up to 7 days after the last drink.
- Commonly encountered problems include infections, bleeding, alcohol withdrawal syndrome (AWS), delirium, heart failure, arrhythmias, aspiration pneumonia, diminished cellular immunity, and exaggerated response to surgical stress.
- Interventions to facilitate cessation of alcohol use in the future can be implemented during the postoperative period, prior to discharge.

31.3 Cocaine

- Cocaine use confers additional risk to patients going for surgery so it is imperative that physicians identify patients who use cocaine and recognize and treat cocaine intoxication, withdrawal and any medical conditions associated with chronic use.
- Cocaine may be injected, snorted or ingested orally and the mode of ingestion can contribute to complications seen in patients (snorting-perforated septum, crack lung).
- Cocaine is a sympathomimetic agent that causes an increase in catecholamine levels by inhibiting the reabsorption of dopamine into sympathetic nerve terminals in the central nervous system. This leads to an increase in dopamine with persistent neuronal stimulation and also causes the addictive properties of cocaine. With long term use patients will develop tolerance as evidenced by increasing doses of the drug as well as increased frequency of use. To prevent withdrawal symptoms and unpleasant side effects that may occur, these patients may use other substances including:
  - Heroin (concurrent use with cocaine is referred to as speedballing) – this enhances the effects of both drugs
  - Cannabis – this drug increases the plasma levels of cocaine
  - Alcohol – along with cocaine leads to the formation of the toxic substance cocaethylene which is more toxic than either alcohol or cocaine alone and has a longer half life.
- Cocaine is rapidly metabolized and its metabolites can be found in urine for several days up to 2 weeks.

31.3.1 Preoperative Evaluation

- Patients requiring urgent or emergent surgery may be in a state of intoxication or withdrawal.
- A thorough history regarding drug use and physical examination for signs and symptoms of cocaine intoxication or withdrawal is important in assessing the patient's status (Table 31.3). Presentation may be nonspecific and subtle in both cases.

Table 31.3 Complications of cocaine use

System	Complications
Cardiovascular	Chest pain Accelerated coronary atherosclerosis Cardiac arrhythmias Heart failure Cocaine induced hypercoagulable state Labile hypertension
Pulmonary	Bronchospasm Pneumonia Hemoptysis Diffuse alveolar hemorrhage Asthma Interstitial pneumonitis BOOP Barotrauma/pneumothorax/pneumomediastinum Chronic rhinitis Osteolytic sinusitis Cough SOB Hoarseness
Central nervous system	Headache Seizures Stroke-ischemic or hemorrhagic Movement disorders, ataxia, tics
GI tract	Delayed gastric emptying Ulcers Intestinal ischemia Colitis Hepatic necrosis
Psychiatry	Insomnia Hallucinations/psychosis Anxiety/panic attacks Weight loss
Renal	Rhabdomyolysis Renal infarction Acute renal failure FSGS
Miscellaneous	Fever Thrombocytopenia Sexual dysfunction Infectious-HepB/C, HIV

Table 31.4 Signs and symptoms of cocaine intoxication and withdrawal

Cocaine intoxication	Cocaine withdrawal
Sense of euphoria	Myalgias
Increased energy	Depressed mood
Decreased appetite	Difficulty sleeping
Increased productivity	Anxiety
Decreased need for sleep	Fatigue
Dilated pupils	Increased need for sleep
Sinus tachycardia	Extrapyramidal symptoms
Fever	Acute psychosis-severe paranoia and bizarre delusions-tactile hallucinations
Hypertension	Strong cravings for cocaine
High doses: Paranoia, violent behavior, auditory hallucinations and tremor	
Over dose: Seizures, acidosis, pulmonary edema, cardiac and/or respiratory arrest	

- Patients who are identified as cocaine users in the perioperative period for elective surgery should be advised to stop taking the drug at least 2 weeks prior to surgery. Concurrent use of other substances should be identified and recommendations be made specifically for those agents to be stopped as well. A UDS is recommended for the morning of surgery.
- Complications of cocaine use depend on route of administration and chronicity of use (see Table 31.4).

31.3.2 Perioperative Management

- For surgical emergencies, in which surgery can still be delayed for an hour or two, patients with recent ingestion of cocaine and symptoms and signs of intoxication can be held in the OR with supportive care until the acute intoxication has passed as the half-life of cocaine is about 30–90 min. Supportive care is recommended during the intoxication phase. Benzodiazepines may be used for hypertension and agitation that may occur during this time. In the postoperative period, cocaine withdrawal should be anticipated and managed early. Supportive care involves placing the patient in quiet surroundings and ensuring that they are eating and sleeping well and are adequately hydrated. Benzodiazepines can be used for severe agitation and psychosis and, if needed, antipsychotics with minimal anticholinergic side effects can be used. Cocaine withdrawal resolves within several days.
- The cardiovascular complications of cocaine are the ones that are frequently encountered in the perioperative setting. The commonest complaint is chest pain.
- Cocaine-induced <u>chest pain</u> mimics the typical cardiac ischemic pain caused by coronary artery disease occlusion. About 50% of patients with cocaine-induced ischemia will have typical anginal chest pain.

  - Cocaine-induced chest pain caused by coronary vasoconstriction may occur in normal or diseased arteries and vasoconstriction may be diffuse or local. Cocaine causes accelerated atherosclerosis as well as induction of a hypercoagulable state.
  - Cardiac ischemia can occur several minutes to 15 h after ingestion of cocaine.
  - Recommended laboratory tests to aid in diagnosis include UDS, cardiac enzymes, and EKG, which may be nonspecific and non-diagnostic.
  - Management includes oxygen therapy, aspirin to decrease thrombus formation, benzodiazepines to decrease the sympathetic drive and thus decrease the myocardial oxygen demand as well as to decrease anxiety and nitrates to relieve chest pain. Currently, it is not recommended to initiate beta blocker use in patients using cocaine. Morphine may be used if needed to relieve pain. Both morphine and nitrates also decrease myocardial demand for oxygen as well as decrease preload. Primary PTCA may be necessary. Second-line treatment considerations include the use of calcium channel blockers (CCB) and phentolamine for management of associated hypertension, and IV heparin, bearing in mind the risk of intracerebral bleeding and aortic dissection in these patients. Thrombolytic agents may be used with caution in patients with STEMI, if angioplasty is not available. Regional anesthesia is recommended as opposed to general anesthesia where possible.

- Labile hypertension and hypertensive crises may be induced by cocaine. Benzodiazepines, nitrates, nitroprusside, hydralazine, CCB, and phentolamine can be used to control BP.
- Cocaine-induced cardiac arrhythmias are generally short lived and usually resolve spontaneously. Sinus tachycardia and bradycardia as well as SVT and VFib may be seen. If the patient becomes hemodynamically unstable, ACLS algorithms are employed. Avoid class Ia antiarrhythmics and beta blockers in these patients. Heart failure is usually systolic dysfunction arising from drug-related interstitial myocardial fibrosis with subsequent LVH and dilated cardiomyopathy. Patients are treated in the same way as those with heart failure of other causes with the exception of the use of beta blockers.

31.4 Opioids

- Opioids may be inhaled, ingested orally, injected or smoked dependent on the preparation. When injected, the drug is most rapid acting and produces the highest concentration of the drug in the body. Tolerance and physical dependence can develop after only 1–2 weeks of daily use. Opioid metabolites may be detected in the urine for 48 h to several days, even longer in chronic users. Heroin has a specific metabolite 6-monoacetylmorphine (MAM), but there may be false-negative screens as not all metabolites of all opioids are detected on routine UDS, and false-positive if the patient is taking fluoroquinolones, rifampin, or poppy seeds.

31.4.1 Preoperative Evaluation

- Elicit the use of any of opiates and once identified, determine the specific drug, route of use, quantity, prescribers, symptoms associated with use or lack of use, and use of other substances. Patients should be assessed for opiate toxicity and withdrawal.
- Ask whether or not the patient is in a maintenance program. If they are, determine which agent is being used, the dose, frequency, and last use (preferably with documentation from the maintenance program). Pain management strategies in the postoperative setting should also be addressed, especially in those patients who are in a maintenance program.
- Patients enrolled in a methadone clinic for heroin addiction provide an additional challenge.
  - Obtain a preoperative EKG to look for QT prolongation.
  - Continue their outpatient dose of methadone up to the morning of surgery.
  - If patient is to be NPO, an opioid analgesic equivalent should be given.
  - Do not titrate the dose of methadone upward for pain control as this may lead to toxicity. Also do not treat with mixed opioid agonist–antagonist (nalburphine), as these agents provide no further benefit and may actually precipitate withdrawal.
- Other medications that patients may be on are:
  - Naltrexone is an opioid antagonist used in the outpatient setting. It should not be given for actively addicted hospitalized patients as it can cause an acute withdrawal.
  - Sublingual buprenorphine (Subutex) is a partial agonist that is used to treat mild to moderate physical dependence. Sublingual buprenorphine is also available in combination with naloxone (Suboxone) in efforts to discourage intravenous abuse. Recommended dose is between 2 and 24 mg/day with a target dose of 16 mg/day. LFT abnormalities may occur.
- Medical complications of chronic opioid dependence should be elicited, and physicians should be aware of the possibility of these complications arising in the perioperative period (Table 31.5).

Table 31.5 Complications of chronic opiate use

Infections	IVDU, HIV, endocarditis, cellulitis, abscess, sepsis, pneumonia, septic emboli, viral hepatitis, necrotizing fasciitis, septic arthritis, thrombophlebitis
Cardiac	Drug induced bradycardia, hypotension, arrhythmias
Pulmonary	Severe or fatal asthma exacerbation, noncardiogenic pulmonary edema, talcosis
Neurologic	Sedation, polyneuropathy, seizures, transverse myelitis
GIT	Ileus, nausea, constipation
GU	Urinary retention, glomerular nephritis
Pregnancy	Pre-eclampsia, neonatal complications

31.4.2 Perioperative Management

- Opioid toxicity affects primarily the central nervous system and the cardiovascular system.
  - Common findings include analgesia, euphoria, lethargy, hypotension, bradycardia, hypothermia, miosis, neurocardiogenic pulmonary edema, and respiratory depression.
  - Management of opioid toxicity involves supportive care-symptom-directed management if the patient is hemodynamically stable, and the use of very small doses of a short-acting opioid antagonist such as Naloxone titrated as appropriate if the patient shows signs of hemodynamic instability – respiratory depression, bradycardia, or hypotension. The patient should be closely monitored.
  - Neurocardiogenic pulmonary edema may be seen 24 h after drug use or naloxone use and is life threatening. NIPPV or intubation along with supportive care is recommended.
- Opioid withdrawal may be noted 4–6 h after last ingestion dependent upon the drug ingested.
  - Withdrawal peaks at 24–48 h (more delayed with methadone) and usually lasts about a week – hence patients are usually admitted for 1 week for detoxification.
  - Look for withdrawal shortly after admission or it may be delayed until after the postoperative analgesics have worn off. Patients may complain of difficulty sleeping, restlessness, nausea, vomiting, diarrhea, diaphoresis, increased lacrimation, myalgias, yawning and abdominal cramping. Mydriasis may be noted on examination.
  - Clonidine, although not approved by the FDA for this use, has been noted to help patients with the GI and autonomic symptoms of opioid withdrawal. It should only be initiated in patients who are deemed compliant. Common side effects include bradycardia, hypotension, and rebound hypertension on abrupt cessation.
  - Perioperative analgesic strategies employ multimodal techniques including anti-inflammatory agents, various "nerve blocks or regional anesthetic/analgesic techniques with continuous infusions of local anesthetics," various nontraditional analgesics/co-analgesics, neuromodulation approaches, and other non-pharmacologic techniques.

31.5 Tobacco

- Tobacco may be smoked or chewed and is usually used in conjunction with other substances.
- Smoking tobacco is a frequent lifestyle risk factor that impacts surgical outcome and is associated with postoperative morbidity.
- Most common perioperative complications related to smoking are cardiopulmonary complications, poor wound and tissue healing, and wound infection.Smoking tobacco results in multiple organ changes that have potential adverse effects on the surgical outcome:

  - Increased levels of carbon monoxide resulting in a decrease in the amount of oxygen available for cellular activity.
  - Increased nicotine levels can cause increased sympathetic activity resulting in tachycardia and hypertension creating an oxygen demand/supply mismatch resulting in relative hypoxia at the wound site and in the heart.
  - Impairment of immune function increasing risk of infection.
  - Impaired production of collagen interfering with wound healing.
  - Reduced pulmonary capacity, increased mucus production, and poor ciliary function leading to perioperative pulmonary complications.
- With abstinence from smoking most of these impairments are corrected: immune competence after 2–6 weeks of abstinence, wound healing after 3–4 weeks, and pulmonary function after 6–8 weeks.
- In the preoperative assessment identify tobacco smoking, quantify it, and inquire whether or not other substances are used.
- Counsel patients to stop smoking for 6–8 weeks prior to surgery. They should be made aware of the benefits and side effects of smoking cessation, how to manage withdrawal symptoms, and offered support for cessation as well as nicotine substitution products.
- Postoperatively monitor patients for cardiopulmonary complications and focus on wound care.

31.6 Marijuana and Metamphetamine

Acute effects of these substances, with or without general anesthesia are listed in Table 31.6.

31.7 Perioperative Management of the Recovering Addict

- Perioperative assessment addresses the patients who are acutely intoxicated with, chronically abusing, or withdrawing from drugs, but there is rarely any consideration for those patients who are recovering from substance abuse. Recovery is a complex process that involves continuous intense personal effort on the part of the patient. It involves abstinence as well as a series of lifestyle changes to maintain sobriety.
- The perioperative period is worrisome for the recovering addict as there is the possibility for relapse and the fear that pain will not be controlled due to a history of addiction. Additionally, the recovering patient may also display abnormal behavioral responses to stress that in turn increase the risk of relapse. Several medications may be used in maintaining sobriety, and these are of importance during the perioperative period because of their effect on the patient and potential to alter response to medications (Table 31.7).
- Although guidelines for management of recovering addicts during the perioperative period are limited, the following are prudent recommendations:

Table 31.6 Acute effects of marijuana and methamphetamine (with or without general anesthesia)

Marijuana	Methamphetamine
• Pupil constriction, conjunctival congestion	• Pupil dilation
• Headache, tremors, ataxia	• Headache, nausea/vomiting, anorexia
• Anxiety, ↑ appetite	• Anxiety, psychosis
• Arrhythmias, orthostatic hypotension	• MI, tachycardia, arrhythmias, chest pain
• Tachycardia (may want to avoid the use of agents such as ketamine, pancuronium) [High doses may lead to bradycardia and hypotension]	• HTN (consider treating with alpha adrenergic blockers; avoid beta-blockers so as not to get unopposed alpha adrenergic stimulation)
• Myocardial depression (May cause additive profound myocardial depression if used with potent inhalation agents)	• Cardiac arrest
• Oropharyngitis with acute upper-airway edema and obstruction (May consider administering dexamethasone as prophylaxis)	• Hyperventilation, pneumothorax, pulmonary edema, cough, wheezing
• Mild tachypnea	• Hyperthermia, rhabdomyolysis
• Upper-airway irritability/bronchospasm; laryngospasm (In the setting of GA – have succinylcholine immediately available)	• Acute renal failure, myoglobinuria, diuresis
• May ↑ sedative effects of drugs like alcohol or diazepam or ↑ the stimulatory effects of drugs like amphetamine or cocaine	• May ↑ Anesthetic Requirements (↓ duration of thiopental, attenuate strength and duration of succinylcholine)

Table 31.7 Medications used in maintenance of sobriety – perioperative implications

Medication	Drug of abuse	Implications
Methadone LAAM Buprenorphine Nalmefene	Opioids	Maintenance dose should be continued in the perioperative setting
Disulfiram Calcium carbimide	Alcohol	Disulfiram should be stopped 10 days preoperatively. There may be altered response to sympathomimetics and alteration in metabolism of medications
Acamprosate	Alcohol	Unsure as to implications in the perioperative period
Naltrexone	Alcohol	Stop this drug 3 days before surgery. It can cause an altered response to opioid antagonists
Antiepileptics	Alcohol Opioids	Prolongation of neuromuscular blockade may occur
SSRIs	Alcohol Benzodiazepines Barbiturates	May cause bradycardia and hypotension but rarely interfere with perioperative management

- Preoperatively, a detailed history of the addiction and recovery will reduce the anxiety about the operative experience.
- Elicit the history of the drug abuse, type, quality and compliance with a recovery program and self-help groups should be elicited.
- Determine how long has the patient been in recovery, if there were relapses, and if so, what were the triggers.
- Note sponsors and counselors and support systems that may be involved in the patients' care, as these are powerful defenses against relapse in the stressful perioperative period.
- Determine if there is end-organ damage from chronic substance abuse that may require further evaluation and management before surgery.
- A urine drug screen (UDS) may be indicated to rule out drug use that may necessitate further referral.
- If needed, anxiolytic agents may be used cautiously.
- Preoperatively, establish a clear plan for postoperative pain control. Patients should be reassured that a history of addiction is not a contraindication to postoperative pain management.

The patient with a history of substance abuse poses many issues during the perioperative evaluation and management of patients. As such, physicians should be comfortable talking about these issues, knowledgeable in assessing patients for complications of substance use, and cognizant of how to treat them.

References

1. Agabio R, Marras P, Gessa GL, Carpiniello B. Alcohol use disorders, and at-risk drinking in patients affected by a mood disorder, in Cagliari, Italy: sensitivity and specificity of different questionnaires. *Alcohol Alcohol.* 2007;42(6):575-581.
2. National Institute on alcohol abuse and alcoholism and National Institute of Health. helping patients who drink too much. Department of Health and Human Services, Public Health Service, National Institutes of Health, 2005; www.niaaa.nih.gov.
3. Saunders JB, Aasland OG, Babor TF, de la Fuente JR, Grant M. Development of the alcohol use disorders identification test (AUDIT): who collaborative project on early detection of persons with harmful alcohol consumption–II. *Addiction.* 1993;88(6):791-804.
4. Reinert DF, Allen JP. The alcohol use disorders identification test: an update of research findings. *Alcohol Clin Exp Res.* 2007;31(2):185-199.
5. Rumpf HJ, Hapke U, Meyer C, John U. Screening for alcohol use disorders and at-risk drinking in the general population: psychometric performance of three questionnaires. *Alcohol Alcohol.* 2002;37(3):261-268.
6. Ewing JA. Detecting Alcoholism. *The CAGE questionnaire JAMA.* 1984;252(14):1905-1907.

The Pregnant Surgical Patient

32

Beth G. Lewis and Michael P. Carson

32.1 Introduction

- The incidence of non-obstetric surgery in pregnant patients is 0.2–1.0%.[1] The most common surgeries are appendectomy (1/2,000 pregnancies)[2] and cholecystectomy (1–6/10,000 pregnancies).
- The ideal time for non-obstetric surgery is during the second trimester, but it can be done in the first or third depending on the indication and urgency.
- The surgical morbidities are generally the same as for non-pregnant patients, and the best fetal outcomes occur when the mother is kept as healthy as possible. The theoretical/potential risks to the fetus are generally outweighed by the evidence supporting the benefits related to treatment of the maternal issue.
- Understanding the physiological, exam, laboratory value, anatomical, and pharmacokinetic changes during normal pregnancy will enable the consultant to provide educated input.

32.2 Physiologic Changes of Pregnancy

32.2.1 Cardiovascular Changes

- Blood Pressure: Decreases in early pregnancy and reaches the nadir around the 20th gestational week after which it slowly climbs to levels seen in the early first trimester.
  - Systolic blood pressure decreases by 10–20 mmHg and diastolic blood pressure decreases by 10 mmHg.

B.G. Lewis (✉)
Saint Peters University Hospital, Drexel University Medical School, New Brunswick, NJ, USA
e-mail: blewis@saintpetersuh.com

S.L. Cohn (ed.), *Perioperative Medicine*,
DOI: 10.1007/978-0-85729-498-2_32, © Springer-Verlag London Limited 2011

  - The decrease is due to a decrease in systemic and pulmonary vascular resistance.

- Heart Rate: Increases 10–20% compared to the non-pregnant state, more in multiple gestations, and plateaus about 32 weeks.
  - Due to blood pooling in the legs and the normal vasodilation of pregnancy, the pulse may be higher when seated than in left lateral decubitus position.

32.2.1.1
Cardiovascular Exam

Cardiac output and stroke volume increase by 50% (peak 16 weeks), and plasma volume increases throughout pregnancy, peaking at 28–32 weeks.

- Most women have an arterial flow murmur heard over the pulmonic area that softens with inspiration as the chest wall moves away from the pulmonary artery.
- Mammary soufflé is heard during late pregnancy and lactation. This is a holosystolic murmur heard over medial aspects of bilateral breasts.
- Pre-existing murmurs will be louder due to increased blood volume, flow, and cardiac contractility.
- S1 is louder and a non-sustained S3 gallop may be a common finding; however, any sustained gallop (S3 or S4) requires echocardiographic evaluation prior to surgery.
- Leg edema is present in one-third of women, although sudden onset of leg edema may be a sign of thromboembolic disease or preeclampsia.

32.2.2
Pulmonary Changes

- Respiratory rate remains normal, but minute ventilation increases due to a progesterone-mediated increase in tidal volume, resulting in respiratory alkalosis. While there may be a subjective sense of breathlessness, tachypnea is not a normal finding.
- In the second/third trimester the gravid uterus exerts pressure on the diaphragm, thus decreasing functional residual capacity (FRC) by up to 70% while supine.
- There is an increase in the anterior–posterior dimensions of the thorax.
- Peak flow and FEV1 (forced expiratory volume at 1 sec) do not change.

32.2.2.1
Abdominal Exam

- Can usually palpate liver if woman takes deep breath, even in late pregnancy. Evaluating the liver for tenderness is important for women who have preeclampsia.
- May have dullness in Traube's space

32.2.2.2
Neurological Exam

- Reflexes are increased, but clonus is not normal.
- Sensory deficits, such as carpal or tarsal tunnel, are common.

32.3
Key Laboratory Changes (Table 32.1)

- Hemoglobin and hematocrit decrease due to a larger increase in plasma volume than in red cell mass resulting in a dilutional anemia: second trimester Hb/(Hct) ~11 g/dL/(33) and third trimester ~10 g/dL/(30). White count increases to about 8–10,000/mcL.
- Albumin and total protein decrease due to increased plasma volume. Normal albumin is ~3 mg/dL and protein ~6 mg/dL.
- Creatinine decreases (usually <0.9 mg/dL) due to an increase in GFR of about 150%. BUN decreases as well. Twenty-four hour urine protein increases (upper limit of normal is 300 mg/24 h).
- TSH decreases in first trimester (some consider upper limit to be 2.5 mIU/L). Due to homology with TSH, HCG stimulates an increase in thyroid hormone output, and the TSH should normalize within the second trimester. Free T4 may be truly elevated with hyperemesis gravidarum, but usually improves without medical intervention. The normal increase in TBG will cause an increase in Total T4 values, but in these settings the Free T4 or Free Thryoixine Index (Total T4 * T3RU) will be normal.
- Respiratory alkalosis is normal. Normal pH ~7.44, because of increased tidal volume, and pCO_2 28–32 mmHg.

32.4
Diagnostic Imaging in Pregnancy

- It is important to make correct diagnoses to treat pregnant women appropriately. Indicated diagnostic tests can be obtained during pregnancy. Do not withhold tests, medications, or procedures from pregnant women if you cannot otherwise make the diagnosis and/or the results will help dictate the treatment plan.
- X-rays: The upper limit of fetal radiation exposure is felt to be 5.0 rads
  - To put this in perspective, background fetal exposure during an average 9-month pregnancy is 0.3–0.9 rads, whereas a transcontinental flight involves about 0.3 rads.
  - Fetal exposure (in rads) for various radiologic studies and the theoretical number of permissible studies based on those exposures are listed in Table 32.2.

Table 32.1 Values of common laboratory tests during pregnancy

Test	Value/effect of pregnancy
Albumin and total protein	Decrease by 1 mg/dL. Dilutional. Albumin ~3.0, total protein ~6.0.
Alkaline phosphatase	Elevated. From the placenta.
Bicarbonate (serum)	Decreased to 20 meq. Other electrolyte levels are normal.
Blood urea nitrogen	Should be $\leq$ 14 mg/dL
Creatinine	Should be $\leq$ 0.8 mg/dL, mean is 0.5 mg/dL
Creatinine clearance	Increases by 50% to about 150 cc/min.
Creatinine Kinase-MB fraction	May be elevated after Cesarean section. CPK-MB makes up 6% of the total enzyme from the uterus and placenta.
D-Dimer	Increased false positive rate during pregnancy. A negative value may be useful as in the non-pregnant population.
Erythrocyte sedimentation rate	Normally elevated. Not useful during pregnancy.
Fibrinogen	High-normal range to elevated.
Hemoglobin	Decreased. Normal is 10–12 g/dL.
Leukocyte count	Slight increase. Mean 8–10 and up to 14×10^9/L after delivery.
pCO_2	Decreased. Normal is 28–32 mmHg as a result of the normal hyperventilation.
pH	Mildly alkalotic. Tends to run 7.44.
Platelets	Typically normal.
Thyroid labs (TSH, Free T4, Free T3)	No change. Normal TSH values during pregnancy are lower than pre-pregnancy, but usually still in the normal range. Free T4 may be elevated during the first trimester in 40% of women with hyperemesis gravidarum.
Transaminases (AST/ALT) and Bilirubin	Normal.
Urine protein – 24 h collection	Up to 300 mg is normal.

– The concerns regarding the potential or theoretical fetal effects of radiation (loss, malformation, or cancer later in life) must be weighed against the concrete benefit of making the proper diagnosis and initiating indicated treatments.

The risk of loss appears to be an all or nothing threshold effect if >10 rad exposure occurs during the first 8 weeks of gestation. However, exposures >10 rads are not encountered in routine medical care. For a woman who, unaware of her pregnancy, underwent radiologic tests and made it to the second trimester, it appears that the risk to the fetus/child is similar to that of other uncomplicated pregnancies.

Table 32.2 Approximate fetal radiation exposure. This table can be used to give clinicians and patients the proper perspective to consider the benefits of an indicated test

Study	Fetal exposure (rads)	Permissible in pregnancy	PubMed ID of reference
Radiation exposure during transcontinental flight	0.015	333	[17411702]
CXR single/abdomen shielding	0.00007 rads	Up to 70,000	[3513577], [10208701]
V/Q scan	0.1–0.2 rads.	50	[3884214]
CT head	≤0.013		
CT chest first trimester	0.002		[12147847]
CT chest helical Third Trimester	0.013		[12147847]
Arteriogram (pulm/coronary) via femoral vessels	0.2–0.4		[a]
MRI		Appears to have no adverse effect on the fetus.	[8475280] [7489290]

[a]Rosene-Montella and Larson[21]

Exposures less than 2 rads do not appear to increase the lifetime risk of cancer in a child who underwent fetal exposure.

Iodinated contrast likely crosses the placenta, but there is no evidence to suggest any fetal harm. While iodine loads will cause a transient decrease in maternal thyroid hormone output, this effect only lasts 24–48 h.

In postpartum women who received iodinated contrast, a reference from the American College of Radiology supports the statement that breastfeeding should not be interrupted.[3]

- Ultrasound:
  - No untoward fetal effects.
- MRI:
  - Guidelines and recommendations from the Safety Committee of the Society for Magnetic Resonance Imaging (SMRI) support obtaining indicated MRI studies during pregnancy.[4-6]
  - MRI may be the diagnostic test of choice for appendicitis in pregnancy if an ultrasound is not diagnostic.[7] It should also be obtained when indicated for new neurological issues.

Gadolinium is generally avoided because it gets into the amniotic fluid and the effects are unknown, but for complex CNS issues it can be considered.

- Nuclear medicine tests
  - Radioactive iodine is contraindicated in pregnancy

    Fetal thyroid gland begins functioning at 12 weeks gestation, and it takes up iodine 400× more avidly than a maternal thyroid gland.
  - V/Q scans should be obtained when indicated during pregnancy (each imparts only 1/50th of the permissible fetal radiation exposure).
  - Nuclear contrast is eliminated renally.

  Because the bladder is next to the gravid uterus it is advisable to hydrate the patient before and after tests to facilitate elimination of the contrast.

32.5 Prescribing Medications During Pregnancy

- FDA categories are oversimplified, and using them as the sole reason for picking a particular medication or advising against its use should be avoided. Rather than considering a medication "safe," determine if the medication is warranted or indicated.
- Most medications used for medical indications, including commonly used antibiotics, blood pressure medications, and unfractionated heparin, were not put on the market based on studies in pregnant women. Therefore, avoiding a medication because it is not "FDA approved during pregnancy" is not the proper approach.
- Accidental exposure does not warrant termination of pregnancy.
- Physicians desire reassurance (evidence) that an intervention is the proper course of action for a patient, and her fetus. Generally, the concerns that clinicians have regarding fetal effects of a medication are theoretical or potentials that have not been supported by evidence.
- Rather than making recommendations to avoid a medication/treatment because you are not familiar with the risks and benefits, utilize a resource (article, textbook, or experienced clinician) dedicated to the care of pregnant women to determine the best plan of action. These sources will not only outline which treatments are indicated but will also point out the potential adverse effects that uncontrolled maternal disease can have on the pregnancy.
  - "Drugs in Pregnancy and Lactation" edited by Gerald Briggs provides summaries of the current data and provides guidance.
  - Medical Care of the Pregnant Patient, Second Edition. Publisher: The American College of Physicians; 2nd edition (May 1, 2007)
  - Websites such as Reprotox , Micromedex, www.otispregnancy.org
- Understand that for commonly used medications, teratogenic effects really do not occur after the first trimester (ACE inhibitors, angiotensin receptor blockers, and doxycycline are exceptions). The majority of fetal development is complete by the end of the first trimester; after this point organs are growing and maturing.

- Most data available is from observation and registries.
- When possible use medications that have been used for many years as there is more data available.

- Ask yourself, and the patient, to consider the consequences of withholding an indicated treatment. This question often gives the clinician and patient the proper perspective.
  - As opposed to the potential fetal effects, the maternal benefits of a medication or treatment are generally very clear, as are the effects if she does not take a necessary medication.
  - Remember that sick mothers affect fetal outcomes. For example, fever and hypoxia have been associated with preterm birth, while treatment of infections and asthma has been shown to improve fetal outcomes.[8]

- Dosing in pregnancy
  - Remember that pharmacokinetics change in pregnancy – renal clearance, volume of distribution, and protein binding are increased.
  - Choose a dose that would be effective for a non-pregnant patient. Avoid underdosing in an effort to "minimize exposure" when the chosen dose will be subtherapeutic.

32.5.1 Antibiotics

- Most antibiotics can be used in pregnancy.
- Penicillins, erythromycins, and cephalosporins are considered very safe, but nitrofurantoin and sulfonamides should be used with caution.[9]
- Most aminoglycosides are safe. Gentamicin can be used but because it could be associated with fetal ototoxicity, avoid once daily dosing.
- Azithromycin is commonly used, but clarithromycin should be avoided due to rabbit data regarding teratogenic effects at serum levels similar to those seen in humans.
- Quinolones have been reported to cause arthropathy in dogs, but no reports of this issue have been reported in humans. A review/meta-analysis did not find an association between quinolones and birth defects. Quinolones are not first-line treatment during pregnancy, but their use can be considered in the setting of infections resistant to other antibiotics, or for patients with severe allergies or intolerance to other antibiotics.[10]
- Tetracyclines should be avoided as they can cause staining of teeth and bone growth depression.

32.5.2 Pain Control

- Opiates should be used when indicated in pregnancy. They do not have teratogenic effects, and they are routinely given to mothers who nurse after cesarean sections without any effects on the newborn. Mothers who are on chronic doses, or who abuse them, should have the neonate monitored for symptoms of withdrawal after birth.

- Acetaminophen is commonly used and is considered safe.
- NSAIDS are generally avoided, but infrequent dosing or use for less than 48 h may be considered. NSAID use for more than 48 h is associated with reversible narrowing of the patent ductus arteriosus. Additionally, use for women with inflammatory disorders such as rheumatoid arthritis can be considered during the first two trimesters.
- Low-dose aspirin (81 mg) has been studied extensively during pregnancy and does not affect the fetus.[11]

32.6 Patient-Related Risk Factors

- Chronic medical problems may improve, worsen, or remain unchanged in pregnancy.
- The physiologic changes normally occurring in pregnancy may increase the risk of various postoperative complications:
  - Pulmonary – airway problems (vocal cord edema), aspiration (decreased gastric motility and gastroesophageal incompetence), hypoxia (positional – decreased FRC when supine)
  - Venous thromboembolism – stasis, increased clotting factors
  - Urinary tract infection – dilatation of the collecting system leading to stasis, presence of urinary catheter
- Potential delays in diagnosis of diseases due to different manner of presentation
- Disease management due to the need to change or adjust a patient's usual medications

32.7 Surgery-Related Risk Factors

- Regarding surgical technique, laparoscopic procedures are preferred over laparotomy as they tend to be better for the mother.[12]
  - Benefits associated with laparoscopy include decreased postoperative pain, lower estimated blood loss, less analgesic use, earlier return to normal function, and shorter hospital stays.[13-15] It is also less stressful for maternal physiology and therefore potentially better for the fetus although no studies have shown a difference in fetal outcomes.
  - Risks of laparoscopic surgery include theoretical risk of trauma to the fetus, risk of maternal absorption of CO_2 from insufflation, and technical difficulty with a large gravid uterus. Consider end-tidal CO_2 monitoring of the mother as maternal hypercarbia may cause uterine contraction.

    Transcutaneous and end-tidal CO_2 correlates with maternal $PaCO_2$.
    Capnography can be used to adjust ventilation and also detect accidental CO_2 insufflation and subsequent pneumothorax and hemorrhage.

Risk of decreased uteroplacental blood flow because of the increased intraperitoneal pressure from insufflation.[16] Limit insufflation pressure to 12–15 mmHg to minimize hemodynamic changes.

Non-obstetric surgery has been associated with intrauterine growth restriction and preterm labor with either approach.

- Although the type of anesthesia used is the decision of the anesthesiologist, consider regional anesthesia when possible to minimize risks of airway management.
- The ideal time for surgery (when possible) is the second trimester. However, concerns for the fetus should not justify delaying indicated maternal surgery. The best situation for a healthy fetus is a healthy mother.
  - Possible issues related to first trimester anesthesia include neural tube defects and hydrocephalus.[17,18] Technical issues for the surgeon in the third trimester relate to the enlarged uterus and potential for preterm labor.
  - Symptomatic cholelithiasis has a high recurrence rate. Delaying cholecystectomy to the post-partum period was associated with more return visits to the hospital, increased operative times, longer hospitalizations, and higher conversion rate to open cholecystectomy.[19]
- Positioning is important as aortocaval compression by the uterus can diminish venous return, cardiac output, and uteroplacental perfusion. Women should be placed in the left lateral decubitus position and a wedge should be placed under the right hip.

32.8 Preoperative Risk Assessment and Perioperative Management

Preoperative evaluation of the pregnant patient is no different from the evaluation for a non-pregnant woman under similar conditions.

- Most pregnant women are low risk for cardiovascular disease.
  - If they have no active cardiac conditions and a functional capacity >4 METS then according to the ACC/AHA guidelines, no cardiac testing is indicated (see Chap. 20). If needed, stress echocardiography is the preferred stress test, but nuclear stress testing or cardiac catheterization can be performed if necessary.
  - Patients with mitral or aortic stenosis should have aggressive pain management, and the heart rate should be kept below 90 beats per minute via judicious use of beta-adrenergic blocking agents.

  Alpha-methyldopa, labetalol, hydralazine, metoprolol, and nifedipine can be used to treat hypertension during pregnancy. Metoprolol is the preferred cardioselective beta-blocker.

- Control reactive airways disease during pregnancy just as one would for the non-pregnant patient.

– Inhaled steroids and short-acting beta agonists are commonly used. Budesonide is the inhaled corticosteroid of choice, but if not available, other forms can be used.
– Oral steroids should be used when indicated.

- Monitor blood sugars as pregnancy is an insulin-resistant state.
- For other organ systems, test if there are known or suspected abnormalities.
- Inquire about personal or family history of bleeding and anesthesia-related complications.

– Low-dose aspirin (81 mg) is commonly prescribed to pregnant women for multiple pregnancy losses or risk for preeclampsia. It was not associated with increased bleeding when epidural anesthesia was used.

32.8.1 Preterm Delivery

- Avoid over-treating contractions. Tocolytic medications can have severe maternal side effects including pulmonary edema, arrhythmias, chest pain, and EKG changes.[20]

32.8.2 Intraoperative Monitoring

- After 24 weeks, use of fetal heart rate (FHR) monitoring should be discussed with the obstetrician or perinatalogist.

– FHR monitoring detects alterations in fetal perfusion and was designed for labor and delivery. It may indicate maternal stress such as hypoxia and hypotension, and correcting maternal stresses in this context will usually correct the FHR readings.

32.8.3 Postoperative Care

- Maintain left lateral decubitus position until ambulatory.
- Continue fetal monitoring if the mother is hemodynamically unstable and/or based on the discretion of the obstetric team.
- Encourage use of incentive spirometry and early ambulation.
- Provide DVT prophylaxis as indicated. Risk of DVT is at least seven times higher than the non-pregnant population, but the additional risk associated with surgery during pregnancy has not been defined.

– Use unfractionated heparin (UFH) or low molecular weight heparin (LMWH) because they do not cross the placenta.

Dosing : UFH 5,000 units subcutaneously three times/day.

Because of the increased clearance, some practitioners give higher dosing: 7,500 units BID in second trimester; 10,000 units BID in third trimester

Enoxaparin 40 mg daily or BID

– Non-pharmacologic methods include compression stockings, pneumatic compression boots, and early ambulation.

• Maintain volume status.

32.8.4 Postoperative Complications

• Urinary tract infection

– Progression to pyelonephritis is more common. Remove the catheter as soon as possible.

• Hypertension

– This may be related to preeclampsia, but pre-existing chronic hypertension, pregnancy-induced hypertension, and pain are other etiologies.
– The syndrome of preeclampsia is diagnosed by documentation of new SBP > 140 or DBP > 90 and proteinuria (>300 mg per 24 h collection OR new proteinuria > "+1" on a urine dipstick.

In the history, ask about a new headache, visual changes, right upper quadrant pain, or new onset edema of the hands or face.
Physical findings include retinal vasospasm, a sustained S3 or S4 gallop, pulmonary edema, tender liver, severe edema, and clonus.
Laboratory abnormalities may include elevated transaminases, thrombocytopenia, proteinuria, hemolysis, or elevated hemoglobin and serum creatinine (>0.9 mg%) from hemoconcentration.
These patients may have intravascular volume depletion from capillary leak.

– Preferred medications:

Labetalol: orally 200 mg BID-TID to a maximum of 2,400 mg/day, or intravenously 20 mg IV bolus; subsequent doses of 40 mg followed by 80 mg IV may be administered at 10–20 min intervals or it may be infused at 1 mg/kg/h. Generally we treat to keep the SBP < 170 and the DBP < 95 mmHg.
Methyldopa (Aldomet): The oldest agent for treatment of chronic hypertension during pregnancy, but no IV formulations.

– Beta-blockers: Metoprolol is preferred because atenolol was associated with mild intrauterine growth restriction when used in randomized trials focusing on the treatment of chronic hypertension during pregnancy.
– Nifedipine: Appears safe in pregnancy. It is occasionally used to treat preterm contractions.

• Be suspicious for pulmonary embolism if patient is newly dyspneic.
• Monitor for noncardiogenic pulmonary edema if tocolytics were administered.

- Emergencies: Maternal cardiac arrest
  - Place the mother in the left lateral decubitus position or, if supine, place a wedge under her right buttocks to tilt the uterus off the vena cava.
  - Use any indicated medication – Fetuses do not live if the mother does not. The sicker the mother, the less time one should spend debating the benefits/risks of a treatment. Support the mother. If ACLS protocols are indicated, follow them. Ephedrine may cause less uterine artery spasm than other pressors.

References

1. Reedy MB, Kallen B, Kuehl TJ. Laparoscopy during pregnancy: a study of five fetal outcome parameters with use of the Swedish Health Registry. *Am J Obstet Gynecol.* 1997;177(3):673-679.
2. Mazze RI, Kallen B. Appendectomy during pregnancy: a Swedish registry study of 778 cases. *Obstet Gynecol.* 1991;77(6):835-840.
3. American College of Radiology Committee on Drugs and Contrast Media. Administration of contrast medium to breastfeeding mothers. *ACR Bull.* 2001;57(10):12-13.
4. Shellock FG, Kanal E. Policies, guidelines, and recommendations for MR imaging safety and patient management. SMRI Safety Committee. *J Magn Reson Imaging.* 1991;1(1):97-101.
5. Kanal E, Gillen J, Evans JA, Savitz DA, Shellock FG. Survey of reproductive health among female MR workers. *Radiology.* 1993;187(2):395-399.
6. Kanal E. Pregnancy and the safety of magnetic resonance imaging. *Magn Reson Imaging Clin N Am.* 1994;2(2):309-317.
7. Pedrosa I, Levine D, Eyvazzadeh AD, Siewert B, Ngo L, Rofsky NM. MR imaging evaluation of acute appendicitis in pregnancy. *Radiology.* 2006;238(3):891-899.
8. Feldkamp ML, Meyer RE, Krikov S, Botto LD. Acetaminophen use in pregnancy and risk of birth defects: findings from the National Birth Defects Prevention Study. *Obstet Gynecol.* 2010;115(1):109-115.
9. Crider KS, Cleves MA, Reefhuis J, Berry RJ, Hobbs CA, Hu DJ. Antibacterial medication use during pregnancy and risk of birth defects: National Birth Defects Prevention Study. *Arch Pediatr Adolesc Med.* 2009;163(11):978-985.
10. Bar-Oz B, Moretti ME, Boskovic R, O'Brien L, Koren G. The safety of quinolones–a meta-analysis of pregnancy outcomes. *Eur J Obstet Gynecol Reprod Biol.* 2009;143(2):75-78.
11. CLASP: a randomised trial of low-dose aspirin for the prevention and treatment of pre-eclampsia among 9364 pregnant women. CLASP (Collaborative Low-dose Aspirin Study in Pregnancy) Collaborative Group. *Lancet.* Mar 12 1994;343(8898):619–629.
12. Sadot E, Telem DA, Arora M, Butala P, Nguyen SQ, Divino CM. Laparoscopy: a safe approach to appendicitis during pregnancy. *Surg Endosc.* 2010;24(2):383-389.
13. Curet MJ. Special problems in laparoscopic surgery. Previous abdominal surgery, obesity, and pregnancy. *Surg Clin North Am.* 2000;80(4):1093-1110.
14. Shay DC, Bhavani-Shankar K, Datta S. Laparoscopic surgery during pregnancy. *Anesthesiol Clin North America.* 2001;19(1):57-67.
15. Akira S, Yamanaka A, Ishihara T, Takeshita T, Araki T. Gasless laparoscopic ovarian cystectomy during pregnancy: comparison with laparotomy. *Am J Obstet Gynecol.* 1999;180(3 Pt 1):554-557.
16. Bhavani-Shankar K, Steinbrook RA, Mushlin PS, Freiberger D. Transcutaneous PCO2 monitoring during laparoscopic cholecystectomy in pregnancy. *Can J Anaesth.* 1998;45(2):164-169.

17. Kort B, Katz VL, Watson WJ. The effect of nonobstetric operation during pregnancy. *Surg Gynecol Obstet*. 1993;177(4):371-376.
18. Kallen B, Mazze RI. Neural tube defects and first trimester operations. *Teratology*. 1990;41(6):717-720.
19. Muench J, Albrink M, Serafini F, Rosemurgy A, Carey L, Murr MM. Delay in treatment of biliary disease during pregnancy increases morbidity and can be avoided with safe laparoscopic cholecystectomy. *Am Surg*. 2001;67(6):539-542. discussion 542–533.
20. Carson MP, Fisher AJ, Scorza WE. Atrial fibrillation in pregnancy associated with oral terbutaline. *Obstet Gynecol*. 2002;100(5 Pt 2):1096-1097.
21. Rosene-Montella K, Larson L. Diagnostic imaging. In: Lee RV, ed. *Medical Care of the Pregnant Patient*. Philadelphia: American College of Physicians; 2000:103-115.

Part IV

Postoperative Complications

Postoperative Fever

33

Barbara A. Cooper* and Nadene C. Fair

33.1 Introduction

- Postoperative fever is defined as a temperature greater than 38°C (100.4° F) and is an elevation of the patients' normal temperature.
- Postoperative fever is common in the first few days following major surgery secondary to physiologic responses from surgery. However, they can also be the result of more serious complications.[1]
- A broad differential must be maintained when evaluating postoperative fevers and special attention must be paid to the timing of the fever, patient risk factors, and specific surgical risks.

33.2 Pathophysology of Postoperative Fever

- Tissue trauma from surgical procedures incites a complex inflammatory response where the body releases cytokines and acute phase reactants. Interleukins (IL1 and 6), tumor necrosis factor alpha (TNF-α), and interferon-gamma (IFN-γ) act on the preoptic area of the hypothalamus which releases fever-inducing prostaglandins.[2]
- Cytokines released by tissue trauma can incite a fever and do not necessarily represent an infection. There are many factors that influence cytokine release, including the magnitude of trauma, genetics, and bacterial endotoxins and exotoxins that may be present in blood during surgery.[2]

*The views expressed in this chapter are those of the author and do not necessarily reflect the official policy or position of the Department of the Army/Navy/Air Force/Marines/Department of Defense, nor the US Government.

B.A. Cooper (✉)
Department of Internal Medicine, Walter Reed Army Medical Center,
6900 Georgia Ave, Washington, DC 20307, USA
e-mail: barbara.ann.cooper1@us.army.mil

S.L. Cohn (ed.), *Perioperative Medicine*,
DOI: 10.1007/978-0-85729-498-2_33, © Springer-Verlag London Limited 2011

33.3 Incidence and Timing

- The frequency of postoperative fever is quite variable, ranging from 12% to 91% depending on the definition of fever used and the type of surgery.
- The timing of fever after surgery is one of the most important diagnostic factors when considering your differential diagnosis
  - Postoperative fever is generally categorized into one of the following:
  - Immediate: during surgery or within 1 h afterward.
  - Acute: more than 1 h to 1 week postoperative.
  - Subacute: 1–4 weeks after surgery.
  - Delayed: more than 1 month after surgery.
- Etiologies in the differential diagnosis of each time period are listed in Table 33.1.

33.4 Assessment of Postoperative Fever

- Though most post-op fevers will resolve spontaneously and most fevers presenting in the first 2 days postop are non-infectious responses to surgery, post-op fever should not be ignored. The timing of a fever in relation to the surgical procedure needs to be considered in narrowing the differential diagnosis. Common sites of infection in the postoperative period include the lungs, bladder, blood, indwelling lines, surgical wound, and any other organ (skin, GI) that is susceptible to nosocomial organisms. The most common medication reactions that cause fever are antimicrobials and heparinoids.
- A targeted history and physical examination must be done in conjunction with appropriate laboratory and radiographic evaluation.

33.5 History

- Besides the timing of the fever, details of the hospital course, both pre- and postoperative, are helpful in determining the cause of postoperative fever. The following are important points to look for in assessing the patient:
  - Specifics of the surgical procedure and intraoperative period (any complications or unanticipated events).
  - Prior history of febrile illnesses/hidden infections (urinary tract infections, pneumonia, wounds)

Table 33.1 Differential diagnosis and the timing of postoperative fever

Timing	Causes
Immediate: (intra-op-1 h postop)	Medication reaction – Malignant hyperthermia – Antibiotic Transfusion reaction Infection present prior to surgery Fulminant surgical site infection Trauma Adrenal insufficiency
Acute: (1 h – 1 week)	Nosocomial infection – Pneumonia – Urinary tract – Surgical site – Catheter-associated Noninfectious – Pancreatitis – Cholecystitis (acalculous) – Myocardial infarction – Pulmonary embolism – Thrombophlebitis – Alcohol withdrawal – Rheumatologic disease (gout)
Subacute: (1–4 weeks)	Surgical site infection Catheter-associated infection Thrombophlebitis Drug fever – Antimicrobials – H2 blockers – Antiseizure medications – Procainamide DVT/PE
Delayed: (>1 month after surgery)	Surgical site infection Cellulitis Infective endocarditis Postpericardiotomy syndrome Blood product transfusion

Data from: Weed and Aronson[3]

- Co morbidities: Past medical history, especially the endocrine disorders (hyperthyroidism, diabetes mellitus, hypoadrenalism), as well as valvular heart disease (endocarditis), and gout.
- Allergies and medications, particularly antibiotics. See Table 33.2 for further listing of common medications causing fever.
- Chemotherapeutic agents and radiation therapy.
- VTE prophylaxis
- Transfusion of blood products
- Recreational drug use, including alcohol, tobacco and all illicit drugs

Table 33.2 Medications associated with fever[3]

Mechanisms	Drug classes
Drug fever • Penicillin, vancomycin	Cardiovascular • Thiazide diuretics, furosemide, spironolactone, hydralazine, quinidine, procainamide, alpha-methyldopa
Inflammatory response • Rifampin, erythromycin, tetracycline	Antimicrobials • Penicillins, cephalosporins, fluoroquinolones, vancomycin, sulfa, nitrofurantoin, amphoterocin B
Hypersensitivity • Captopril, hydralazine, labetalol	Anticonvulsants • Phenytoin
Pyrogen release • Ranitidine, cimetidine	Miscellaneous • Heparin, salicylates, NSAID, allopurinol, immunoglobulins, iodides, propyluracil, hydroxyurea, mycophenolate mofetil
Endogenous pyrogen release • Interferon	

- Trauma (release of cytokines) or tissue destruction with resultant necrosis and possible infection.
- Associated symptoms that can narrow down which organ system may be a potential source for the fever (for example, cough, shortness of breath, chest pain, wound pain, sinusitis, skin breakdown, rashes, diarrhea or abdominal pain, etc.)
- Presence of catheters – type, location, duration, and method of insertion; presence of nasogastric tube (NGT).
- Nurses notes (often overlooked) which can provide information about bowel function skin breakdown, and mental status.

33.6 Physical Examination

- A targeted physical examination should be done looking for signs that will confirm or rule out diagnoses being considered from the history and that denote an unstable condition that needs urgent management.
- After noting the vital signs and trends, the physician's examination should include the following items:
  - Operative site assessment for erythema, dehiscence, drainage-pus, cellulitis and odor;
  - Catheter sites for erythema and thrombophlebitis
  - Skin, subcutaneous tissue (abscesses, necrotizing fasciitis, gas gangrene, rash, ecchymoses, injection site erythema, and hematoma)

- Chest examination for signs of pneumonia, effusion or consolidation.
- Cardiovascular examination for tachycardia (nonspecific but may suggest sepsis, pulmonary embolus, malignant hyperthermia) or a new murmur (endocarditis).
- Abdominal examination should look for tenderness, rebound, guarding, and bowel sounds.
- Pelvic examination is warranted if there is lower abdominal tenderness and surgery that could involve a complication in this region – abscess, hematomas, etc.
- CNS examination for mental status (delirium may indicate sepsis or drug reaction), neck stiffness (meningitis), and any focal neurologic deficit (stroke).
- Skeletal examination for tenderness and swelling over bony prominences or joints suggestive (acute arthritis, gout)
- Lower extremities for evidence of DVT. Graft sites should be assessed for warmth and erythema suggestive of infection.

33.7 Laboratory Workup

- There are no mandatory lab tests for evaluation of post-op fever. The history and physical examination and the immune status of the host will help direct laboratory testing. Post-op fever workups, particularly within the first 48 h after surgery, are usually of low clinical yield.

  - HEMATOLOGY: The white blood cell count (WBC) should be done if an infectious cause is suspected, with attention being paid to the differential (left shift for infection, eosinophilia for allergic reaction). The white cell count may be depressed in overwhelming sepsis. The platelet count may be increased with stress and decreased in DIC and TTP.
  - CHEMISTRY: Elevated BUN and creatinine may be seen in sepsis with renal failure. Abnormal liver function tests may indicate hepatitis, cholecystitis, or severe sepsis. The blood glucose and lactic acid may also be elevated in sepsis.
  - An ABG may be abnormal with respect to oxygenation in the case of pneumonias or acid–base disorders in septic shock.
  - CARDIAC ENZYMES can be done if myocardial damage is suspected and may be elevated in the case of myocardial inflammation, ischemia, and inflammation. They may also be elevated with PE.
  - SERUM AMYLASE/LIPASE: if pancreatitis is suspected as it may complicate abdominal surgeries.
  - BACTERIOLOGICAL ASSESSMENT: This is dependent on the history, physical, and any initial laboratory workup that may suggest an infectious process and include where appropriate:Blood, urine and sputum cultures, wound swab and culture, culture of intravascular catheter tips upon removal, aspiration and culture of pleural and peritoneal fluids and CSF analysis.
  - IMAGING: This is also dependent on the history, physical and initial lab work.

33.8 Management of Postoperative Fever

- The aim of treatment in postoperative fever is to treat underlying cause, if found, to decrease the elevated hypothalamic set point, to facilitate heat loss, and to decrease the body's demand for oxygen. For every increase of 1°C greater than 37°C, there is a 13% increase in oxygen consumption. The physician should discontinue all unnecessary treatments.
- If the initial assessment suggest a non-infectious case then it is recommended to NOT GIVE ANTIBIOTICS ROUTINELY:
  - ANTIBIOTICS: should be administered once infection is highly suspected. They should be broad spectrum pending sensitivity and then tailored based on results. Empiric therapy should also be based on the patient's age, weight, renal and liver function, allergies and severity of the potential infection. One must also always remember the potential toxicity of the antibiotics being given and drug–drug interactions. Empiric therapy should theoretically not progress beyond 48 h. Persistent fever despite identification of organism and treatment with appropriate antibiotic should prompt a search for occult infection, fungal infections, or a diagnosis of drug fever.
- CONSIDER ANTIPYRETICS IF TEMPERATURE >39°C
  - ANTIPYRETICS: Choices include aspirin and NSAIDs as well as acetaminophen. They all work by inhibiting cyclo-oxygenase and causing a decrease in prostaglandins and increasing the hypothalamus set point. NSAIDS may also decrease cytokine release. Treatment of the non-infectious cause usually leads to resolution of the fever.
- ADMINISTER SUPPORTIVE CARE
  - FLUIDS AND OXYGEN: Should be administered while attempting to control the systemic infection. It is key to identify the source of infection and where necessary, eliminate it by draining abscesses, removing diseased organs, changing or discontinuing catheters and drains. Antipyretics may be given especially if patients are shivering. This will help to lessen patient discomfort and the physiologic stress and metabolic demand of fever and shivering.

33.8.1 Surgery-Specific Approach

- The cause of postoperative fever may be related to the type of surgery performed. Below are issues to consider for patients who have undergone specific surgical procedures:

33.8.1.1
Cardiothoracic Surgery

- Fever is common in first few days after CT surgery so work up is probably not indicated until POD3.
- Risk factors for sternal wound infection include prolonged or emergent surgery, internal mammary artery grafting, diabetes, renal failure, and cigarette smoking.
- Evidence of instability or inflammation warrants imaging or re-exploration to rule out mediastinitis and sternal osteomyelitis.
- Pneumonia may be seen in 5% of patients and is correlated with prolonged mechanical ventilation, reintubation, hypotension, neurologic dysfunction, and transfusion of more than three units of blood products during surgery.
- Pleural effusions (transudates) are common after CT surgery, and thoracentesis is rarely required as they tend to resolve spontaneously within a week.
- Fever after heart valve surgery should prompt consideration of infective endocarditis, typically with Staphylococcus.

33.8.1.2
Neurosurgery

- Meningitis, either bacterial or chemical, may cause fever after neurosurgery. Classic symptoms and signs (headache, photophobia, and nuchal rigidity) cannot distinguish between these etiologies, and examination of CSF is key for these patients. Findings suggestive of chemical meningitis include fever less than 39.4°C, CSF – WBC <7,500/μL, glucose >10 mg/dL, no delirium, seizure or surgical site inflammation.
- Empiric antibiotic coverage for suspected bacterial meningitis after neurosurgery should cover *S. aureus* (vancomycin) and hospital-acquired gram-negative bacilli inclusive of pseudomonas aeruginosa.
- Surgeries involving the hypothalamus may lead to disorders of thermoregulation resulting in fever postoperatively.
- DVT is a non-infectious cause of fever that is more frequently seen after neurosurgery because patients have limited mobility and there is less aggressive VTE prophylaxis so as not to cause bleeding at the surgical site.

33.8.1.3
Vascular Surgery

- Diagnosis of graft infection can be difficult. Imaging (CT, MRI, or nuclear scintigraphy) can be helpful. CT scanning is usually the best first test as it can detect fluid collections for aspiration. However, negative findings on imaging studies do not rule out a graft infection.
- After endovascular repair of aortic aneurysms with endoluminal stent graft a post-implantation syndrome of fever, leukocytosis, elevated CRP, with perigraft gas, and negative blood cultures, may occur. Fever resolves spontaneously in this case.

- Arterial embolization or blue toe syndrome is a non-infectious cause of fever similar to emboli from infected graft. Of note, vascular graft infections are more common after upper leg and inguinal surgery.

33.8.1.4
OB-GYN Surgery

- The differential diagnoses to consider are UTI (patient may complain of dysuria), cellulitis, necrotizing fasciitis, superficial abscess, deep abscess, endometritis (purulent vaginal discharge) and pelvic thrombophlebitis, especially after C-section. CT/MRI may be helpful in diagnosis, and treatment may include antibiotics and heparin.
- Without localizing features, fever 1–2 days after gynecologic surgery does not require empiric antibiotics or further testing and usually resolves spontaneously. However, ongoing re-evaluation of the patient is necessary.

33.8.1.5
Abdominal Surgery

- Fever presenting early in the postoperative period may be an indication of peritonitis.
- Other etiologies of fever after abdominal surgery include abscesses, hematomas, pancreatitis, and acalculous cholecystitis.
- CT scanning may be falsely negative in the early postoperative period and may need to be repeated if the patients' clinical condition warrants.
- Three indicators have been proposed for postoperative abdominal infections: WBC < 5,000 or > 10,000/μL, fever after postop day 2, and BUN > 15 mg/dL.
- Empiric antimicrobial treatment should cover aerobic gram-negative bacilli and anaerobes.

33.8.1.6
Urologic Surgery

- Etiologies include UTI, prostatitis, and perinephric abscess.
- Urinalysis and culture are the initial diagnostic tests, but imaging studies may be warranted.

33.8.1.7
Orthopedic Surgery

- Fever after orthopedic surgeries is common and usually self-limited.
- Persistent fever may suggest surgical site infections, infection of a prosthesis, hematoma, or DVT.

- For prosthetic infections, repeated clinical assessment imaging and sometimes needle aspiration is needed. If the prosthetic joint becomes infected soon after surgery, virulent organisms such as *S. aureus* should be considered.

33.8.1.8
Transplantation

- These patients are immunosuppressed and warrant special considerations.
- Fever in this setting may either be infectious or non-infectious, although immunosuppressive medications can mask fever.
- Infectious causes may be determined based upon the timing of the fever:
  - In the first 4 weeks postoperatively, fever may be caused by the usual bacterial infections such as UTI, surgical site infections, and pneumonias. Reactivation of HSV is also common during this period.
  - Fever after 4 weeks up to 6 months may be indicative of opportunistic infections such as CMV, fungi (aspergillosis, candidiasis), toxoplasmosis, pneumocystis, and nocardia.
- The non-infectious causes include organ rejection, lymphoproliferative disease, and drug reactions.

References

1. Garibaldi RA, Brodine S, Matsumiya S, Coleman M. Evidence for the non-infectious etiology or early postoperative fever. *Infect Control.* 1985;6:273.
2. Pile JC, Weed HG. Postoperative complications. In: Cohn SL, Smetana GW, Weed HG, eds. *Perioperative Medicine: Just the Facts.* New York: McGraw-Hill Companies; 2006:275-281.
3. Weed HG, Aronson MD. Postoperative fever. In: Collins KA, ed. *Up To Date.* Waltham: UpToDate; 2010.

Postoperative Hypertension/Hypotension 34

Steven L. Cohn and Brian Harte

34.1 Introduction

- Despite its high prevalence, hypertension remains undiagnosed, untreated, or uncontrolled in many patients.
- Hypertension is also one of the most commonly encountered medical problems in surgical patients, both preoperatively and postoperatively.
- Preoperative hypertension is discussed in Chap. 20. This chapter reviews the causes of postoperative hypertension and hypotension, contributing factors, and guidelines for management.

34.2 Incidence

- The frequency of postoperative hypertension varies due to a lack of standard definition, but the reported incidence ranges from 3% to 91% depending on the definition of hypertension and the type of surgery.[1]
  - Intracranial neurosurgery: 57–91%; vascular surgery (carotid, aortic, cardiac): 10–75%; radical neck dissection: 10–20%; elective general surgery: 3–20%

S.L. Cohn (✉)
Internal Medicine-Medical Consultation Service,
SUNY Downstate - Kings County Hospital Center,
450 Clarkson Ave, Box 68, Brooklyn, NY 11203, USA
e-mail: steven.cohn@downstate.edu

S.L. Cohn (ed.), *Perioperative Medicine*,
DOI: 10.1007/978-0-85729-498-2_34, © Springer-Verlag London Limited 2011

34.3 Risk Factors

- Patients with uncontrolled hypertension, in general, tend to experience more perioperative blood pressure (BP) lability than non-hypertensive patients or those with controlled hypertension. The presence of antihypertensive medication "on board" may decrease this lability to some degree.
- A history of severe uncontrolled hypertension predicts postoperative hypertension more reliably than the BP just before surgery ("admit BP").[2]
  - An elevated BP on admission may be due to anxiety, rebound from discontinued medications, or the white coat effect.
  - A diastolic BP >110 mmHg preoperatively predicts postoperative hypertension.
- The risk of postoperative hypertension is greatest after vascular procedures, including peripheral vascular surgeries and aortic aneurysm surgery, because of fluid overload (IV fluid challenges more likely) and decreased renal perfusion.[2] Major intrathoracic and intraperitoneal procedures are also more likely to be associated with postoperative hypertension than less invasive procedures.

34.4 Timing and Causes

- Hypertension can occur throughout the perioperative period:
  - Preoperatively – upon admission to the hospital or entry into the operating room.
  - Intraoperatively – during induction of anesthesia with laryngoscopy and intubation, with surgical manipulation, or after extubation.
  - Postoperatively – early, in the recovery room, or 1–2 days later in the postoperative period.
- The causes of postoperative hypertension differ based on timing after surgery[3] (see Fig. 34.1).

34.4.1 Immediate Postoperative Period

- Reversal of anesthesia reduces the vasodilatory effect of the anesthetic agents. The subsequent increase in the peripheral vascular resistance combined with volume overload from intraoperative intravenous fluids leads to BP elevation.
- Postoperative pain and hypoxia are sympathetic stimuli that elevate norepinephrine levels increasing systemic vascular resistance and BP.
- Hypothermia decreases catecholamine reuptake, thus increasing catecholamine levels, and shivering can also increase BP postoperatively.

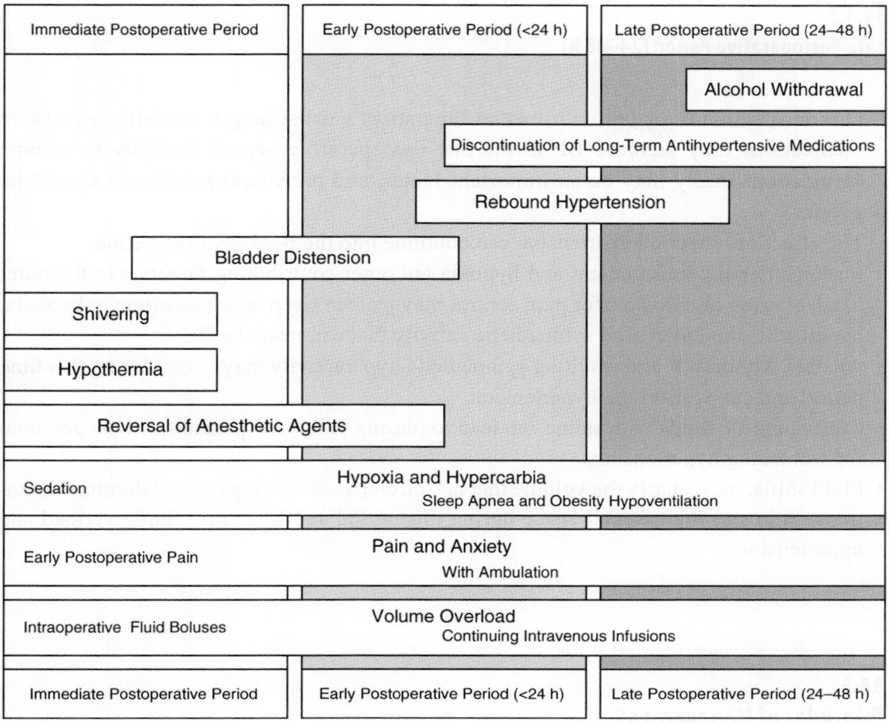

Fig. 34.1 Causes of postoperative hypertension based on time of occurrence (Reproduced with permission from Shafi et al.[4] Copyright © 2006, The McGraw Hill Companies, Inc.)

34.4.2
Early Postoperative Period (<24 h)

- Discontinuation of the epidural anesthesia reduces the peripheral vasodilation leading to a return of fluid into the central circulation and an elevation of BP.
- Rebound hypertension may be seen due to abrupt withdrawal of beta-blockers or centrally acting sympatholytic agents (e.g., clonidine).
  - Patients on chronic therapy with both these classes of drugs are especially susceptible if the sympatholytic agent is withdrawn and the beta-blocker is continued. The ensuing hyperadrenergic withdrawal state is similar to the pheochromocytoma crisis. Selective beta-blockade with unopposed alpha-receptor stimulation by the circulating catecholamines can cause severe BP elevation.
- Pain, ventilatory problems (hypercarbia, hypoxia), and bladder distension may also contribute to the elevated BP.

34.4.3
Late Postoperative Period (24–48 h)

- Discontinuation of or failure to restart the patient's usual long-term antihypertensive medications may increase BP in the late postoperative period. Inability to resume medications orally may be an important factor, and parenteral substitutes should be given.
- The effect of rebound hypertension can continue into the postoperative period.
- Inadequate pain management and hypoxia are other contributing factors. On the other hand, overuse of narcotics for pain control may worsen sleep apnea resulting in hypoxia, hypercarbia, and increased sympathetic activity that can raise the BP.
- Alcohol withdrawal and resulting sympathetic hyperactivity may occur during this time period and can worsen the hypertension.
- Continuing IV fluids with saline can lead to plasma volume expansion and the potential for worsening hypertension.
- Fluid shifts, particularly the volume that is "third-spaced" during intra-abdominal operations returns to the vascular space during this period and can cause fluid overload and hypertension.

34.5
Principles of Management

- Continue most antihypertensive medications perioperatively, including on the morning of surgery to minimize the risk of postoperative hypertension (see Chap. 3)

34.5.1
Adaptation to Longstanding Uncontrolled Hypertension

- Patients with longstanding uncontrolled hypertension adapt to chronic elevations of arterial pressure by the development of arteriolar hypertrophy. This phenomenon occurs in both cerebrovascular and other vascular beds as well. As a result, they are able to tolerate arterial pressures that would cause complications in a normotensive individual.
  - A patient with previously well-controlled hypertension may become symptomatic with acute elevation of BP, and in this case, one should lower the BP relatively quickly to prevent acute target organ injury and encephalopathy.
  - On the other hand, a hypertensive individual with poor BP control prior to surgery may be completely asymptomatic at much higher pressures. In this circumstance,

sudden lowering of the BP with short-acting agents may precipitate acute cerebral, renal, and myocardial ischemia.

34.5.2 BP Treatment Thresholds

- There is no absolute BP threshold for treatment. When treating acute BP elevations, take into account the overall condition of the patient and baseline BP, rather than the level of BP.
- Drug trials evaluating the efficacy of individual agents in treating postoperative hypertension have either used a fixed threshold (e.g., systolic BP > 160 mmHg, or diastolic BP > 90 mmHg, or mean BP > 110 mmHg) or a relative change from baseline (e.g., an increase in systolic BP or diastolic BP > 20%).[3] However, most of these trials were designed to compare the BP lowering efficacy of a newer agent compared to an older established drug rather than to determine an optimal treatment threshold.
- Studies of intraoperative changes in BP demonstrate an increase in postoperative cardiac and renal complications with a 20% change in the mean BP compared to the preoperative level.[5]
  - In the absence of good evidence, the goal of treatment should be to maintain the BP within 20% of the preoperative BP level. Initiate treatment if the postoperative BP is >20% above the preoperative BP level.
  - When acute BP lowering is necessary, do not acutely lower the mean arterial pressure by more than 20% or to less than 160/100 mmHg.

34.5.3 Patient Evaluation and Decision Making

- Evaluate the patient with an elevated postoperative BP to determine whether it represents an urgent or emergent situation.
- Initiate or intensify treatment based on the presence and severity of target organ damage such as chest pain, pulmonary edema, worsening renal failure, encephalopathy, retinal hemorrhages, or exudates, or papilledema.
- Progressive target organ damage indicates a hypertensive emergency. Patients at excessive risk of hemorrhage from suture lines and vascular anastomoses also have hypertensive emergencies. These patients will need treatment in an intensive care unit with parenteral antihypertensive agents. A number of short-acting antihypertensive agents are available for this purpose (Table 34.1).
- If a hypertensive emergency is not present, evaluate the likely etiology of the hypertension, and reverse any precipitating factors before resorting to antihypertensive medications.

Table 34.1 Short-acting antihypertensive agents

Drug	Dose	Effect	Comments
Sodium Nitroprusside	Initial: 0.25 mcg/kg/min Titrate: Double dose every 5 min Max: 10 mcg/kg/min	Onset:30 s–2 min Duration:1–3 min	• Coronary steal • Cyanide/thiocyanide toxicity with prolonged infusion, renal insufficiency, high infusion rate • Reflex tachycardia • ↑ Intracranial pressure
Nitroglycerin	Initial: 5–10 mcg/min Titrate: 5–10 mcg/min every 3–5 min. If no response at 20 mcg/min, titrate by 10–20 mcg/min Max: 100 mcg/min	Onset:2–5 min Duration:3–5 min	• Coronary vasodilatation • Tolerance with prolonged use • Can ↑ intracranial pressure
Hydralazine	Initial: 10 mg IV bolus over 3–5 min, increase 5–10 mg every 20–30 min Usual dose: 10–20 mg IV every 4–6 h Max: 50 mg IV per dose	Onset:10–20 min Duration: Unpredictable 3–8 h	• Reflex tachycardia • Safe in pregnancy
Nicardipine	Initial: 5 mg/h Titrate: 1–2.5 mg/h every 5–15 min Max: 15 mg/h	Onset:5–10 min Duration:1–4 h	• Long elimination half life • Phlebitis at IV site • Reduced cerebral vasospasm in subarachnoid hemorrhage
Clevidipine	Initial: 1–2 mg/h IV Titrate: dose may be initially doubled at 90-second intervals. Max: 21 mg/h	Onset:1–2 min Duration: 5–15 min	• Fever in 19% • Rapid titration; as target BP neared, reduce titration rate to 5–10 min
Enalaprilat	Initial: 0.625–1.25 mg IV every 6 h Titrate: Double dose every 6 h Max: 5 mg every 6 h	Onset:15–30 min Duration:6 h	• Long residual effect • First dose hypotension with volume depletion • May reset cerebral blood flow autoregulation
Fenoldopam	Initial: 0.1 mcg/kg/min (or 0.03–0.1 mcg/kg/min) Titrate: 0.05–0.1 mcg/kg/min every 15–20 min Max: 1.6 mcg/kg/min	Onset:5–15 min Duration: 10–15 min	• ↑ renal blood flow and natriuresis • No coronary steal • Can transiently ↑ intracranial pressure • Can be used in renal failure • Infusion can be abruptly discontinued • Contraindicated with glaucoma

(continued)

Table 34.1 (continued)

Drug	Dose	Effect	Comments
Esmolol	Initial: Bolus 500 mcg/kg IV for 1 min, followed by 25–100 mcg/kg/min for 4 min. Titrate: Repeat bolus if inadequate response after 5 min, ↑ rate in increment of 50 mcg/kg/min to max of 300 mcg/kg/min	Onset:1–2 min Duration: 10–20 min	• Rapid, controllable onset • Short duration • Easily titratable
Labetalol (IV)	Initial bolus: 20 mg IV over 2 min Titrate: Repeat bolus dose of 40–80 mg every 10–15 min up to max of 300 mg per 24 h Infusion: 0.5–2.0 mg/min	Onset:5–10 min Duration:3–6 h	• Does not ↑ intracranial pressure • Prolonged action • Not easily titratable
Clonidine (Oral)	Initial: 0.1–0.2 mg PO every 1 h (max 0.6 mg) Usual dose: 0.2–1.2 mg/day PO in 2–4 divided doses Max: 2.4 mg/day	Onset:30–60 min Duration:6–10 h	• Prolonged unpredictable effect • Rebound hypertension with abrupt cessation • Sedation, dry mouth and bradycardia
Captopril (Oral)	Initial: 6.25–12.5 mg Usual dose: 12.5–50 mg every 8 h Max: 450 mg/day	Onset:10–15 min Duration:4–6 h	• Long residual effect • First dose hypotension with volume depletion • May reset cerebral blood flow autoregulation
Labetalol (Oral)	Initial:200–400 mg, repeat every 2–3 h Instructions post IV: 200 mg, followed in 6–12 h by 200–400 mg; titrate at 1 day interval Max: Total dose 2.4 g/day divided BID or TID	Onset:30 min–2 h Duration:8–12 h	• Does not ↑ intracranial pressure • Prolonged action

Source: Modified from Shafi et al.,[4] with permission

- Treat pain, anxiety, hypervolemia, and hypothermia.
- Treat ventilatory abnormalities (hypoxia, hypercarbia).
- In elderly men, make sure that bladder distension is not present.
- Evaluate for rebound hypertension and restart the patient's usual antihypertensive medications. If NPO, consider parenteral alternatives.

• If BP improves (reduced by approximately 20%), observe and continue usual BP medications and monitoring. If response is inadequate, increase the medication dose, add another agent, or consider the use of parenteral agents.

34.6 Postoperative Hypotension

- Hypotension and shock in the immediate perioperative setting and in the days following surgery is a predictor of postoperative cardiac complications and requires a rapid and comprehensive assessment to distinguish among the various clinical entities that may contribute to unstable hemodynamics.
  - These include fluid shifts and blood loss, physiological and inflammatory changes which accompany surgery, the various pharmacological agents used perioperatively including anesthetics, sedatives, antiemetics, and narcotics, potential surgical complications, and manifestations of chronic medical pathology. In addition, hypotension is regarded as a risk factor for postoperative cardiac events in patients with pre-existing hypertension.[6]
- In general, hypotension or shock can be classified as distributive, hypovolemic, or cardiogenic. Note however that any clinical scenario may involve multiple contributing etiologies.

34.7 Hypovolemic Hypotension

- Hypovolemia refers to inadequate intravascular volume.
- Most commonly, it is due to hemorrhage, which may be intraoperative or a postoperative complication, or to isotonic fluid losses (or inadequate fluid replacement), either intraoperatively, or such as due to diarrhea, burns, or vomiting, or "third-spacing."[7]
- In addition, conditions which limit cardiac output due to obstruction of flow can also manifest in a similar manner. While unusual, these conditions are life-threatening and demand prompt treatment: cardiac tamponade, pulmonary embolism, and tension pneumothorax.

34.8 Distributive Hypotension

- Distributive shock refers to the inability to support appropriate vital organ perfusion due to peripheral vasodilation and a drop in the systemic vascular resistance (SVR).
- Most commonly, distributive shock is due to infection with sepsis.[8] Wound infections generally occur more than 48 h after surgery, but consideration should also be reserved for line and urinary catheter-related infections.
- Patients with a history suggestive of corticosteroid dependence may develop acute adrenal insufficiency after surgery if appropriate "stress-dosing" of steroids is not administered.[9] While ACTH stimulation testing can be diagnostic, the turnaround time is usually several days, and immediate administration of stress doses of corticosteroids should not be delayed.

- Anaphylactic shock can be induced by any number of agents, including antibiotics, iodinated contrast, and nonsteroidal anti-inflammatory drugs.
- Neurogenic shock is rare, and induced by spinal trauma, with subsequent loss of autonomic and sympathetic reflexes.
- In addition, many pharmacological agents reduce SVR or cardiac preload, including inhaled anesthetics, and spinal anesthesia causes peripheral vasodilatation and may cause a decrease in blood pressure and perfusion.[10]

34.9 Cardiogenic Hypotension

- Cardiogenic shock is defined as hypotension resulting from an inadequate cardiac output due to cardiac pump failure. Common causes include:
  - Cardiac ischemia, which causes a reduction in myocardial contractility and can induce acute congestive heart failure. Myocardial infarction can be complicated by ventricular wall rupture, arrhythmias, or acute valvular incompetence.
  - Inhalational anesthetic agents, which also reduce myocardial contractility.
  - Pre-existing ventricular dysfunction or valvular disease, which may acutely decompensate due to ischemia, fluid shifts, or pharmacological agents.
  - Brady- or tachyarrythmias.

34.10 Assessment

- Physical examination should focus on manual verification of blood pressure and a search for the etiology of the hypotension – infection, cardiopulmonary status, and bleeding.
- Check medication history including recent pharmaceuticals and allergies.
- Review fluid intake and output.
- Order focused laboratory and ancillary studies including EKG and chest films.

34.11 Intervention

- Initial intervention should focus on resuscitation and stabilization:
  - Intravenous fluids through large-bore intravenous lines
  - Foley catheter (if not already present)
  - Administration of epinephrine or stress-dose corticosteroids may be appropriate (see distributive etiologies, above).
- Subsequent treatment should be directed at the appropriate etiology, and may include:

- Blood product transfusion and/or surgical re-exploration
- Transfer to monitored setting if condition warrants
- Urgent or emergent therapy for tamponade, pneumothorax, or myocardial infarction
- Vasopressors may be required for inotropic and/or blood pressure support

References

1. Kaplan N. *Kaplan's Clinical Hypertension*. 8th ed. Philadelphia: Lippincott Williams and Wilkins; 2002.
2. Goldman L, Caldera DL. Risks of general anesthesia and elective operation in the hypertensive patient. *Anesthesiology*. 1979;50:285-292.
3. Haas CE, LeBlanc JM. Acute postoperative hypertension: a review of therapeutic options. *Am J Health Syst Pharm*. 2004;61:1661-1673.
4. Shafi T, Cohn SL. In: Cohn SL, Smetana GW, Weed HG, eds. *Hypertension/Hypotension in Perioperative Medicine – Just the Facts*. New York: McGraw Hill; 2006.
5. Charlson ME, MacKenzie CR, Gold JP, Ales KL, Topkins M, Shires GT. Intraoperative blood pressure. What patterns identify patients at risk for postoperative complications? *Ann Surg*. 1990;212(5):567-580.
6. Charlson ME, MacKenzie CR, Gold JP, Ales KL, Topkins M, Shires GT. Preoperative characteristics predicting intraoperative hypotension and hypertension among hypertensives and diabetics undergoing noncardiac surgery. *Ann Surg*. 1990;212:66-81.
7. Baskett PJF. ABC of major trauma. Management of hypovolaemic shock. *Br Med J*. 1990;300:1453.
8. Hinshaw LB. Sepsis/septic shock: participation of the microcirculation: an abbreviated review. *Crit Care Med*. 1996;24(6):1072-1078.
9. Bouachour G et al. Hemodynamic changes in acute adrenal insufficiency. *Intensive Care Med*. 1994;20:138.
10. Prys-Roberts C, Meloche R, Foex P. Studies of anaesthesia in relation to hypertension. I. Cardiovascular responses of treated and untreated patients. *Br J Anaesth*. 1971;43:122-137.

Postoperative Arrhythmias

35

Barbara Slawski and Kurt Pfeifer

35.1 Introduction

- Arrhythmias are common events after surgical procedures.
- Supraventricular and ventricular arrhythmias predict perioperative cardiac events.[1]
- Generally, postoperative arrhythmias are associated with increased morbidity and longer hospital stays.[2,3]
- New-onset atrial fibrillation after coronary artery bypass grafting (CABG) is predictive of long-term mortality.[4]

35.2 Incidence

- Cardiac surgeries have the highest incidence of postoperative arrhythmias.[3,5-7]
  - CABG

    Atrial fibrillation up to 27%
    Ventricular Tachycardia (VT) 1.2%
    Bradyarrhythmias 1%
    Pacemaker placements 1–3%[6]
  - Valve surgeries (particularly aortic and mitral valve)

    Atrial fibrillation: 35–50%
    Bradyarrhythmias: 10%
    Mobitz I heart block: 3%

B. Slawski (✉)
General Internal Medicine and Orthopaedic Surgery, Medical College of Wisconsin, 9200 W. Wisconsin Ave, Milwaukee, WI 53226, USA
e-mail: slawski@mcw.edu

S.L. Cohn (ed.), *Perioperative Medicine*,
DOI: 10.1007/978-0-85729-498-2_35,

- Noncardiac surgeries have a lower incidence of arrhythmias, but disease burden is higher due to number of surgeries performed.[1,3,8]
  - Atrial fibrillation: 0.37–26%
  - Colorectal surgeries: 13–26%
  - Reentrant supraventricular tachycardias: 6%

35.3 Timing

- Some arrhythmias are exacerbated by the high postoperative adrenergic state and are of limited duration.
- Atrial fibrillation incidence is highest on postoperative days 2–4.[7]
- Bradyarrhythmias usually occur immediately after surgery due to increased vagal tone.
- Heart block and bundle branch blocks also occur immediately postoperatively.

35.4 Causes

- Arrhythmias in the perioperative setting may unmask underlying cardiac conditions.
- In every case, search for an underlying precipitating cause while treating.
- Consider new medications or medication withdrawal as precipitating factors.
- Rapid ventricular rates may produce cardiac ischemia by increasing myocardial oxygen demand.
- Common universal causes
  - Electrolyte imbalance
  - Hypoxia/ischemia
  - Postoperative catecholamine excess (tachycardias)
  - Mechanical disruption (cardiac surgery)
- Causes of specific postoperative arrhythmias (in addition to universal causes noted above) are listed in Table 35.1.

35.5 Diagnosis

- Basic evaluation
  - Establish urgency based on evidence of hemodynamic compromise and symptoms
  - Physical Exam

Table 35.1 Causes of specific postoperative arrhythmias

Arrhythmia	Causes
Sinus tachycardia[2,3]	Stimulant exposure, enhanced catecholamine state, pain; hypo-/hypervolemia; anemia; hypoxia/hypercarbia; substance or medication withdrawal; pulmonary emboli; fever/infection/sepsis; acute coronary syndrome; congestive heart failure (CHF); hyperthyroidism
Atrial fibrillation	Atrial injury/inflammation; myocardial ischemia; atrial stretch/increased volume state
Multifocal atrial tachycardia[5]	Pulmonary disease; theophylline toxicity; digitalis toxicity
Ventricular tachycardia (VT)[5]	Polymorphic VT: ischemia; polymorphic VT in the setting of a prolonged QT interval is often torsades de pointes triggered by QT interval prolonging drugs (expansive list) Monomorphic VT: underlying structural heart disease/scarring
Bradycardias[5,7]	Sinus bradycardia may be physiologic (sleep, young patients, athletes) Increased vagal tone: spinal/epidural anesthesia; nausea/vomiting; eye surgery; laryngoscopy, orotracheal suctioning; increased intracranial pressure; obstructive sleep apnea Medications
Heart blocks[5,6]	Mechanical disruption of the conduction system during cardiac procedures; increased vagal tone; drugs that suppress the AV node; right ventricular infarct/ischemia; Mobitz I heart block is usually benign but may occur due to myocardial infarction (MI), increased vagal tone, medications

Assess ventricular rate, blood pressure, peripheral perfusion
Identify

Congestive heart failure and ischemia
Findings suggestive of cardiovascular disease
Evidence of AV dissociation

– Diagnostic Testing

12 lead EKG (essential as opposed to telemetry); review telemetry strips
Electrolytes
CXR if indicated
Drug levels if indicated
Consider assessing LV function (particularly atrial fibrillation, VT)

– Diagnosis of Specific Arrhythmias (see Table 35.2)

Table 35.2 Diagnostic features of common arrhythmias

Arrhythmia	Diagnostic features
Sinus tachycardia	Rate greater than 100 P waves have appropriate sinus morphology Gradual onset and offset
Atrial fibrillation	P waves absent or may appear chaotic RR intervals are irregularly irregular
Multifocal atrial tachycardia	Rate greater than 100 3 or more different p wave morphologies
Reentrant supraventricular tachycardia	Narrow complex unless aberrantly conducted Abrupt onset and termination P waves are usually consistent with sinus morphology
Atrial flutter	A subset of reentrant supraventricular tachycardias Biphasic "sawtooth" f waves Atrial rate regular at 300 bpm Ventricular rate often 150 bpm (2:1 block)
Ventricular tachycardia	NSVT=3 or more consecutive beats of ventricular origin Sustained VT=30s or symptomatic ECG features consistent with VT: QRS complex >120 ms in duration AV dissociation is pathognomonic, present in about 50% of patients with VT Fusion and capture beats are diagnostic
Heart blocks	Progressive PR interval prolongation precedes nonconducted p wave
Mobitz I (Wenckebach)	Unchanging PR interval with a p wave that suddenly fails to conduct
Mobitz II heart block Complete heart block	No atrial impulses are conducted to the ventricle

35.6 Treatment

- Unstable tachyarrhythmias should be treated with direct current cardioversion (DCCV).[1]
- Adenosine may be diagnostic in addition to therapeutic value in some arrhythmias.
- When urgent heart rate control is required or use of oral agents is not possible, use IV medications.
- Beta blockers are useful in multiple postoperative arrhythmias due to the ability of these medicines to decrease the effect of catecholamine excess in the postoperative period.

- Treatment of Specific Arrhythmias
  - Sinus tachycardia

    Evaluate and treat underlying causes.
    Rate control with medications is rarely indicated.

  - New-onset atrial fibrillation

    Most guidelines are based on cardiac surgery patients and can be cautiously extended to noncardiac surgery patients.
    Carefully consider the usually self-limited duration of new postoperative atrial fibrillation and weigh the risks/benefits of treatment.[1,2,5,7]
    Some evidence suggests beta blockers (best evidence), statins, and steroids may prevent postoperative atrial fibrillation after cardiac surgery.[5,6]
    Major goals of therapy (see Fig. 35.1):

      Ventricular rate control
      Prevent embolism. Stroke risk in the general surgery population is 0.08–0.2% (CABG up to 3.8%).[9]
      Convert to normal sinus rhythm (NSR).

    Rate Control[2,3]

      First line agent – beta blockers.
      Second line – calcium channel blockers (usually diltiazem).
      Digoxin is usually not effective due to high adrenergic tone in the postoperative state.
      Consider amiodarone in patients when other measures are unsuccessful or contraindicated.
      Patients with atrial fibrillation and an accessory pathway – IV procainamide or ibutilide are alternatives.

    Anticoagulation [1-3,10]

      No randomized trials of new-onset postoperative atrial fibrillation/anticoagulation exist.
      Consider the concurrent use of antiplatelet agents when considering risk/benefit of anticoagulation for new-onset atrial fibrillation in the postoperative period.
      Cardiac surgery patients

        In selected patients with new-onset atrial fibrillation after CABG, discharge on warfarin is associated with a decrease in long-term mortality.[4]
        In optimally selected patients with atrial fibrillation (chronic or rhythm is likely to persist postoperatively), anticoagulation with warfarin is advised.
        In high-risk patients, such as those with history of transient ischemic attack or stroke, heparin use should be considered.

      Noncardiac surgery patients

        No standard new-onset postoperative atrial fibrillation guidelines.
        It is reasonable to use the CHADS2 score when considering postoperative treatment with aspirin or warfarin in this group.
        Carefully weigh risks and benefits of bridging anticoagulation.

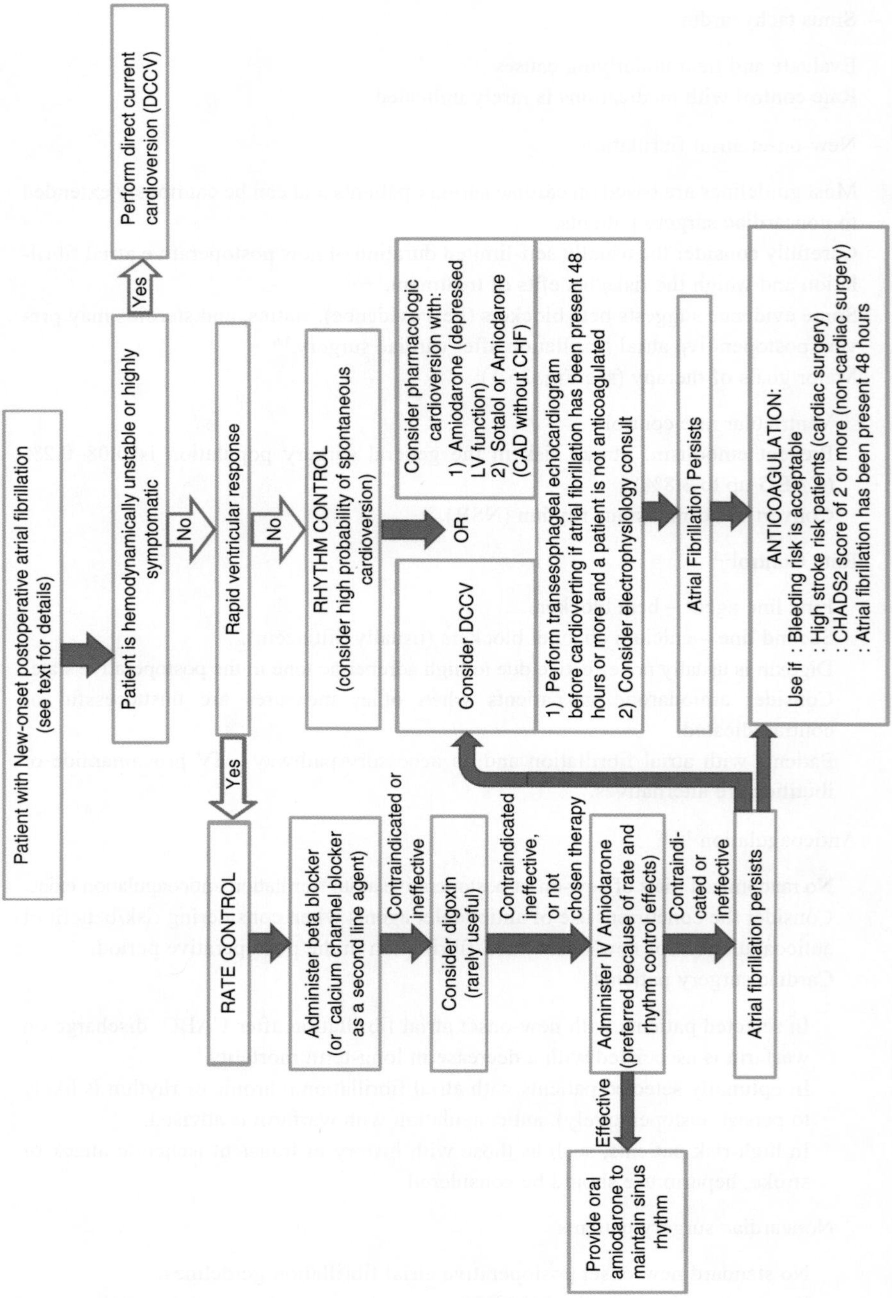

Fig. 35.1 Treatment of new-onset atrial fibrillation

Because of continued impaired atrial contraction after conversion to NSR, consider continuing anticoagulation for 1 month after patient converts to NSR if bleeding risk is acceptable.

If amiodarone is used, consider decreasing the warfarin dose by 25–40% due to drug interactions.

Rhythm control

Rhythm control strategies are used in the majority of post-CABG patients.

Amiodarone is recommended for patients with depressed LV function.

Sotalol may be used in patients with coronary artery disease who do not have CHF (available PO only). Amiodarone is also an option.

Most protocols recommend continuing antiarrhythmics for 4–6 weeks following surgery without evidence from randomized trials.

– Chronic Atrial Fibrillation

Rate control

Continue chronic therapy.

Additional agents/increased doses of chronic agents may be required postoperatively for rate control due to high adrenergic tone.

Anticoagulation for atrial fibrillation patients on chronic warfarin (see guidelines for recommendations regarding valvular disease and VTE)[8]

Postoperative bridging is recommended until INR is therapeutic.

High Risk – bridging anticoagulation with therapeutic-dose subcutaneous LMWH or IV UFH

CHADS2 score = 5–6

Stroke or TIA within the last 3 months

Rheumatic valvular disease

Moderate risk – bridging anticoagulation with therapeutic-dose subcutaneous LMWH, therapeutic-dose IV UFH, or low-dose subcutaneous LMWH

CHADS2 score = 3–4

– Multifocal Atrial Tachycardia[5]

Control rate while searching for and treating a cause.

Cardioversion is not effective.

Rate control with beta blockers and calcium channel blockers.

Amiodarone may be useful.

– AV nodal reentrant tachycardias

Vagal maneuvers

Adenosine

Beta blockers, calcium channel blockers, and class 1a and 1c antiarrhythmics may decrease recurrence.

- Atrial flutter (a subset of reentrant tachycardias)

  Management of rate and anticoagulation is similar to atrial fibrillation, although rate control is more challenging.

  Rhythm control

  Atrial overdrive pacing, ibutilide may produce cardioversion.

  Radiofrequency ablation may be necessary.

- Ventricular Tachycardia

  Evaluation

  Assess hemodynamics.

  NSVT in patients with an EF of 35% or less warrants cardiology evaluation for potential ICD.

  Polymorphic VT – consider additional need to evaluate for ischemia/MI.[5]

  Assess LV function.

  Treatment[1,5]

  Unstable VT (polymorphic or monomorphic) – DCCV

  PVCs, ventricular couplets, and NSVT are not associated with complications after noncardiac surgery and do not require therapy unless they result in hemodynamic compromise or ischemia.[1]

  NSVT is a risk for long-term sustained ventricular arrhythmias. Refer to a cardiologist.

  For an uncertain diagnosis of VT vs. SVT, treatment of presumed VT is suggested[6] and may restore sinus rhythm in SVT.

  Stable patients – pharmacologic therapy

  Beta blockers are effective in suppression of ventricular ectopy, arrhythmias, and sudden cardiac death.[4]

  Monomorphic VT

  Consider amiodarone IV (do not bolus rapidly for patients with a pulse/BP).

  Alternatives are lidocaine and procainamide.

  Polymorphic VT

  Antiarrhythmic therapy similar to monomorphic VT.

  If ischemia is felt to be the cause, treat unstable angina and obtain urgent cardiology evaluation.

  Coronary revascularization and balloon pump may be required.

  After conversion, give amiodarone or lidocaine for arrhythmia suppression.

  Torsades de pointes – give magnesium IV and identify underlying cause (medications).

  Patients with sustained VT and depressed EF may benefit from an ICD.

- Bradycardia/Heart Blocks[1,5,6]

  For unstable patients with bradycardia consider atropine. Use transcutaneous pacing for high-degree heart blocks. Consider epinephrine and dopamine while waiting for pacing.

- Sinus bradycardia
  - Transient/hemodynamically stable bradycardia does not usually require treatment.
- New Heart Blocks
  - Search for reversible causes. Many cardiac surgery patients require only temporary pacing.
  - Mobitz I does not usually require treatment.
  - New bundle branch blocks.
    - Often rate related in the postoperative period.
    - New left bundle pattern may be indicative of ischemia – rule out MI.
  - High grade/third degree heart block
    - Persistent heart blocks – EP consult for possible permanent pacemaker

References

1. Fleischer LA, Beckman JA, Brown KA, et al. 2009 ACCF/AHA focused update on perioperative beta blockade incorporated into the ACC/AHA 2007 guidelines on perioperative cardiovascular evaluation and care for noncardiac surgery. *J Am Coll Cardiol.* 2009;54(22): e13-e118.
2. Epstein AE, Alexander JC, Gutterman DD, et al. American College of Chest Physicians guidelines for the prevention and management of postoperative atrial fibrillation after cardiac surgery. *Chest.* 2005;128(2 suppl):1S-5S. 24S-27S.
3. Jongnarangsin K, Oral H. Postoperative atrial fibrillation. *Med Clin North Am.* 2008;92(1): 87-99.
4. El-Chiami MF, Kilgo P, Thourani V, et al. New-onset atrial fibrillation predicts long-term mortality after coronary artery bypass graft. *J Am Coll Cardiol.* 2010;55(13):1370-1376.
5. Heintz KM, Hollenberg SM. Perioperative cardiac issues: postoperative arrhythmias. *Surg Clin North Am.* 2005;85(6):1103-1114. viii.
6. Merin O, Ilan M, Oren A, et al. Permanent pacemaker implantation following cardiac surgery: indications and long-term follow-up. *Pacing Clin Electrophysiol.* 2009;32(1):7-12.
7. McClennen S, Zimetbaum PJ. Perioperative complications: arrhythmias. In: Cohn SL, Smetana GW, Weed HG, eds. *Just the Facts in Perioperative Medicine*. New York: McGraw Hill; 2006:290-296.
8. Douketis JD, Berger PB, Dunn AS, et al. The perioperative management of antithrombotic therapy: American College of Chest Physicians Evidence-Based Clinical Practice Guidelines (8th Edition). *Chest.* 2008;133(6 Suppl):299S-339S.
9. Vink R, Rienstra M, van Dongen CJJ, et al. Risk of thromboembolism after general surgery in patients with atrial fibrillation. *Am J Cardiol.* 2005;96(6):822-824.
10. Estes M, Halperin JL, Calkins H, et al. ACC/AHA/Physician Consortium 2008 clinical performance measures for adults with nonvalvular atrial fibrillation or atrial flutter: a report of the American College of Cardiology/American Heart Association Task Force on Performance Measures and the Physician Consortium for Performance Improvement (Writing Committee to Develop Clinical Performance Measures for Atrial Fibrillation): developed in collaboration with the Heart Rhythm Society. *Circulation.* 2008;117(8):1101-1120. Epub 2008 Feb 18.

Perioperative Chest Pain/Dyspnea 36

Kalpana R. Prakasa and Leonard S. Feldman

This chapter focuses on the diagnosis and management of perioperative chest pain and dyspnea in noncardiac surgery patients. An internal medicine consultant should evaluate patients in the perioperative period who are suspected to have ischemic chest pain and/or heart failure. Postcardiac surgery patients are typically managed by cardiothoracic surgeons and cardiologists.

36.1 Incidence

- One hundred million adult patients, 25% of whom have known or occult CAD, undergo noncardiac surgery worldwide each year.[1]
- The overall incidence of perioperative nonfatal MI, nonfatal cardiac arrest, and cardiovascular death in high-risk populations is about 5–7%.[2]
  - The incidence of myocardial infarction following major noncardiac surgery ranges between 1% and 26%, while rates of myocardial ischemia range between 15% and 41%.
  - The incidence of myocardial infarction increases as patients exceed 80 years of age.[3]

36.2 Timing and Pathophysiology

- Most postoperative myocardial infarctions occur within 48 h after surgery and do not present with chest pain.[4]
- Myocardial ischemia is caused by a mismatch between oxygen demand and supply. This can be due to plaque rupture and thrombosis, a fixed obstruction, or inadequate collateral circulation.

L.S. Feldman (✉)
Johns Hopkins University, Baltimore, MD, USA
e-mail: lf@jhmi.edu

S.L. Cohn (ed.), *Perioperative Medicine*,
DOI: 10.1007/978-0-85729-498-2_36, © Springer-Verlag London Limited 2011

- The stress response to surgery results in release of various hormones including ACTH and cortisol, epinephrine and norepinephrine, vasopressin, and endorphins. These elicit various physiological changes:
  - Cytokine-mediated inflammatory changes that last approximately 24 h.
  - Catecholamine elevations and sodium retention that return to baseline in 3–5 days.
  - Impaired free water excretion lasting up to 5–7 days.
- Myocardial ischemia may result from this increased sympathetic activity producing tachycardia and hypertension as well as fluid and electrolyte changes. Other precipitating factors for ischemia and heart failure are listed in Table 36.1.
- Plaque rupture and coronary thrombosis, the leading cause of MI in perioperative patients, leads to MI in patients with pre-existing but not necessarily obstructive coronary artery disease.
  - Two-thirds of cases of fatal myocardial infarction in nonoperative setting as well as in postoperative setting are due to plaque rupture, hemorrhage, and thrombosis.[5]
  - Plaque rupture and occlusion commonly occurs in vessels with nonflow limiting stenoses of less than 50%.
- Angiographic studies of survivors of perioperative myocardial infarction suggest that infarction can be due to inadequate collateralization around pre-existing occlusions.
- Most perioperative myocardial infarctions are non-ST segment elevation and non-Q wave events.[6]
- Prevention and treatment strategies for perioperative myocardial infarction mimic non-perioperative myocardial infarctions strategies.
- Heart failure tends to occur either immediately after surgery or 1–3 days later.

Table 36.1 Risk factors for postoperative MI and heart failure

Myocardial ischemia/infarction	Heart failure/pulmonary edema
History of CAD/angina/MI	*Early (within hours)*
Tachycardia	Iatrogenic fluid overload
Hypertension	MI/ischemia
Volume overload	Hypertension/hypotension
Hypotension/blood loss	Tachycardia
Hypercoagulability/platelet activation	Hypoxia
Hyperthermia (fever)	Cessation of positive pressure ventilation
Decreased pulmonary function	*Later (postoperative days 1–3)*
Altered pain perception (failure to recognize)	Reabsorption of interstitial fluid
	Ischemia
	Failure to restart usual medications

- Postoperative pulmonary edema, with mortality rates for the elderly as high as 65%,[7] can be cardiac or noncardiac in origin.
- Cardiac etiologies for pulmonary edema include:
  - Left ventricular failure as a result of volume overload, myocardial ischemia, uncontrolled hypertension, or severe valvular disease (aortic or mitral)
  - Heart failure with a preserved ejection fraction as a result of age-related increases in arterial stiffening, systolic hypertension, left ventricular hypertrophy, and impaired cardiac relaxation
  - Perioperative transient left ventricular apical ballooning syndrome (Takotsubo cardiomyopathy)

    Characterized by transient left ventricular dysfunction in the absence of obstructive coronary artery disease that was preceded by an episode of emotional and physiological stress.
    Presents in the postoperative period with acute chest pain, pulmonary edema, electrocardiographic changes similar to myocardial infarction, and mildly elevated cardiac enzymes.
    It is more common in postmenopausal women.[8]

- Noncardiac pulmonary edema may be due to:
  - Re-expansion of a collapsed lung following thoracentesis or chest tube placement
  - Rarely due to naloxone therapy

36.3 Differential Diagnosis of Perioperative Chest Pain/Dyspnea

- The differential diagnosis appears in Table 36.2 and should be tailored based on the history and physical. Further testing will depend on this information.
- Remember to rule out likely high-stakes diagnoses first: MI, aortic dissection, pulmonary embolism, pneumothorax, cardiac tamponade, etc.

36.4 Diagnosis of Ischemia

- The triad of chest pain, electrocardiographic changes (ST changes or new Q waves), and positive cardiac enzymes (cardiac Troponin I) confirm myocardial infarction in over 90% of patients.
- Characteristic pain (crushing, substernal, pressure-like, same as previous pain diagnosed as myocardial infarction), that radiates (to jaw, neck, shoulder, or arm), lasts for more than 20 min, and is associated with shortness of breath, sweating, and nausea can point toward ischemic chest pain.

Table 36.2 Differential diagnosis of perioperative chest pain

Cardiac/vascular	Pulmonary	Gastrointestinal	Other
Ischemic chest pain	Pulmonary embolism	Gall bladder or biliary pathology	Wound infection
Heart failure – systolic or preserved	Atelectasis	Gastrointestinal reflux	Musculoskeletal pain
Pericarditis/pericardial effusion	COPD/Asthma exacerbation	Esophageal spasm	
Cardiac arrhythmias	Pneumonia	Peptic ulcer disease	
Transient left ventricular apical ballooning syndrome	Pleural effusion	Pancreatitis	
Uncontrolled hypertension	Hemothorax		
Aortic dissection	Pneumothorax		

- Cardiogenic shock presents with hypotension, tachycardia, cool and clammy extremities, and respiratory distress.
- Hypotension, clear lungs, elevated jugular venous pressure, Kussmaul's sign (inspiratory increase in jugular venous pressure), and a prominent x descent help to identify a right ventricular infarction.
- Rupture of the interventricular septum as a result of ischemia presents with hypotension, new harsh and loud holosystolic murmur heard at lower left sternal border, and a thrill.
- Troponin T and I are more useful than creatinine kinase for diagnosing postoperative ischemia.
- Echocardiography is useful to assess left ventricular function and wall motion changes.
  - Transesophageal echocardiography can be used emergently to determine cause of life threatening hemodynamic instability (Class IIa – Level C)
- The likelihood of mortality from ischemia-induced chest pain is increased if the following factors are present: chest pain prolonged over 20 min, pulmonary edema, dynamic ST changes $\geq$1 mm, new or worsening mitral regurgitation murmur, hypotension, and/or heart failure.

36.5 Diagnosis of Heart Failure

- Heart failure patients can present with dyspnea, tachypnea, and a cough with pink frothy sputum. Physical examination signs include jugular venous distention, S3 gallop, rales, and pedal edema.

- Diagnostic testing can include pro-brain natriuretic peptide level, chest x-ray findings, electrocardiography, arterial blood gas levels, pulmonary artery and central venous pressure measurements if available.
- Echocardiography is a diagnostic mainstay to assess left ventricular function and wall motion changes.

36.6 Screening for Cardiac Complications

- During intraoperative screening, prolonged ST segment depression precedes and predicts overt myocardial infarction.
  - ST segment changes noted in two precordial leads (V2, V3, V4) have the maximum sensitivity.[9]
  - Continuous 12-lead electrocardiographic monitoring is more sensitive than two leads monitoring for detection of prolonged ischemia, sensitivity (12%), specificity (98%), positive predictive value (40%), and negative predictive value (90%).[10]
  - ST segment monitoring is useful in patients with coronary artery disease undergoing vascular surgery (Class IIa – Level B).
  - Consider using ST segment monitoring in patients with ≥1 coronary artery disease risk factors (Class IIb – Level B).
- Half of ischemic ST segment changes occur during surgery and the rest occur within 72 h postoperatively.
- Screening for ischemia appears to be cost-effective for *high-risk* patients.
  - Obtain electrocardiograms preoperatively, immediately postoperatively, and on the first 2 postoperative days.
  - Myocardial ischemia is rare after 3 days.[11]
  - Monitor for ischemia beyond postoperative day 3 only in patients who present with early ischemia.[12]
- Screening with Troponin I
  - Troponin I should be obtained when symptoms or electrocardiography suggests acute coronary syndrome (Class I – Level C).
  - The utility of Troponin I is unclear in asymptomatic vascular surgery and intermediate surgery patients (Class IIb – Level C).
  - Do not obtain Troponin I in asymptomatic stable patients after low-risk surgery (Class III – Level C).
  - In a prospective cohort study in 229 vascular surgery patients, Troponin I was obtained immediately after surgery and on postoperative days 1, 2, and 3. Twelve percent of patients had positive cardiac Troponin I over 1.5. Patients with an elevated Troponin I had an increase in their 6-month mortality.
  - There is a dose–response relationship between increasing levels of Troponin I elevation and future mortality.[13]

- Screening with postoperative pro-brain natriuretic peptide (pro-BNP)
  - In a prospective cohort study in 218 vascular surgery patients, a pro-BNP over 860 pg/mL on postoperative day 3–5 was associated with an increase in nonfatal myocardial infarction, percutaneous coronary intervention (PCI), coronary artery bypass surgery, or cardiac death.[14]
- Right heart catheterization
  - ACC/AHA 2007 guidelines for noncardiac surgery

    Pulmonary artery catheterization may be reasonable for select patients and surgical procedures when hemodynamic instability is expected (Class IIb – Level B).

    Routine use is not recommended (Class III – Level A).
  - A large randomized controlled trial of pulmonary artery catheterization directed therapy versus standard therapy in 1994 surgical patients over 60 years old with an ASA class of III/IV showed no difference in rates of myocardial infarction, congestive heart failure, or mortality.[15]

36.7 Management Plans

- Continue antiplatelet agents (if possible), statins, beta-blockers, and antihypertensive agents (see Chap. 20).
- Acute Treatment of Ischemia and MI (Table 36.3)
  - Thrombolytics are contraindicated in postoperative patients due to increased risk of bleeding.
  - Pain control

    Opioids can reduce catecholamine surge and hypercoagulability. Opioids may also reduce adhesion and migration of neutrophils, and may be directly cardioprotective in patients susceptible to ischemia.[16]
    Music can reduce pain, lower stress hormones, lower the anxiety, and reduce morphine use based on the study involving 75 patients underwent open hernia repair.[17] Personalized music helped even more.[18]
  - Primary PCI is the treatment of choice in patients with high risk of bleeding.
  - Primary PCI should be considered in patients with severe heart failure and symptom duration >3 h.
  - Advantages of primary PCI include reduced reocclusion rates; good TIMI-3 flow rate; early risk stratification; reduced mortality, stroke, and reinfarction; reduced risk of intracranial hemorrhage; and shorter length of hospitalization.
  - Stents should be placed during primary PCI when coronary anatomy is favorable.

Table 36.3 Pharmacologic therapy for myocardial infarction

Agent	Clinical effect/indication	ACC/AHA recommendation
Aspirin 162–325 mg	Improve survival, decrease reinfarction	Class I
Clopidogrel 300–600 mg loading dose at the time of PCI, 75 mg daily	Decrease death and MI	Class I
Glycoprotein IIb/IIIa inhibitors in patients having primary PCI	Decrease death, MI	Class IIa
Unfractionated heparin for patients having PCI	Decrease death and MI	Class I
Low-molecular-weight heparin alternative to heparin	Reduce cardiac events	Class IIb
Direct thrombin inhibitors	For heparin-induced thrombocytopenia	Class IIa
Beta-blockers	Improve survival, reduce infarct size, arrhythmias, and recurrent ischemia	Class I
ACE inhibitors within 24 h of MI	Improve survival, decrease heart failure, and LV dysfunction	Class I
ARB	Intolerant to ACE inhibitors	Class I
Nitroglycerin for the first 48 h for chest pain, heart failure, and hypertension	Decrease death and MI	Class I
Statins within 24 h of MI	Decrease death and MI	Class I
Calcium channel blockers alternative to beta-blockers	No survival benefit	Class II
Warfarin	Reduce embolic stroke in LV thrombus and dysfunction	Class I
Magnesium to patients on diuresis	Improve reperfusion	Class IIa

MI myocardial infarction, *PCI* percutaneous coronary intervention, *LV* left ventricle, *ACE* angiotensin converting enzyme, *ARB* angiotensin receptor blocker

- Patients with left main stenosis >60% and triple vessel disease should be referred for coronary artery bypass grafting.
- Aspirin 162–325 mg should be given at presentation and continued indefinitely thereafter.
- Clopidogrel or ticlopidine should be administered for aspirin insensitive patients. Clopidogrel added for 1 month after PCI with bare metal stent and for 1 year after drug eluting stent.
- Beta blockers should be given to all patients with acute myocardial infarction.

Consider alpha-2 agonists to treat perioperative myocardial ischemia and infarction when beta adrenergic blockade is contraindicated

- Angiotensin converting enzyme inhibitors (ACEI) should be given to all patients within 24 h after myocardial infarction. Angiotensin receptor blockers can be given to patients intolerant to ACEI.
- Nitroglycerin given to relieve ischemic chest pain except in patients with hypotension and right ventricular infarction.
- Verapamil or diltiazem can be given to patients to control heart rate in arrhythmias after myocardial infarction in the absence of heart failure, left ventricular dysfunction, and AV block. The short-acting dihydropyridine, nifedipine, should not be used in acute myocardial infarction.
- Magnesium replacement should be considered to treat hypomagnesemia and torsades de pointes.
- HMG-CoA reductase inhibitors should be initiated with a LDL target of 70 mg/dL.
- Warfarin should be prescribed for postmyocardial infarction patients with atrial fibrillation and/or left ventricular thrombus.

• There are five major complications of acute myocardial infarction

- Cardiogenic shock managed with intra-aortic balloon pump counterpulsation, positive inotropes (dobutamine and dopamine), and diuretics as needed.
- Right ventricular infarction managed with reperfusion, intravenous fluids. Drugs that decrease right ventricular preload (diuretics, nitrates, and morphine) should be avoided.
- Acute mitral valve regurgitation caused by posteromedial papillary muscle dysfunction from underlying left ventricular ischemia and infarction. Treated with reperfusion and surgery in case of papillary muscle rupture.
- Ventricular septal rupture can be apical and simple or basal and complex. It is managed by surgical closure.
- Rupture of left ventricular free wall is always fatal, managed with emergency surgery.

• Discharge

- Close follow-up after discharge is needed as patients with postoperative myocardial ischemia have a 2.2-fold increase in the rate of subsequent cardiac complications over next 2 years.[19]
- Hospital discharge planning should therefore include strategies to modify future risk such as the initiation of preventative therapies and plans for additional cardiac testing and cardiology follow-up. Furthermore, the physician assuming primary care of the patient must be fully informed.
- Elderly patients with postoperative myocardial ischemia are 10 times more likely to die within 30 days of surgery and 15 times more likely to die within 1 year of surgery.[20]

36.8
Acute Treatment of Heart Failure

- Manage precipitating factors such as acute ischemia, hypertension, and atrial fibrillation.
- Oxygen therapy.
- Diuretics, fluid, and salt restriction are the primary treatment of fluid retention.
- ACE inhibitors are recommended for all patients with heart failure and reduced left ventricular ejection fraction, unless contraindicated.
  - Treat with ARBs in patients intolerant to ACEIs.
- Consider adding an aldosterone antagonist in selected patients with heart failure and reduced left ventricular ejection fraction who can be carefully monitored for preserved renal function and normal potassium concentration. Creatinine should be ≤2.5 mg/dL in men or ≤2.0 mg/dL in women. The potassium should be <5.0 mEq/L.
- Routine combined use of an ACEI, ARB, and aldosterone antagonist is not recommended.
- Beta-blockers (using 1 of the 3 proven to reduce mortality, i.e., bisoprolol, carvedilol, and sustained release metoprolol succinate) are recommended for all stable patients, unless contraindicated.
- Consider the addition of a combination of hydralazine and a nitrate for persistent symptoms, patients with renal insufficiency and patients with intolerance to ACEI and ARB. This treatment has been studied most extensively in African-Americans.
- Digitalis can be beneficial to decrease hospitalizations for heart failure.
- Avoid nonsteroidal anti-inflammatory drugs, antiarrhythmic drugs, and calcium channel blocking drugs.
- Add positive inotropic agents in patients with hypotension.
- Use intubation and ventilation with positive end expiratory pressure as needed.
- Refer for valve repair in patients with valvular (mitral, aortic) disorders.

36.9
Conclusion

- Postoperative ischemic chest pain typically afflicts patients with preexisting coronary artery disease or with cardiac risk factors. It is rare in patients with no cardiac risk factors who are undergoing low-risk surgery.
- Emergency surgery, vascular surgery, thoracic and upper abdominal surgery, and prolonged intraoperative hypotension are associated with the greatest risk of postoperative cardiac complications.

- The diagnosis and management of postoperative ischemic chest pain and heart failure is similar to nonoperative settings.
- Patients with postoperative ischemia need close follow-up after discharge. Communication with the primary care physician is crucial.

References

1. Devereaux PJ, Beattie WS, Choi PT, et al. How strong is the evidence for the use of perioperative beta blockers in non cardiac surgery? Systematic review and meta-analysis of randomized controlled trails. *BMJ*. 2005;331(7512):313-321.
2. POISE Study Group. Effects of extended-release metoprolol succinate in patients undergoing non-cardiac surgery (POISE trial): a randomized controlled trial. *Lancet*. 2008;371: 1839-1847.
3. Hamel MB, Henderson WG, Khuri SF, et al. Surgical outcomes for patients aged 80 and older: morbidity and mortality from major noncardiac surgery. *J Am Geriatr Soc*. 2005;53:424-429.
4. Landesberg G. The pathophysiology of perioperative myocardial infarction: facts and perspectives. *J Cardiothorac Vasc Anesth*. 2003;17:90-100.
5. Dawood MM, Gupta DK, Southern J, et al. Pathology of fatal perioperative myocardial infarction: implications regarding pathophysiology and prevention. *Int J Cardiol*. 1996;57:37-44.
6. Priebe HJ. Triggers of perioperative myocardial ischemia and infarction. *Br J Anaesth*. 2004;93:9-20.
7. Roche JJ, Wenn RT, Sahota O, et al. Effect of comorbidities and post operative complications on mortality after hip fracture in elderly people: prospective observational cohort study. *BMJ*. 2005;331:1374.
8. Liu S, Dhamee MS. Perioperative transient left ventricular apical ballooning syndrome: Takatsubo cardiomyopathy: a review. *J Clin Anesth*. 2010;22:64-70.
9. Landesberg G, Mosseri M, Wolf Y, et al. Perioperative myocardial ischemia and infarction: identification by continuous 12-lead electrocardiogram with online ST-segment monitoring. *Anesthesiology*. 2002;96(2):264-270.
10. Martinez EA, Kim LJ, Faraday N, et al. Sensitivity of routine intensive care unit surveillance for detecting myocardial ischemia. *Crit Care Med*. 2003;31:2302-2308.
11. Polancyk C, Rhode L, Goldman L, et al. Right heart catheterization and cardiac complications in patients undergoing noncardiac surgery: an observational study. *JAMA*. 2001;286: 309-314.
12. Mangano D, Wong M, London M, et al. Perioperative myocardial ischemia in patients undergoing noncardiac surgery – II: incidence and severity during the 1st week after surgery. *J Am Coll Cardiol*. 1991;17:851-857.
13. Kim L, Martinez E, Faraday N, et al. Cardiac troponin I predicts short term mortality in vascular surgery patients. *Circulation*. 2002;106:2366-2371.
14. Mahla E, Baumann A, Rehak P, et al. N-terminal pro-brain natriuretic peptide identifies patients at high risk for adverse cardiac outcome after vascular surgery. *Anesthesiology*. 2007;106:1088-1095.
15. Sandham JD, Hull RD, Brant RF, et al. A randomized, controlled trial of the use of pulmonary-artery catheters in high-risk surgical patients. *N Engl J Med*. 2003;348:5-14.
16. Fleisher LA, Beckman JA, Brown KA, et al. ACC/AHA 2007 guidelines on perioperative cardiovascular evaluation and care for noncardiac surgery: executive summary: a report of the American College of Cardiology/American Heart Association Task Force on Practice Guidelines (Writing Committee to Revise the 2002 Guidelines on Perioperative Cardiovascular

Evaluation for Noncardiac Surgery) Developed in collaboration with the American Society of Echocardiography, American Society of Nuclear Cardiology, Heart Rhythm Society, Society of Cardiovascular Anesthesiologists, Society for Cardiovascular Angiography and Interventions, Society for Vascular Medicine and Biology, and Society for Vascular Surgery. *J Am Coll Cardiol*. 2007; 50(17):1707–32. Erratum in: *J Am Coll Cardiol*. 2008; 52(9): 794–7.
17. Nilsson U, Unosson M, Rawal N. Stress reduction and analgesia in patients exposed to calming music postoperatively: a randomized controlled trial. *Eur J Anaesthesiol*. 2005;22(2):96-102.
18. Leardi S, Pietroletti R, Angeloni G, et al. Randomized clinical trial examining the effect of music therapy in stress response to day surgery. *Br J Surg*. 2007;94:943-947.
19. Mangano D, Browner W, Hollenberg M, et al. Long term cardiac prognosis following noncardiac surgery. *JAMA*. 1992;268:233-239.
20. Oscarsson A, Eintrei C, Anskar S, et al. Troponin T values provide long term prognosis in elderly patients undergoing non-cardiac surgery. *Acta Anaesthesiol Scand*. 2004;48: 1071-1079.

Postoperative Pulmonary Complications 37

Ibironke Oduyebo and Leonard S. Feldman

37.1 Introduction

- Postoperative pulmonary complications (PPCs) is an umbrella term encompassing a heterogeneous collection of respiratory problems after surgery. PPCs can include atelectasis, pneumonia, bronchospasm, acute respiratory distress syndrome, and postoperative respiratory failure (RF). Definitions of PPCs often vary in scholarly articles, and this chapter focuses on pneumonia and atelectasis.
- PPCs are as common as postoperative cardiac complications, but incidence varies widely based on the definitions used.
- PPCs accounted for the largest increase in hospital cost and prolongation of length of stay after surgery in a large academic hospital study.[1] Pneumonia and failure to wean from the ventilator were the leading causes of PPCs in that study.

37.2 Causes of PPCs

- Many PPCs are related to disruption of normal pulmonary physiology arising from preexisting lung disease or from surgical, anesthetic, and/or from pharmacologic interventions.
- These disruptions predispose to PPCs by decreasing lung volumes, producing hypoventilation, and altering the lung defense mechanism, leading to atelectasis and pneumonia (Table 37.1).

L.S. Feldman (✉)
Johns Hopkins University, Baltimore, MD, USA
e-mail: lf@jhmi.edu

S.L. Cohn (ed.), *Perioperative Medicine*,
DOI: 10.1007/978-0-85729-498-2_37,

Table 37.1 Mechanism for PPCs

Physiologic change	Etiology	Result
Decrease in functional residual capacity	• Can be produced by surgical trauma to chest wall muscles during thoracic and upper abdominal surgery	• Produces regional atelectasis
Diaphragmatic dysfunction	• Caused by a decrease in central nervous system output to phrenic nerves mediated by anesthetic agents	• Produces hypoventilation
Impairment in gas exchange	• Mediated by residual effects of anesthesia and anesthetic inhibition of hypoxic pulmonary vasoconstriction	• V/Q mismatch created by respiratory muscle dysfunction
Alteration in lung defense mechanism	• Endotracheal intubation, ciliary damage by inhalation anesthetics, and hyperoxic gas mixtures • Narcotic use or inadequate control of postoperative pain	• Impairment in mucociliary clearance • Inhibition of coughing

37.3 Disease-Specific Review

37.3.1 Pneumonia

37.3.1.1 Incidence

- Postoperative infections are a major cause of morbidity and mortality in patients undergoing surgery. Postoperative pneumonia ranks as the third most common postoperative infection behind urinary tract infections and surgical site infections.[2]
- The incidence of postoperative atelectasis <u>and</u> pneumonia was 22.5% in a multicenter observational study of **abdominal** surgery patients.[3]
- In a large multicenter observational study of postoperative pneumonia in patients undergoing **major** surgery in Veterans Affairs medical centers, the incidence of postoperative pneumonia was 1.5%.[2]

37.3.1.2 Timing

- Pneumonia can occur at any time in the postoperative period.
- Ventilator-associated pneumonia occurs more often in the first week of ventilation and may be divided into early (<72 h since intubation) or late (≥72 h) since the pathogens vary.

37.3.1.3
Risk Assessment (see Chap. 21)

- Similar to perioperative cardiac risk indexes, various studies have attempted to produce a validated risk index for predicting postoperative pneumonia.
- In one of the largest prospective studies, Arozullah et al.[2] enrolled 160,805 patients undergoing major noncardiac surgery at 100 Veterans Affairs Medical Centers to develop a preoperative risk model utilizing 14 risk factors including patient-specific risk factors as well as surgery-specific risk factors for predicting postoperative pneumonia.
  - Surgical procedures and patient risk factors associated with a higher risk include abdominal aortic aneurysm and thoracic surgery and patient's age, poor functional status, weight loss >10% in the past 6 months, history of COPD, impaired sensorium, history of CVA, BUN <8 mg/dL and >30 mg/dL, steroid use for chronic condition, and smoking within the past year.
  - The risk index incorporates basic medical information that is readily available to practitioners. However, the disadvantages of this risk index are that it incorporates a large number of risk factors, 14, and that most of the patients in the cohort were men, decreasing its generalizability. In addition, a significant portion of the veterans who receive care at Veterans Affairs medical centers have multiple comorbid illness, and the model might not be generalizable to healthier populations.
- Johnson et al.[4] in 2007 updated the study above by including patients at the VA and private sector academic centers with women making 20% of the study population. They developed a respiratory risk index (RRI) to be used as a predictive model for postoperative respiratory failure (RF) defined as postoperative mechanical ventilation for longer than 48 h or unplanned reintubation. Very similar to the above risk model they identified a large number of variables, 28 in this study, that were independently associated with RF. Very similar to above, older patients, patients with a higher ASA classification, elevated creatinine, and smokers were at higher risk for postoperative RF.
- Brooks-Brunn[5] prospectively validated a six factor index in 276 abdominal surgery patients. The factors included impaired cognitive function, BMI >27, incision location, history of smoking in the past 8 weeks, history of cancer, and age >60 years of age. However, this risk index had a low positive predictive value in a split sample validation group, although the negative predictive value was slightly better. In the same study, incision length >30 cm, history of angina, and ASA status 3, 4, or 5 were identified as additional risk factors in the validation sample.
- These indexes highlight the need for more studies to validate pulmonary risk models, and unlike the revised cardiac risk index, these indexes are not ready for routine use in clinical practice.

37.3.1.4
Etiology

- Most cases of postoperative pneumonia are bacterial and they may be polymicrobial (Table 37.2).

Table 37.2 Potential pathogens for postoperative pneumonia[6]

Non-MDR organism	• *Streptococcus pneumonia* • *H. influenza* • *MRSA* • Antibiotic sensitive *E. coli, K. pneumoniae*, Enterobacter species, Proteus species, and *Serratia marcescens*
MDR organisms	• Drug-resistant gram-negative organisms such as *P. Aeruginosa*, K. pneumoniae (ESBL), and *Acinetobacter* species • MRSA • *Legionella pneumophilia*

- *Streptococcal pneumonia*, *Moraxella pneumonia,* and other pathogenic causes of community acquired pneumonia are common causes of early onset postoperative pneumonia. Other pathogens like aerobic gram-negative rods such as *Pseudomonas aeruginosa*, *Escherichia coli*, *Klebsiella pneumionae,* and *Acinetobacter* species and gram-positive organisms such as methicillin resistant *Staphylococcus aureus* (MRSA) are causes of late onset postoperative pneumonia.[7]
- Multidrug resistant (MDR) organisms are more commonly associated with the following factors: recent antibiotic therapy in the preceding month 30 to 90 days, current hospitalization or long-term hospital stay or chronic dialysis within 30 days, immunocompromised state from disease or drugs, structural lung disease, or early onset after hospitalization.
- Prevalence of MDR organisms varies by patient population and hospital, underlying the importance of surveillance cultures and knowing your own institution's antibiogram.

37.3.1.5 Diagnosis

- Criteria for diagnosing pneumonia differ in the literature. Some employ physician diagnosis alone, and others take into account clinical, laboratory, radiologic features, or various combinations of all three.
- In practice, a physician diagnosis alone is not an acceptable criterion for the diagnosis of postoperative pneumonia. All patients need at least <u>two serial</u> chest radiographs demonstrating infiltrate or cavitation to make the diagnosis.
- The Centers for Disease Control and National Health Safety Network (CDC/NHSN)[8] have published guidelines for the definition of health care-acquired pneumonia. They have three different definitions for pneumonia, with one arm being a clinical definition based on objective signs and symptoms, and the other two arms are defined with the addition of positive cultures from the blood, sputum, or pleural fluid.
- The CDC/NHSN minimal criteria for the definition of postoperative pneumonia include demonstrating an infiltrate or cavitation on at least two serial chest x-rays and a combination of abnormal vital signs and presence of clinical symptoms with a cough, sputum, or rales on exam (see Table 37.3).
- Although the basic diagnosis of pneumonia above does not require microbiologic or histologic conformation from cultures or samples, having that information can help with narrowing antibiotic choice and further confirming the diagnosis.

Table 37.3 CDC/NHSN diagnosis of postoperative pneumonia[8]

Radiology: Two or more serial radiographs with at least one of the following: • New or worsening infiltrate • Consolidation • Cavitation
Signs/Symptoms: At least one of the following: • Fever (>38°C) with no other recognized cause • Leukopenia or leukocytosis • For adults >70 years, altered mental status with no other recognized cause
AND At least two of the following: • New sputum or change in sputum production or increased suctioning requirements • Abnormal breath sounds from baseline • New onset or worsening of cough or dyspnea • Worsening hypoxia

- The guidelines support obtaining a blood culture, pleural fluid culture, or quantitative cultures from minimally contaminated lower respiratory tract specimen (e.g., BAL or specimen brushings) for bacteriologic confirmation. An endotracheal aspirate is not a minimally contaminated specimen.
- There are diagnostic strategies that include obtaining expectorated sputum from nonintubated patients and semiquantitative cultures from endotracheal aspirate for bacteriologic studies. Using these strategies, more patients receive antibiotics in a timely manner but antibiotics are overused as compared to strategies that rely on cultures from lower respiratory tract specimen. You should take into consideration what diagnostic testing is readily available at your institution for quick bacteriologic diagnosis.
- Patients who are immunocompromised require one symptom to be clinically significant for pneumonia.
- To diagnose candidal infection, matching cultures from blood and expectorated sputum are necessary. Otherwise, BAL or protected specimen brushing specimen are required.
- Elderly patients might not have the typical signs of pneumonia. Altered mental status may be the only manifestation.
- Patients on a ventilator within the 48-h period before the onset of the diagnosis of pneumonia have ventilator associated pneumonia (VAP).
- For ventilated patients, distinguish between tracheal colonization and upper respiratory tract infections such as tracheobronchitis.

37.3.1.6
Treatment

- Choice of antimicrobial agent is largely determined by the likelihood of MDR organisms (Table 37.4).
  - For patients with no risk factors for MDR organisms, the empiric regimen should have a limited spectrum coverage and be based on the organism of suspicion.

Table 37.4 Empiric antibiotic treatment for postoperative pneumonia

Non-MDR	Suspected MDR
Ceftriaxone	Broad spectrum antipseudomonal agent (cephalosporin or carbapenem or beta lactam/lactamase inhibitor)
Or	*plus*
Moxifloxacin	Antipseudomonal fluroquinolone
Or	*plus*
Ampicillin/sulbactam	MRSA coverage (if risk factors are present or there is a high incidence locally)
Or	
Ertapenem	

  - For patients with risk factors for MDR organisms, treat with broad spectrum antibiotics determined to be effective against MDR bacteria based on your hospital microbial profile. The antibiotic regimen should then be narrowed based on culture data when available.
  - Combination therapy is common in the treatment of MDR suspected nosocomial pneumonia. Treat with a combination therapy only to provide broad spectrum coverage that is likely to be active against the etiologic agent. Do not use combination therapy for a synergistic effect as the data does not support this.[7]
- Duration of therapy should not be prolonged.
  - Patients usually improve in 3–5 days and prolonged therapy can lead to colonization by drug-resistant organisms.[7]
- Duration of therapy can be as short as 7 days provided that the patient has a good clinical response with resolution of clinical symptoms.
- Extend the duration of therapy up to 14 days in patients with *P. aeruginosa* pneumonia.[7]

37.3.2 Atelectasis

37.3.2.1 Incidence

- Atelectasis refers to collapse or loss of lung volume.
- Postoperative atelectasis is the most common complication of surgery, but it is often clinically insignificant.
- Depending on the definition, the incidence can vary from a few percent to >80%.
  - Subsegmental atelectasis is usually minor and transient.
  - Segmental and lobar atelectasis are usually significant and cause hypoxemia.

37.3.2.2
Timing

- Atelectasis tends to occur in the first 48 h after surgery and is often subclinical. When it is present after that, it is more likely to be clinically relevant.

37.3.2.3
Etiology

- Obstructive from airway obstruction by mucus or an aspirated material.
- Compressive from anesthetic-induced diaphragmatic relaxation or surgical trauma to chest wall muscles.
- Adhesive from anesthetic-induced surfactant impairment.[9]

37.3.2.4
Diagnosis

- The diagnosis is suggested by clinical signs and symptoms such as respiratory distress or hypoxemia in a patient with risk factors for atelectasis.
- Fever is not a sign of atelectasis (i.e., atelectasis does not cause fever but may occur concomitantly).
- Confirmation is by chest x-ray.
  - Increased opacification of the airless lobe or long segment.
  - Displacement of fissures (lobar atelectasis).
  - Larger areas of atelectasis may result in displacement of hilar structures, cardiomediastinal shift toward the side of collapse, ipsilateral hemidiaphragm elevation, narrowing of the ipsilateral intercoastal spaces, and hyperlucency of the remaining aerated parts of the lung.

37.3.2.5
Treatment

- Employ techniques that increase aeration of the lung and that encourage the patient to inspire deeply ("lung expansion maneuvers").
- Techniques such as incentive spirometry, intermittent positive-pressure breathing, and chest physiotherapy have been shown to have equal efficacy in reversing and preventing atelectasis.

37.4 Prevention of Postoperative Pulmonary Complications (See Chap. 21)

- There is a large amount of literature studying modifiable risk factors to prevent PPCs.
- A meta-analysis reviewed the literature to determine evidence-based prevention strategies and concluded that ***postoperative lung expansion techniques*** to be the only modality with benefit for the prevention of PPCs. Strategies with probable benefit included selective postoperative nasogastric decompression and use of shorter acting neuromuscular blocking agents, but smoking cessation and neuraxial blockade were of indeterminate value.
- Smoking cessation deserves a special comment. All studies on risks of PPCs have identified smoking as an important risk factor for the development of PPCs. One could infer from this that smoking cessation would decrease the risk of PPCs. However, there are several conflicting studies on this point. In the ACP guideline meta-analysis, the benefit of smoking cessation is rated as indeterminate. However, with the knowledge of the significant health risks associated with smoking, physicians need to encourage smoking cessation during any possible patient contact. More studies are needed on the optimal timing for smoking cessation prior to surgery.

References

1. Dimick JB, Chen SL, Taheri PA, et al. Hospital costs associated with surgical complications: a report from the private-sector National Surgical Quality Improvement Program. *J Am Coll Surg*. 2004;199:531-537.
2. Arozullah AM, Khuri SF, Henderson WG, Participants in the National Veterans Affairs Surgical Quality Improvement Program, et al. Development and validation of a multifactorial risk index for predicting postoperative pneumonia after major noncardiac surgery. *Ann Intern Med*. 2001;135:847-857.
3. Brooks-Brunn JA. Predictors of postoperative pulmonary complications following abdominal surgery. *Chest*. 1997;111:564-571.
4. Johnson RG, Arozullah AM, Neumayer L, et al. Multivariable predictors of postoperative respiratory failure after general and vascular surgery: results from the patient safety in surgery study. *J Am Coll Surg*. 2004;6:1188-1198.
5. Brooks-Brunn JA. Validation of a predictive model for postoperative pulmonary complications. *Heart Lung*. 1998;27:151-158.
6. Lawrence VA, Cornell JE, Smetana GW, American College of Physicians. Strategies to reduce postoperative pulmonary complications after noncardiothoracic surgery: systematic review for the American College of Physicians. *Ann Intern Med*. 2006;144:596-608.
7. American Thoracic Society and Infectious Diseases Society of America. Guidelines for the management of adults with hospital-acquired, ventilator-associated, and healthcare-associated pneumonia. *Am J Respir Crit Care Med*. 2005;171:388-416.
8. Horan TC, Andrus M, Dudeck MA. CDC/NHSN surveillance definition of health care-associated infection and criteria for specific types of infections in the acute care setting. *Am J Infect Control*. 2008;36:309-332.
9. Duggan M, Kavanagh BP. Pulmonary atelectasis: a pathogenic perioperative entity. *Anesthesiology*. 2005;102:838-854.

Postoperative Venous Thromboembolism (DVT and PE) 38

David G. Paje and Scott Kaatz

38.1 Introduction

38.1.1 Definitions

- **Venous Thromboembolism** (VTE) clinically manifests with either **deep vein thrombosis** (DVT) or **pulmonary embolism** (PE), or both.
- DVT may occur in the upper or lower extremities.
  - Upper extremity DVT (UEDVT) refers to thrombosis of the axillary and/or subclavian vein. It is most commonly associated with central venous catheterization.
  - Lower extremity DVT may be classified as either **proximal** or **distal**. Proximal DVT is located in or superior to the popliteal vein, which is the confluence of the tibial and peroneal veins. This includes the superficial femoral vein, which is actually a deep vein and is more appropriately referred to as the femoral vein. Distal DVT is found inferior to the popliteal vein, which includes the tibial and peroneal veins and their tributaries.
- PE refers to the occlusion of any part of the pulmonary arterial bed, which in most cases is a consequence of embolization of DVT.

38.1.2 Epidemiology

- Without adequate thromboprophylaxis, the incidence of objectively confirmed DVT is as high as 60% among hospitalized surgical patients, depending on patient-related

D.G. Paje (✉)
Hospital Medicine, Henry Ford Hospital, Wayne State University School of Medicine, 2799 West Grand Boulevard, CFP-413, Detroit, MI 48202 USA
e-mail: dpaje1@hfhs.org

S.L. Cohn (ed.), *Perioperative Medicine*,
DOI: 10.1007/978-0-85729-498-2_38, © Springer-Verlag London Limited 2011

individual risk factors and on the type of surgery,[1] and most of these events are asymptomatic. Important clinical predictors include prior VTE, presence of malignancy, advancing age, and certain high-risk procedures such as invasive neurosurgery, total hip arthroplasty, major vascular surgery, and radical cystectomy[2] (see Chap. 7).

- Almost half (44%) of symptomatic VTE occur during the relatively short period of time when patients remain in the hospital after surgery, which makes it the highest risk period for postoperative VTE. The risk remains elevated for 2–3 months after surgery, and the majority (56%) of all surgery-related VTE is diagnosed after hospital discharge.[2]
- Among patients who develop symptomatic VTE following surgery, as many as 50% present with clinically overt PE.[3]

38.1.3 Pathophysiology

- The current recognized predisposing risk factors for VTE reflect the underlying pathophysiologic processes that Rudolph Virchow first proposed in 1884. He acknowledged that thrombosis is the result of at least one of three underlying etiologic factors, which are listed below in relation to surgery-specific issues:
  - **Alterations in normal blood flow** – Immobility during surgery and the postoperative period may result in venostasis especially in the lower extremities.
  - **Disruption or injury to the vascular endothelium** – Direct trauma or as a result of surgical dissection may lead to disruption of the venous endothelial lining such as damage to the popliteal vein during knee arthroplasty or damage to the pelvic veins during abdominal hysterectomy.
  - **Alterations in the constitution of blood** – Tissue trauma and the resultant reparative process activate hemostasis and elicit both local and systemic inflammatory responses that may lead to a hypercoagulable state.
- An individual patient may have a preoperative subclinical or intrinsic thrombosis risk as a result of underlying **genetic** (e.g., anticoagulant deficiencies, factor V Leiden, prothrombin G20210A) or **acquired** (e.g., prior VTE, malignancy, age, varicose veins, obesity, hormone treatments) risk factors; the subsequent trauma or surgery may sufficiently elevate the risk above the threshold for thrombosis.
- The consequences of DVT include PE, recurrent VTE, and **postthrombotic syndrome** (PTS). PTS may cause chronic debilitating swelling and pain of the affected extremity, and in severe cases it may lead to venous ulcers. The risk of PTS is about 20–50% following an acute DVT.[4]
- The key clinical sequelae of acute PE are primarily hemodynamic. Less severe episodes of PE may result in complete resolution of perfusion defects or in **chronic thromboembolic pulmonary hypertension**. Alternatively, the abrupt increase in pulmonary vascular resistance may be sufficiently severe to result in acute right ventricular (RV) failure that may present with sudden death from electromechanical dissociation or with syncope from systemic hypotension, which can progress to shock and death.

38.2 Diagnosis

- VTE is often unrecognized and sometimes difficult to diagnose. Various clinical trials have shown that it is usually clinically silent. Its initial manifestation may be massive PE or sudden death from PE. Thus, the optimal use of effective preventive strategies is the best approach against VTE. Perioperative VTE prevention is discussed in detail in Chap. 7.

38.2.1 Clinical Presentation

- DVT typically presents with pain, tenderness, warmth and swelling of the involved extremity, as well as edema distal to the area of thrombosis. However, physical findings are usually unreliable especially in the postoperative period or when there is concomitant trauma or injury to the limb.
- PE often presents atypically in the postoperative period. In most cases, it is suspected when patients complain of dyspnea or chest pain. PE may also manifest with tachypnea, tachycardia, hemoptysis, and syncope. In severe PE, shock or arterial hypotension may be present. Lastly, sudden death may be the first clinical manifestation of massive PE.
- As with DVT, signs and symptoms of PE may be confused with other perioperative complications. Individual clinical findings have limited accuracy in the diagnosis of VTE, but when evaluated together with predisposing factors, the likelihood of DVT or PE can be determined, and this is particularly important to the selection of an appropriate diagnostic strategy and to the subsequent interpretation of diagnostic test results. For this reason, clinical prediction rules have been developed for both DVT and PE (Tables 38.1 and 38.2).[5,6] However, these rules were derived and validated in studies involving the general outpatient population. They cannot be relied upon in the immediate postoperative period during which the risk of VTE is higher.

38.2.2 Differential Diagnosis

- Various perioperative complications mimic signs and symptoms of VTE, and make it more difficult to recognize.
  - DVT may be hard to distinguish from **cellulitis,** which presents with pain, swelling, erythema, and warmth. **Large hematomas** especially in the thighs may present with leg swelling, skin discoloration, warmth, and tenderness. **Baker's cysts**, which are located in the popliteal fossa, may rupture and produce sudden severe pain, swelling, erythema, and leg tenderness similar to signs and symptoms of DVT. Also, leg swelling may result from chronic venous insufficiency, immobilization, reflex sympathetic dystrophy, renal failure, end stage liver disease, heart failure, or pregnancy.

Table 38.1 Clinical model for predicting pretest probability for deep-vein thrombosis

Clinical feature	Score
Active cancer (treatment ongoing or within previous 6 months or palliative)	1
Paralysis, paresis, or recent plaster immobilization of the lower extremities	1
Recently bedridden for more than 3 days or major surgery, within 4 weeks	1
Localized tenderness along the distribution of the deep venous system	1
Entire leg swollen	1
Calf swollen by more than 3 cm when compared with the asymptomatic leg (measured 10 cm below tibial tuberosity)	1
Pitting edema (greater in the symptomatic leg)	1
Collateral superficial veins (nonvaricose)	1
Previously documented deep-vein thrombosis	1
Alternative diagnosis at least as likely as deep-vein thrombosis	–2

Source: Reproduced from Wells et al.,[5] with permission

A total score of 2 or higher indicates that deep-vein thrombosis is likely; a score of less than 2 indicates that deep-vein thrombosis is unlikely. In patients with symptoms in both legs, the more symptomatic leg is used. **This model has limited clinical utility in the immediate postoperative period, particularly in the inpatient setting**

- PE in the postoperative period may be mistaken for atelectasis, analgesia-induced hypoventilation, pleurisy, and pneumothorax.
- **Pulmonary congestion and edema** due to fluid overload, especially in patients with renal dysfunction or limited cardiac reserve, may cause dyspnea and hypoxemia simulating PE. Measuring the B-type natriuretic peptide (BNP) is most useful if the level is low, in which case heart failure is less likely. On the other hand, an elevated BNP level has poor specificity since PE may also increase BNP secretion as a result of RV overload.
- **Myocardial ischemia and infarction** are common in the postoperative setting and may also manifest with dyspnea and chest pain similar to PE. Cardiac enzymes, particularly troponins, may not distinguish between PE and acute coronary syndromes because the former may cause significant strain on the right ventricle, which also increases troponin release.

38.2.3 Diagnostic Evaluation

- Once DVT or PE is suspected, diagnostic evaluation begins with a thoughtful appraisal of the patient's clinical findings using validated clinical prediction rules to estimate the likelihood of either DVT or PE (Tables 38.1 and 38.2).[5,6] However, these rules have limited utility in the immediate postoperative period, particularly in the inpatient setting. A diagnostic test is then selected, and the result is interpreted in the light of the pretest probability.

Table 38.2 Clinical model for predicting pretest probability for pulmonary embolism[6]

Clinical feature	Points
Clinical signs and symptoms of DVT (minimum of leg swelling and pain with palpation of the deep vein)	3
An alternative diagnosis is less likely than PE	3
Heart rate greater than 100	1.5
Immobilization or surgery in the previous 4 weeks	1.5
Previous DVT/PE	1.5
Hemoptysis	1
Malignancy (on treatment, treated in the last 6 months or palliative)	1
Clinical probability (3 levels)	**Total**
Low	0–1
Intermediate	2–6
High	≥7
Clinical probability (2 levels)	
PE unlikely	0–4
PE likely	>4

Source: Adapted from Writing Group for the Christopher Study Investigators,[7] with permission.
This model has limited clinical utility in the immediate postoperative period, particularly in the inpatient setting
DVT deep vein thrombosis, *PE* pulmonary embolism

- **D-dimer** is a degradation product of fibrin and is used as a laboratory marker for thrombosis. In the outpatient setting, a negative D-dimer reliably excludes VTE if the pretest clinical probability is low but not if it is intermediate to high. However, in hospitalized patients, particularly in the postoperative period, D-dimer testing has limited utility because the pretest probability of VTE is high and because it is very unlikely to find a negative D-dimer in this population.[8]
- Whenever DVT is suspected, the most useful test in the postoperative period is lower extremity **compression ultrasonography** (CUS). Thrombosis is diagnosed by noncompressibility of the vein under gentle pressure using the ultrasound transducer; this suggests venous hypertension due to outflow obstruction by the thrombus. Sometimes, thrombi may also be visualized and collateral circulation may be identified. CUS has a sensitivity of 89–96% and a specificity of 94–99% in detecting symptomatic proximal DVT. In asymptomatic patients, the veins may not be completely obstructed, resulting in less venous hypertension, and thus remain compressible. Because of this, the sensitivity declines (47% and 62%) for the diagnosis of thrombi in proximal veins of asymptomatic patients. Sensitivity is also diminished in patients who have distal DVT, both symptomatic (73–93%) and asymptomatic (50%).[9]

- Since CUS is less sensitive for DVT limited to the calf, a negative result does not rule out DVT. If the clinical suspicion is high, a CUS may be repeated after 1 week or contrast venography may be considered.
- If postoperative PE is suspected, diagnostic imaging is essential. Current options include **ventilation-perfusion scan** (V/Q), multidetector **computed tomography angiogram** (CTA), and conventional pulmonary angiography.
- CTA is usually the most readily available test, and it also has the advantage of providing alternative or concomitant diagnoses which may account for the patient's clinical presentation. The usual limitation of CTA arises from the fact that it requires intravenous iodinated contrast; this is especially a concern for those at risk for contrast-induced nephropathy including patients with underlying renal disease. While current literature has lagged behind rapid advances in CT technology, the estimated sensitivity and specificity of CTA for the diagnosis of PE are at least 90% and 95%, respectively.[9] If the CTA is negative and the clinical probability is high, further testing is required, and a pulmonary angiogram may be considered. CUS may also be a useful option in this scenario; a positive test may rule in PE (specificity of 99% and likelihood ratio of 42.2), but a negative test does not rule out PE (sensitivity of 39%).[10]
- V/Q scan is usually preferred in patients who have contraindications to CTA because of allergy to iodinated contrast dye or renal dysfunction. The results are reported according to criteria established in the PIOPED[11] trial into four categories: normal or near-normal, low, intermediate (nondiagnostic), and high probability of PE. A normal perfusion scan has a likelihood ratio of 0.10 and safely excludes PE in most cases. On the other hand, a high-probability V/Q scan establishes the diagnosis of PE with a high degree of certainty especially in a patient with a high clinical probability. All other combinations of V/Q scan result and clinical probability require further testing.[12]
- As soon as PE is suspected and while diagnostic evaluation is in progress, it is essential to concurrently stratify the severity of PE and promptly identify high-risk patients who can benefit from more intensive management. Various models of prognostic stratification have been proposed and validated; some are more useful for identifying low-risk patients who may be discharged early or treated in the outpatient setting.[13] The European Society of Cardiology (ESC) guidelines suggest a risk-stratification scheme based on expected PE-related mortality rate (Tables 38.3 and 38.4).[12] In this model, patients are classified as having either high-risk PE, intermediate-risk PE, or low-risk PE.

  - **High-risk PE** must be suspected in patients presenting with shock or hypotension. This is a distinct clinical entity associated with a very high rate of short-term mortality and requiring immediate aggressive treatment. Differential diagnosis includes cardiogenic shock, acute valvular dysfunction, tamponade, and aortic dissection. A bedside echocardiogram may demonstrate signs of RV overload or dysfunction, which may point to PE as the etiology for the hemodynamic derangement.
  - **Intermediate-risk PE** is diagnosed when PE results in RV dysfunction but without systemic hypotension. Normotensive patients with PE should be evaluated for signs

Table 38.3 Principal markers for risk stratification in acute pulmonary embolism[12]

Clinical markers	Shock Hypotension[a]
Markers of RV dysfunction	RV dilatation, hypokinesis, or pressure overload on echocardiography RV dilatation on spiral computed tomography BNP or NT-proBNP elevation Elevated right heart pressure on RHC
Markers of myocardial injury	Cardiac troponin T or I positive[b]

Source: From Torbicki et al.,[12] with permission

BNP B-type natriuretic peptide, *NT-proBNP* N-terminal proBNP, *RHC* right heart catheterization, *RV* right ventricle

[a]Defined as systolic blood pressure <90 mmHg or a pressure drop of ≥40 mmHg for >15 min if not caused by new-onset arrhythmia, hypovolemia or sepsis

[b]Heart-type fatty acid binding protein (H-FABP) is an emerging marker in this category, but still requires confirmation

Table 38.4 Risk stratification according to expected PE-related early mortality rate

PE-related early mortality risk		Risk markers			Potential treatment implications
		Clinical (shock or hypotension)	RV dysfunction	Myocardial injury	
High >15%		+	(+)[a]	(+)[a]	**Thrombolysis or embolectomy**
Nonhigh	**Intermediate** 3–15%	–	+ + –	+ – +	**Hospital admission**
	Low <1%	–	–	–	**Early discharge or home treatment**

Source: From Torbicki et al.,[12] with permission

PE pulmonary embolism, *RV* right ventricle

[a]In the presence of shock or hypotension it is not necessary to confirm RV dysfunction/injury to classify as high risk of PE-related early mortality

of RV dysfunction and myocardial injury; this may be achieved by performing an **echocardiogram** and by measuring cardiac **troponin** levels. Patients who are found to have RV dysfunction are at risk for subsequent hemodynamic instability and death from right heart failure.

– **Low-risk PE** is characterized by hemodynamic stability and by the absence of signs of RV dysfunction and myocardial injury. These patients have a low PE-related early mortality risk of less than 1% and they may be discharged early and can be safely treated at home.

38.3 Treatment

38.3.1 Initial Treatment

- As soon as VTE is suspected, particularly if the clinical probability is high, immediate anticoagulation should be considered unless the patient is actively bleeding or if the risk of bleeding outweighs the benefit of anticoagulant therapy.
- Current pharmacologic options for initial treatment of acute VTE include the following parenteral anticoagulants (see Table 38.5 for dosing regimens):

Table 38.5 Anticoagulant regimens for initial treatment of venous thromboembolism[14]

Unfractionated Heparin (UFH)[a] – preferred if CrCl<30 mL/min • **Monitored intravenous** – 80 U/kg or 5,000 U IV bolus, followed by 18 U/kg/h or 1,300 U/h continuous infusion; aPTT monitored every 6 h and adjusted to 1.5–2.5 times control (0.3–0.7 IU/mL factor Xa inhibition) • **Monitored weight-based subcutaneous** – 250 U/kg or 17,500 U SC bid; aPTT monitored every 6 h and adjusted to 1.5–2.5 times control (0.3–0.7 IU/mL factor Xa inhibition) • **Fixed-dose weight-based subcutaneous** – 333 U/kg SC once, then 250 U/kg SC bid
Low-molecular-weight heparin (LMWH)[b] • **Enoxaparin** 1 mg/kg SC bid or 1.5 mg/kg SC daily; if CrCl<30 mL/min, reduce dose to 1 mg/kg SC daily or consider UFH as an alternative • **Dalteparin** 100 IU/kg SC bid or 200 IU/kg SC daily; adjust if CrCl<30 mL/min • **Tinzaparin** 175 IU/kg SC daily; if CrCl<30 mL/min, consider UFH as alternative
Fondaparinux[c] – contraindicated if CrCl<30 mL/min • BW<50 kg: 5 mg SC daily • BW 50–100 kg: 7.5 mg SC daily • BW>100 kg: 10 mg SC daily
Initiate VKA at 2.5–10 mg/day on the first treatment day and overlap with any of the above parenteral anticoagulants for at least 5 days until the INR is ≥2.0 for 24 h

CrCl creatinine clearance, *IV* intravenous, *SC* subcutaneous, *aPTT* activated partial thromboplastin time, *bid* twice daily, *BW* body weight, *VKA* vitamin K antagonist, *INR* international normalized ratio

[a]Monitor platelet count at baseline and every other day from day 4 to day 14 or until heparin is stopped

[b]Monitor platelet count at baseline and every 2–4 days from day 4 to day 14 or until heparin is stopped

[c]No routine platelet monitoring is necessary

- **Unfractionated Heparin** (UFH) binds to antithrombin and inhibits thrombin (factor IIa) and other coagulation enzymes (factors Xa, IXa, XIa, and XIIa). It has a relatively short half-life and is usually preferred in patients with severe renal disease.

  Monitored intravenous UFH is most useful in the immediate postoperative period, because its effect may be completely reversed by protamine sulfate (given at 1–1.5 mg intravenously per 100 units of heparin) in case significant bleeding complications arise. It is also particularly useful in the setting of massive PE presenting with shock or hypotension as well as in other situations where there is concern about subcutaneous absorption, or in patients for whom thrombolytic therapy is being considered.

  Monitored weight-based subcutaneous UFH is an effective and safe option for hospitalized patients who have difficult venous access.[14]
  Fixed-dose weight-based subcutaneous UFH is another alternative that may be used in the outpatient or ambulatory setting.[14]

- **Low-molecular-weight heparin** (LMWH), such as enoxaparin, dalteparin, and tinzaparin, are administered subcutaneously using a fixed dose that is based on actual body weight. Their limited protein binding confers predictable pharmacokinetics and anticoagulant response, and thus monitoring is usually unnecessary. In patients undergoing coronary artery bypass or orthopedic procedures, LMWH is ten times less likely to cause heparin-induced thrombocytopenia (HIT) when compared to UFH. More importantly, LMWH is preferred in patients with active cancer, but it must be used with caution in patients who are obese or who have renal dysfunction.
- **Fondaparinux** is a synthetic pentasaccharide that indirectly inhibits factor Xa through antithrombin. It is contraindicated in patients with renal impairment.
- Several new oral medications are in phase III trials but are not yet FDA approved. These include factor Xa inhibitors (rivaroxaban, apixaban) and direct thrombin inhibitors (dabigatran) although the latter was recently approved for stroke prevention in atrial fibrillation.

• If therapeutic anticoagulation is not possible, **inferior vena cava** (IVC) filters may be used in patients with acute proximal DVT to prevent further embolization to the pulmonary arterial bed. Retrievable IVC filters are available and are best suited for patients who have temporary contraindications to anticoagulation, such as those recovering from central nervous system surgery who may be at high risk for bleeding complications during the first few postoperative days. It is important to remember that the need for anticoagulation does not change with the insertion of a filter; thus once the risk of bleeding resolves, therapeutic anticoagulation should be initiated.[15]

• For high-risk PE presenting with cardiogenic shock or persistent arterial hypotension, the first-line treatment is immediate systemic thrombolysis. However, this is contraindicated within 3 weeks of major trauma, surgery, or head injury. The alternative therapeutic option in this setting or when thrombolysis has failed is surgical pulmonary embolectomy.

38.3.2 Maintenance Treatment

- Warfarin, a **vitamin K antagonist** (VKA), is started on the first treatment day unless the VTE is related to HIT, in which case, it is started once the platelet count has substantially improved (usually above 150,000/μL). The dose of VKA is adjusted to maintain a target INR of 2.5 (INR range, 2.0–3.0).[14,16]
- Therapeutic parenteral anticoagulation is continued for at least 5 days **and** until the INR is ≥2.0 for at least 24 h.[14]
- Postoperative VTE is considered provoked or due to a transient reversible risk factor. In this case, the recommended duration of treatment with a VKA is 3 months.[14]
- However, if the VTE is cancer-related, LMWH is the recommended anticoagulant for the first 3–6 months. This may be subsequently followed by long-term therapy with either VKA or LMWH indefinitely or until the cancer is resolved.[14]
- The use of **compression stockings** has been shown to markedly reduce the incidence of PTS after acute DVT (odds ratio, 0.3).[17] Current guidelines recommend the use of an elastic compression stocking with an ankle pressure gradient of 30–40 mmHg as soon as feasible after starting anticoagulant therapy for symptomatic proximal DVT; this should be continued for a minimum of 2 years or longer if symptoms of PTS are present.[14]

38.4 Conclusion

- Postoperative patients are at a high risk for VTE.
- The best strategy against this potentially life-threatening surgical complication is optimal use of perioperative VTE preventive measures.
- A high index of suspicion is essential since VTE is often difficult to recognize particularly in surgical patients who are also at risk for other complications that have similar manifestations.
- Certain laboratory markers, such as BNP and D-dimer, have limited clinical value in postoperative patients.
- Clinical prediction rules are useful in determining the clinical probability of VTE, which is important in both the selection and the interpretation of diagnostic tests. However, during the immediate postoperative period, these rules have limited clinical utility.
- When PE is suspected, prognostic risk stratification is performed to rapidly identify patients with a very high risk of death and who may benefit from more aggressive interventions and intensive support.
- Parenteral anticoagulation should be initiated promptly when VTE is suspected, especially when the clinical probability is high.
- Retrievable IVC filters are best suited for patients with transient contraindications to therapeutic anticoagulation.
- Surgery-related VTE requires 3 months of anticoagulant treatment.

References

1. Geerts WH et al. Prevention of venous thromboembolism: American College of Chest Physicians Evidence-Based Clinical Practice Guidelines (8th edition). *Chest.* 2008;133(6 suppl): 381S-453S.
2. White RH, Zhou H, Romano PS. Incidence of symptomatic venous thromboembolism after different elective or urgent surgical procedures. *Thromb Haemost.* 2003;90(3):446-455.
3. Arcelus JI et al. Clinical presentation and time-course of postoperative venous thromboembolism: results from the RIETE registry. *Thromb Haemost.* 2008;99(3):546-551.
4. Kahn SR, Ginsberg JS. The post-thrombotic syndrome: current knowledge, controversies, and directions for future research. *Blood Rev.* 2002;16(3):155-165.
5. Wells PS et al. Evaluation of D-dimer in the diagnosis of suspected deep-vein thrombosis. *N Engl J Med.* 2003;349(13):1227-1235.
6. Wells PS et al. Derivation of a simple clinical model to categorize patients probability of pulmonary embolism: increasing the models utility with the SimpliRED D-dimer. *Thromb Haemost.* 2000;83(3):416-420.
7. Writing Group for the Christopher Study Investigators. Effectiveness of managing suspected pulmonary embolism using an algorithm combining clinical probability, D-Dimer testing, and computed tomography. *JAMA.* 2006;295(2):172-179.
8. Righini M et al. D-Dimer for venous thromboembolism diagnosis: 20 years later. *J Thromb Haemost.* 2008;6(7):1059-1071.
9. Qaseem A et al. Current diagnosis of venous thromboembolism in primary care: a clinical practice guideline from the American Academy of Family Physicians and the American College of Physicians. *Ann Intern Med.* 2007;146(6):454-458.
10. Le Gal G et al. A positive compression ultrasonography of the lower limb veins is highly predictive of pulmonary embolism on computed tomography in suspected patients. *Thromb Haemost.* 2006;95(6):963-966.
11. Value of the ventilation/perfusion scan in acute pulmonary embolism. Results of the prospective investigation of pulmonary embolism diagnosis (PIOPED). The PIOPED Investigators. *JAMA.* 1990; 263(20): 2753–9.
12. Torbicki A et al. Guidelines on the diagnosis and management of acute pulmonary embolism: the Task Force for the Diagnosis and Management of Acute Pulmonary Embolism of the European Society of Cardiology (ESC). *Eur Heart J.* 2008;29(18):2276-2315.
13. Aujesky D et al. A prediction rule to identify low-risk patients with pulmonary embolism. *Arch Intern Med.* 2006;166(2):169-175.
14. Kearon C et al. Antithrombotic therapy for venous thromboembolic disease: American College of Chest Physicians Evidence-Based Clinical Practice Guidelines (8th edition). *Chest.* 2008;133(6 suppl):454S-545S.
15. Ingber S, Geerts WH. Vena caval filters: current knowledge, uncertainties and practical approaches. *Curr Opin Hematol.* 2009;16(5):402-406.
16. Warkentin TE et al. Treatment and prevention of heparin-induced thrombocytopenia: American College of Chest Physicians Evidence-Based Clinical Practice Guidelines (8th edition). *Chest.* 2008;133(6 suppl):340S-380S.
17. Kolbach DN, et al. Non-pharmaceutical measures for prevention of post-thrombotic syndrome. *Cochrane Database Syst Rev.* 2004; 1: CD004174.

Postoperative Fluid, Electrolyte, and Acid/Base Disorders

39

Ross Kerridge and Paul J. Primeaux

39.1 Introduction

This chapter will review common disorders of fluids, electrolytes, and pH seen postoperatively, particularly in the Intensive Care Unit (ICU), or the Post Anesthesia Care Unit (PACU). These common disorders range in sequelae from mild, self-limited conditions to those associated with major organ dysfunction, severe morbidity, and in extreme cases, mortality. Identifying patients at risk for these disturbances and preventing their development is clearly preferable to treating the conditions after they occur. Nevertheless, despite our best efforts, patients will continue to develop these conditions postoperatively, and we must understand the physiological basis of these disturbances, how they may be correctly diagnosed, and the principles of effective treatment.

39.2 Key Principles

39.2.1 Fluid Volumes and Compartments

- Total Body Water comprises about 60% of body mass in normal adults.
  - Of this, two-thirds is intracellular fluid (ICF), and one-third extracellular fluid (ECF). Of ECF, about a quarter comprises plasma volume, and the remainder is interstitial fluid (ISF).
- In a 70-kg human, TBW is 42 L; 28 L ICF including RBC; 11 L ISF and 3 L PV. Plasma volume (PV) and ICF in red blood cells make up the circulating volume of about 5 L.

R. Kerridge (✉)
John Hunter Hospital & Royal Newcastle Centre,
University of Newcastle, Callaghan, NSW 2308, Australia
e-mail: ross.kerridge@hnehealth.nsw.gov.au

S.L. Cohn (ed.), *Perioperative Medicine*,
DOI: 10.1007/978-0-85729-498-2_39,

39.2.2
Distribution of Electrolytes (Table 39.1)

- Note that sodium is 90% extracellular and potassium is more than 95% intracellular. This gradient is maintained by an energy-dependent Na/K exchange pump.

39.2.3
Colloid Osmotic Pressure

- Proteins within the plasma exert a form of osmotic pressure known as colloid osmotic (or oncotic) pressure. Due to their large size, proteins cannot easily cross the semipermeable membrane walls of capillaries. As a result, these proteins exert a force that counteracts the tendency of fluid to leak from the capillaries into the interstitium.
- A loss of circulating protein (e.g., low albumin) tends to favor fluid extravasation into peripheral tissues and results in edema formation. Some disease states such as septic shock or systemic inflammatory response syndrome (SIRS) or major burn injury result in disruption of the semipermeable membrane, allowing increased leakage of proteins and fluids out of the circulating volume into the interstitial space.

39.2.4
Approximate Daily Fluid and Electrolyte Requirement (for Adults)

- Sodium 1–1.5 mmol/kg/day, e.g., 50–100 mmol/day
- Potassium 1 mmol/kg/day, e.g., 40–80 mmol/day
- Water 1.5–2.5 L/day[1]
- Urine output: Normal healthy adults may pass less than 0.5 ml/kg/h of urine overnight

39.2.5
The Surgical Stress Response

- This includes a range of physiological mechanisms used by the body to attempt to maintain homeostasis after surgical trauma or other injury:
  - Activation of the rennin-angiotensin-aldosterone system, secretion of antidiuretic hormone (ADH), and the release of endogenous catecholamines.
  - Salt and water are retained and oliguria results. This occurs even in the presence of volume overload.[1]

Table 39.1 Distribution of electrolytes

Electrolytes	Intracellular meq/L	Extracellular meq/L
Sodium	13	140
Potassium	140	4
HCO_3	10	24
Chloride	3	110
Magnesium	7	1.1

39.2.6
The 'Third Space'

- Major tissue damage can be accompanied by leakage and 'trapping' of fluid from plasma into a nonphysiological 'compartment' of the interstitial space. This volume can be considerable in some settings (major surgery, trauma, burns, sepsis) and needs to be replaced to maintain PV.
- Recent work has suggested that losses into this 'third space' may have been overestimated, particularly for modern surgery. The concept is thus controversial.

39.2.7
Components of Common IV Fluids (Table 39.2)

- Note that Lactated Ringers is slightly hypotonic.
- 0.9% saline has approx 45 mmol/L of chloride more than plasma, which may cause hyperchloremic acidosis.

39.2.8
Maintenance and Perioperative Intravenous Fluids

- There is increasing recognition that common hospital practice has been to give excessive salt and water in 'maintenance' regimes. In surgical patients, the modern techniques of minimally invasive surgery, reduced fasting times, and less use of inappropriate bowel preparation regimes, together with recognition of the dangers of excess salt and water, are leading to a reassessment of appropriate intravenous therapies.
- In uncomplicated moderate surgery, 1.5–2 L of near-isotonic fluid (e.g., Lactated Ringers) is appropriate, with 2–3 L in major surgery.
- Fluid requirements are reduced 24 h postoperatively.

Table 39.2 Components of common IV fluids, Meq/L (Approximate)

Fluids	Osmol	pH	Na (meq/L)	K (meq/L)	Ca (meq/L)	Mg (meq/L)	Cl (meq/L)	HCO_3 (or equiv)	Glucose (g/L)
0.9% Saline	308	6.0	154	0	0	0	154	0	0
Lactated Ringer's	273	6.5	130	4	2	0	109	27	0
0.45% Saline	154	6.0	77	0	0	0	77	0	0
5% Dextrose	252	4.5	0	0	0	0	0	0	50
Plasmanate, 5% Albumin	330	7.4	140	2	2	1	95	25	0
Normosol	269	7.4	140	5	0	3	98	50	0
Hetastarch	308	6	154	0	0	0	154	0	0

39.3 Fluid Derangements

39.3.1 Hypovolemia

39.3.1.1 Etiology

- The most important cause of hypovolemia in a postoperative patient is ongoing surgical blood loss. Bleeding may be easily identifiable when inspecting the surgical site, or it may be confined to an internal space and therefore unnoticeable upon visual inspection.
- **Unrecognized internal blood loss should be suspected in any patient presenting with hypotension in the postoperative period.**
- Perioperative sodium and water loss is common and is often compounded by poor preoperative nutritional status (preoperative starvation aimed at reducing aspiration risk).
- Other important sources of fluid loss (besides blood loss) include gastrointestinal loss (nasogastric suction, preoperative bowel preparation, perioperative vomiting or diarrhea, fluid within the intestinal lumen), insensible loss (respiratory and intraoperative evaporative losses), and renal loss (increased with diuretics, renal dialysis with aggressive fluid removal, transient diabetes insipidus in patients undergoing neurosurgical procedures).
- Patients who have experienced significant blood loss replaced with crystalloids or colloids may experience redistribution of fluid to extravascular compartments.
- Redistributive fluid losses secondary to vasodilation and capillary leak can be dramatic in those patients with the Systemic Inflammatory Response Syndrome, burns, or other causes of increased capillary permeability. Remember, these patients may be edematous and hypovolemic.
- Hypothermic patients will vasodilate on re-warming which contributes to hypovolemia.

39.3.1.2 Diagnosis

- Volume status can be difficult to assess, but a systematic history and physical exam will often provide the diagnosis. Hypovolemia is a clinical diagnosis (Table 39.3).

What to Look for

- Symptoms: increased thirst, postural dizziness
- Clinical signs: such as poor peripheral circulation, cool peripheries, dry mucous membranes, slow capillary refill, poor skin turgor; hypotension (often worsened with orthostatic changes); tachycardia (postoperative pain may also increase heart rate). A significant drop

Table 39.3 Postoperative fluid assessment

• Preop – Preexisting conditions – Indications for surgery – Preop volume status
• Intraop events – Procedure performed – Duration of surgery – Blood loss estimate (often difficult to accurately assess) – Fluid shifts/third space loss (also difficult to assess) – Method of anesthesia (regional, general, neuraxial, combined) – Fluids given (types and amounts of each) – Hemodynamic monitoring employed – Intraoperative events/trends
• Postop status – Physical exam – Lab results – Imaging (CXR, echo) – Hemodynamic parameters

in blood pressure associated with narcotics to relieve pain may be an important clue that the patient is hypovolemic.

- Decreasing urine output: Look for a minimum of 0.5 ml/kg/h and pay attention to the rate of change.
- Laboratory findings
  - Urinary hyperosmolality: Well-functioning kidneys will increase urine osmolality to >400 mOsm/kg in the setting of hypovolemia.
  - Increased BUN: Remember BUN:Creatinine ratio greater than 20:1 suggests prerenal cause of azotemia
  - Fractional excretion of sodium (FENa) <1% suggests renal reabsorption of sodium to control hypovolemia
- The assessment of volume status becomes more difficult in the setting of renal dysfunction or diuretic administration, which render measurements of urine volume and electrolytes less helpful. In more difficult cases, the measurement of various hemodynamic parameters may be necessary to assess volume status adequately. These include:
  - Analysis of variation in stroke volume during the ventilatory cycle. In patients with arterial pressure monitoring, this can be estimated by visual observation of the pressure trace.
  - Monitors are now on the market utilizing a variety of different flow-based modalities of measurement.
  - Echocardiography to estimate volume status and myocardial function.

- Central venous pressure and pulmonary artery catheters provide useful information, which must be interpreted by a practitioner with considerable expertise. A single reading is very unreliable – the response to therapy is more meaningful.
- **The 2008 British consensus guidelines provide the following valuable advice on the diagnosis of hypovolemia:**

When the diagnosis of hypovolaemia is in doubt and the central venous pressure is not raised, the response to a bolus infusion of 200 ml of a suitable colloid or crystalloid should be tested. The response should be assessed using the patient's cardiac output and stroke volume measured by flow-based technology if available. Alternatively, the clinical response may be monitored by measurement/estimation of the pulse, capillary refill, CVP and blood pressure before and 15 minutes after receiving the infusion. This procedure should be repeated until there is no further increase in stroke volume and improvement in the clinical parameters.[1]

39.3.1.3 Treatment

- Once the diagnosis of hypovolemia is made, the treatment is intuitive and rather obvious: **give volume** (fluids).
  - For patients with ongoing bleeding packed red blood cells should be considered. Isotonic balanced salt solutions or colloids should be given until blood becomes available. Remember, the decision to give blood in a briskly bleeding patient is made clinically; the fall in hematocrit will lag behind the loss of blood and requires interstitial fluid to diffuse into the intravascular space as the patient compensates for the loss of intravascular volume.
  - Patients with massive blood loss may require fresh frozen plasma, platelets, and other therapies as both platelets and coagulation factors are depleted and other derangements occur.
  - In most cases, isotonic crystalloid solutions (Ringers lactate or normal saline) can be used for the volume resuscitation of hypovolemic patients. Note: Recent evidence suggests that normal saline may be associated with hyperchloremic acidosis when given in large amounts. Normal saline may also be associated with renal dysfunction.[2]
  - The controversy regarding the use of colloid solutions (e.g., albumin or hetastarch) continues despite a multitude of studies. Colloids are claimed to remain within the plasma compartment, so that less volume of colloid is needed to achieve equal circulating volume expansion. However, no clear survival benefit of either colloids or crystalloids has been proven.[3] The use of colloids for volume expansion is an appropriate option in selected patients but is more expensive than crystalloid to administer.
  - The presence of renal or cardiac dysfunction should not preclude the administration of fluids to a hypovolemic patient. In these cases, more sophisticated monitoring of volume status, as described above, may be necessary to determine the proper endpoint of therapy.

39.3.2 Hypervolemia

39.3.2.1 Etiology

- Patients with end stage renal, liver, or cardiac disease may present to the operating room with some degree of volume overload.
- Large intraoperative fluid shifts (especially common in septic patients, in open abdominal cases, and in the setting of substantial blood loss) often require intravascular volume expansion despite hypervolemia of the interstitial space.
- Inadvertent perioperative administration of excessive volumes of intravenous fluids.

39.3.2.2 Diagnosis

- Like hypovolemia, the diagnosis of hypervolemia is made clinically (Table 39.3).

What to Look for

- Symptoms: dyspnea, orthopnea, nausea, confusion, restlessness, leg swelling.
- Clinical signs: dependent crackles on auscultation (CXR will show signs of interstitial and/or alveolar fluid), jugular or other venous distension and plethora, dependent edema (although intravascular fluid volume may be low, normal, or high), hypertension (although volume overloaded patients may display low systemic pressures if cardiac failure coexists or is developing).
- Note that these signs and symptoms are nonspecific and may leave the practitioner without a clear understanding of volume status.

39.3.2.3 Treatment

- Restrict sodium intake in IV or oral fluids.
- Diuresis – loop diuretics or dialysis to remove excess fluid.
- Intubation and mechanical ventilation in patients with respiratory distress/failure secondary to hypervolemia.
- Inotropic support as well as after-load reduction in order to provide adequate renal perfusion and subsequent diuresis for patients with heart failure.

39.3.3 Hyponatremia

- Postoperative hyponatremia (defined as a serum sodium concentration <135 meq/L) is a common condition and can be asymptomatic or cause significant morbidity.
- Acute reductions in serum sodium concentration lead to cerebral swelling as water diffuses across the blood–brain barrier and can result in seizures, lethargy, and coma. Hyponatremia should be suspected in any postsurgical patient with delayed emergence from anesthesia.

39.3.3.1 Etiology

- Increased antidiuretic hormone secretion is a part of the physiological response to surgical stress. The resulting water reabsorption and concentrated urine dilutes serum sodium.
- Iatrogenic administration of hypotonic fluids (D5W, ¼ NS, etc.) to postoperative patients is a common cause of hyponatremia.
- Systemic absorption of irrigating solution in transurethral resection of the prostate (TURP) results in rapid hyponatremia.
- Patients with advanced liver, cardiac, or renal disease commonly present with hyponatremia.
- Renal salt wasting can result from thiazide diuretics, SIADH, and cerebral salt wasting (CSW), a condition similar to SIADH also seen in neurosurgical patients.

39.3.3.2 Diagnosis

- Review the history for preexisting conditions commonly associated with hyponatremia (cirrhosis, CHF). TURP or neurosurgical patients are at higher risk.
- Review fluid administration records.

What to Look for

- Clinical manifestations: nausea/vomiting, headache, lethargy, seizures, coma, delayed emergence from anesthesia, malignant arrhythmias (in severe cases).

Labs

- Serum sodium and creatinine
- Urine sodium and creatinine
- Calculate FENa (%): (urine Na × plasma creatinine/plasma Na × urine creatinine) × 100

Differential Diagnosis

- CSW, diuretics, SIADH associated with urine Na>40 meq/L and FENa >1%
- TURP syndrome typically low urine sodium (<25 meq/L) and FENa <1%

39.3.3.3
Treatment

- The general principle is to treat acute hyponatremia quickly but chronic hyponatremia slowly.
- Restrict free water in asymptomatic patients with Na^+ >125
- IV normal saline (0.9%) and furosemide in patients with mild symptoms (furosemide will promote relatively dilute urine compared to normal saline which will aid in increasing serum sodium)
  - Aim for increase in serum sodium of 0.5 meq/L/h (faster rises in sodium concentration risk osmotic demyelination syndrome)
- Three percent saline may be necessary in cases of acute hyponatremia in which symptoms such as seizures, lethargy, or coma are present or serum sodium concentrations are <115–120 meq/L. Target the increase in sodium to 1 meq/L/h and slow the rate of increase to 0.5 meq/L/h upon clinical improvement.

39.3.4
Hypernatremia

- Hypernatremia is a deficit of free water relative to total body sodium content. It is defined as serum sodium concentration >145 meq/L.

39.3.4.1
Etiology

- Inadequate water intake: Often a result of impaired thirst mechanism and/or extreme preoperative restrictions of oral intake in combination with prolonged perioperative isotonic fluid administration.
- Excessive water loss: Can result after the administration of mannitol and furosemide in neurosurgical patients to reduce intracerebral fluid volume. A hypotonic osmotic diuresis may also result from diabetic ketoacidosis.
- Lack of ADH (vasopressin): Central or nephrogenic diabetes insipidus may be seen in postoperative patients.
- Excess sodium intake: Due to hypertonic saline infusion.

39.3.4.2
Diagnosis

- When hypernatremia develops slowly over a long period of time, few symptoms may develop. However, when the process develops acutely, the following signs/symptoms may be seen.

What to Look for

- Symptoms: excessive urine output, severe thirst
- Clinical signs: confusion/stupor/coma, convulsions, intracranial hemorrhage

Lab Analysis

- Serum sodium >145 meq/L
- Urine osmolality: Patients with diabetes insipidus will have dilute urine with low osmolality (typically <300 mOsm/L) due to the lack of ADH and a loss of the ability to reabsorb free water.

Assess volume status (may be hypo-, eu-, or hypervolemic).

39.3.4.3
Treatment

- In diabetes insipidus, correct the lack of ADH with desmopressin.
- If the patient is able to take fluids orally, increase the amount of free water ingested.
- If hypovolemic, give isotonic fluids to replace fluid deficit and then treat hypernatremia.
- Hypotonic saline or D5W should be administered intravenously along with diuretic given to remove excess sodium.
- Be careful to avoid too rapid correction of serum sodium concentration.
  - Limit reduction in serum sodium to no more than 0.5–0.7 meq/L/h.

39.3.5
Hypokalemia

This condition is commonly seen in postoperative patients and is typically mild and asymptomatic.

39.3.5.1
Etiology

- Reduced potassium intake
- GI losses: nasogastric suctioning, vomiting/diarrhea

- Renal losses
  - Excess mineralocorticoids or high dose glucocorticoids, diuretics
- Intracellular shift of potassium
  - Insulin therapy, acute alkalosis, stress-induced catecholamines, beta-2 agonists
- The surgical stress response (renin/angiotensin, aldosterone, cortisol, catecholamines)

39.3.5.2
Diagnosis

- Patients typically asymptomatic

What to Look for

- If severe, may have generalized weakness, cramps

Lab Analysis

- Serum potassium <3.5 meq/L
- Check magnesium levels: hypomagnesemia tends to promote renal potassium loss.
- EKG: flattening of T waves, depression of the ST segment, and prominence of U waves; arrhythmias (including atrial fibrillation and PVCs) or other EKG abnormalities seen with potassium levels 2.0–2.5 meq/L

39.3.5.3
Treatment

- Give intravenous potassium to those patients unable to take oral supplements or to those who are symptomatic.
  - Limit IV administration to 20 meq/h via central venous lines or 10 meq/h through peripheral intravenous lines.
  - Monitor patients receiving IV potassium with continuous EKG monitoring.
  - Recheck serum potassium after 60–80 meq have been given.
- In asymptomatic cases, oral administration is the mainstay of therapy.
  - Give 40 meq twice daily (larger doses are associated with GI discomfort).
  - Generally 100–200 meq of potassium will increase potassium by 1 meq/L in adults.
  - Replace magnesium stores in hypomagnesemic patients.

39.3.6 Hyperkalemia

- Hyperkalemia is a common and often life-threatening condition seen in postoperative patients. Like hypokalemia, most patients with this condition will be asymptomatic.

39.3.6.1 Etiology

- Iatrogenic:
  - KCL supplementation in IV fluids
  - Drugs associated with increased potassium: ACE inhibitors/angiotensin receptor blockers (ARBs), potassium-sparing diuretics (amiloride, spironolactone, triamterene), pentamidine, succinylcholine, trimethoprim, NSAIDs, digoxin, cyclosporine, tacrolimus, heparin.
  - Large volume blood transfusion (as stored red blood cells lyse they release significant amounts of potassium)
  - Renal Failure
  - Acidosis: As extracellular H^+ concentration rises, intracellular K^+ is exchanged for extracellular H^+ as the body attempts to restore homeostasis.
  - Rhabdomyolysis, crush injury, or other cause of cell breakdown
  - Burns
  - Malignant hyperthermia (classically associated with the use of volatile anesthetics or succinylcholine).
  - Succinylcholine use in association with upregulation of the number of neuromuscular junctions as seen in severe multiple sclerosis, burns, ALS, muscular dystrophy, or other causes of paralysis may cause extremely rapid hyperkalemia.

39.3.6.2 Diagnosis

What to Look for

- Patients are typically asymptomatic (except those with marked metabolic acidosis who may be tachypneic as they attempt to compensate by removing respiratory acid)

Lab Analysis

- Serum potassium levels >5.5 meq/L (not hemolyzed)
- EKG findings
  - Narrow, symmetrical, peaked T waves with potassium levels >6.5 meq/L

- Widened QRS, decreased P wave amplitude, prolonged PR interval, A-V block (with potassium 7–8 meq/L), progressing to asystole (sometimes preceded by “sine waves”) with potassium levels of 8–10 meq/L or greater

39.3.6.3 Treatment

- Hyperkalemic patients should immediately be placed on continuous EKG monitoring
- Three types of treatment may be implemented
  - Stabilization of cardiac membranes by the administration of intravenous calcium chloride (500 mg–1 g in adults)
  - Change the relationship of intra to extracellular potassium, shifting potassium into the cells:
    - Raise the pH by giving sodium bicarbonate or increasing the ventilation rate in intubated patients
    - Give inhaled beta-2 agonists (albuterol)
    - Administer insulin: 10–20 units of IV insulin with one 50 ml ampule of D50 (50% dextrose)
  - Speed elimination of potassium:
    - Dialysis in severe cases, especially those complicated by renal failure
    - Loop diuretics (furosemide 20–40 mg intravenously)
    - Sodium polystyrene sulfonate (Kayexalate): Remember that this requires potassium sequestration in the gut and elimination in fecal matter

39.4 Acid/Base Disorders

Acid/base abnormalities are extremely common in postoperative patients especially immediately after surgery. Mild hypercarbia and the slight respiratory acidosis that results should be expected in patients receiving narcotics, benzodiazepines, propofol, and other commonly administered anesthetic agents that depress respiration. More severe acid/base disturbances are also common and can be life threatening. This section will describe the four basic categories – respiratory acidosis, metabolic acidosis, respiratory alkalosis, metabolic alkalosis – which may occur alone (simple disorder) or in combination (as a mixed disorder).

39.4.1 Respiratory Acidosis

- Definition: arterial pH <7.35 and a coexisting $PaCO_2$>45 mmHg.
- Note that over time the kidneys will compensate for this acidosis by reabsorbing bicarbonate in an attempt to return the pH to normal (7.4).

39.4.1.1 Etiology

- Impaired removal of respiratory acids (CO_2):
  - Depressed respiratory drive due to anesthetic agents (propofol, narcotics, benzodiazepines) and incomplete reversal of neuromuscular blockade
  - Airway obstruction – obstructive sleep apnea, morbid obesity
  - COPD, atelectasis, pulmonary infection, pleural effusion, pneumothorax, other pulmonary or chest wall pathology
  - Pulmonary edema
  - Pain impairing ventilation (e.g., upper abdominal, chest wall)
  - Neuromuscular disease
  - Ascites or other cause of raised intra-abdominal pressure
  - Low perfusion states (impaired delivery of CO_2 to the pulmonary capillaries)
  - Uncommonly, aggressive oxygen therapy in patients with chronic hypercarbia

- Increased CO_2 production
  - Shivering
  - Sepsis, SIRS, or other cause of increased metabolic rate
  - Malignant hyperthermia
  - After laparoscopic or endoscopic procedures (due to absorption of the CO_2 used for insufflation)

39.4.1.2 Diagnosis

What to Look for

- CNS effects: confusion, anxiety, somnolence.
- Hypoventilation: apnea during sleep, increased pCO_2 causing cerebral vasodilation and increasing ICP; hypoxemia.
- Cardiovascular effects: increased sympathetic output with resulting tachycardia, hypertension, and dysrhythmias.

Lab Analysis

- Arterial blood gases (ABG) showing $PaCO_2$ >45 mmHg and pH <7.35
- Check oxygenation for desaturation that often accompanies hypercarbia in post-op hypoventilatory states.
- Hyperkalemia due to intracellular potassium being exchanged for hydrogen ion.

39.4.1.3
Treatment

- Increase minute ventilation.
  - Postoperative patients with respiratory acidosis and either dyspnea or mental status changes may require immediate intubation and mechanical ventilation for impending respiratory failure.
  - If already intubated, adjust ventilator settings (increase TV or RR).
- In patients with milder problems, sitting the patient up, chest physiotherapy, and optimization of pain relief may improve the patient dramatically.
- A trial of continuous positive pressure–assisted ventilation (CPAP) with a face mask or BIPAP may appropriate.
- Treat impaired respiratory drive. If appropriate, reverse drugs that may cause respiratory depression (narcotics, benzodiazepines) or nondepolarizing neuromuscular blockers. Avoid or minimize the further use of respiratory depressing agents.
- Treat hypoxemia. Provide supplemental oxygen (especially in those patients with concomitant arterial oxygen desaturation).
- Treat hyperkalemia as described earlier (if increased K^+ is due to respiratory acidosis, then reducing $PaCO_2$ will correct the K^+ disturbance).

39.4.2
Metabolic Acidosis

Patients predisposed to this disturbance are those with active infections, poor postoperative perfusion, or active bleeding.

39.4.2.1
Etiology

- Can be divided into two groups based on calculation of the anion gap
  - Increased anion gap

    Lactic acidosis (typically due to inadequate tissue perfusion)
    Renal failure
    Diabetic ketoacidosis
  - Normal anion gap

    Hyperchloremic metabolic acidosis due to large volumes of 0.9% saline administration
    Renal tubular acidosis
    GI losses (prolonged diarrhea, bilious drainage)

39.4.2.2
Diagnosis

What to Look for

- Cardiovascular effects: impaired contractility, hypotension, arrhythmias
- CNS effects: confusion, somnolence, tachypnea
- Fever
- Hyperkalemia as H^+ moves intracellular in exchange for K^+
- Generalized weakness, decreased muscle strength

Lab Analysis

- pH <7.35 with bicarbonate <20–24 meq/L on ABG
- Base deficit <−5 on arterial blood gas
- Investigation and workup for infection or sepsis.

39.4.2.3
Treatment

- Treat the underlying cause of the acidosis if known (e.g., antibiotics for infection).
- Ensure adequate tissue oxygenation.
  - Correct hypovolemia.
  - Transfuse red cells in significant anemia.
  - Ensure perfusing cardiac output and blood pressure (may require both volume administration as well as inotropes/vasopressors).
- Reduce metabolic work: Intubation and mechanical ventilation may be required for patients with metabolic acidosis and severe dyspnea or mental status changes.
- pH <7.2 and renal failure, consider hemodialysis. Administration of sodium bicarbonate is generally not beneficial.

39.4.3
Respiratory Alkalosis

Respiratory alkalosis is defined as an arterial pH >7.45 and $PaCO_2$ <35 mmHg. Severe hypocapnia can lead to marked intracranial vasoconstriction resulting in cerebral ischemia in patients with cerebral blood flow limitations.

39.4.3.1
Etiology

- Enhanced removal of respiratory acids (hyperventilation)
  - Over ventilation of mechanically ventilated patients, pain, anxiety, metabolic acidosis, hypoxemia, pregnancy
- Decreased metabolic rate
  - Hypothermia, general anesthesia

39.4.3.2
Diagnosis

What to Look for

- Tachypnea, arrhythmias, dizziness, confusion, seizures

Lab Analysis

- pH >7.45 with $PaCO_2$ <35 mmHg on arterial blood gas
- Hypokalemia (potassium shifts intracellular in exchange for H^+; will self-correct with correction of pH toward 7.40)

39.4.3.3
Treatment

- Treat underlying cause (pain, anxiety, acidosis)
- Decrease minute ventilation in mechanically ventilated patients
- Give supplemental oxygen if hypoxemia is present

39.4.4
Metabolic Alkalosis

Metabolic alkalosis and its associated hypoventilation and hypercarbia may complicate weaning from mechanical ventilation.

39.4.4.1
Etiology

- Increased bicarbonate intake/retention
  - Renal retention of bicarbonate in response to hypovolemia (contraction alkalosis)
  - Massive blood transfusion: citrate used as an anticoagulant in stored packed RBCs is metabolized to bicarbonate
  - Sodium bicarbonate administration
- Loss of H^+ and Cl^- ions
  - HCL losses from GI tract seen in vomiting or nasogastric tube suction
  - Renal loss or thiazide or loop diuretics

39.4.4.2
Diagnosis

What to Look for

- Most patients with metabolic alkalosis will be asymptomatic.
- Hypoventilation and decreased respiratory drive (caution with the concomitant use of drugs that depress respiration).

Lab Analysis

- pH of >7.45 and bicarbonate > 28 meq/L on arterial blood gas
- Base excess >+5 on arterial blood gas
- Urinary chloride< 10 mmol/L helps define Cl^- loss as the etiology of metabolic alkalosis.
- Hypokalemia due to intracellular potassium movement.
- Increased lactate levels (resolves spontaneously with correction of the alkalosis).

39.4.4.3
Treatment

- 0.9% saline infusion for GI/Cl^- losses
- Potassium chloride or calcium chloride if volume replacement is contraindicated; in extreme cases, hydrogen chloride may be used.
- Acetazolamide may be given to increase renal bicarbonate loss (careful in hypokalemia as potassium loss will also occur).

References

1. Powell-Tuck J, Gosling P, Lobo DN, Allison SP, Carlson GL, Gore M, et al. British consensus guidelines on intravenous fluid therapy for adult surgical patients GIFTASUP 2008. Available at: http://www.bapen.org.uk/pdfs/bapen_pubs/giftasup.pdf
2. O'Malley CM, Frumento RJ, Hardy MA, et al. A randomized, double-blind comparison of lactated Ringer's solution and 0.9% NaCl during renal transplantation. *Anesth Analg.* 2005;100:1518-1524.
3. Finfer S, Bellomo R, Boyce N, et al. SAFE study investigators: a comparison of albumin and saline for fluid resuscitation in the intensive care unit. *N Engl J Med.* 2004;350:2247-2256.

Suggested Reading

Ganter MT, Hofer CK, Pittet JF. Postoperative intravascular fluid therapy. In: Miller R, ed. *Miller's Anesthesia*. 7th ed. Philadelphia: Churchill Livingstone; 2009: chap 88.

Kaye AD, Riopelle JM. Intravascular fluid and electrolyte physiology. In: Miller R, ed. *Miller's Anesthesia*. 7th ed. Philadelphia: Churchill Livingstone; 2009: chap 54.

Postoperative Management. Chapter 14.7. Essential surgical care manual. Online edition. Published by World Health Organization. Available at: http://www.steinergraphics.com/surgical/introduction.html

Postoperative Renal Failure

40

Adam C. Schaffer and Mihaela S. Stefan

40.1 Introduction and Definitions

- Renal failure is a common problem in hospitalized patients. Postoperative patients are at elevated risk of renal failure, accounting for 9–25% of cases[1] with an associated increase in mortality up to 26%.[2]
- The term acute kidney injury (AKI) is starting to replace the term acute renal failure. AKI is an umbrella term including various degrees of acute renal dysfunction, which are defined by the RIFLE criteria. The RIFLE criteria, given in Table 40.1, provide a uniform definition of AKI and allow for meaningful comparisons among different studies.[3]
- The RIFLE criteria predict mortality in patients who have undergone both cardiac and noncardiac surgery. In a systematic review, the relative risk of death for patients in the risk category was 2.40 and those in the failure category it was 6.37.[4]

40.2 Risk Factors and Epidemiology

- Risk factors for postoperative AKI can be separated into patient- and procedure-specific risk factors (see Chap. 26).[5,6]
- Some of the most important patient-specific risk factors are as follows:
  - Preoperative chronic kidney disease (CKD)
  - Older age
  - Diabetes mellitus on insulin
  - Congestive heart failure

A.C. Schaffer (✉)
Department of Medicine, Brigham and Women's Hospital/Harvard Medical School,
75 Francis Street, Boston, MA 02115, USA
e-mail: aschaffer1@partners.org

S.L. Cohn (ed.), *Perioperative Medicine*,
DOI: 10.1007/978-0-85729-498-2_40, © Springer-Verlag London Limited 2011

Table 40.1 RIFLE definitions

	GFR criteria	Urine output criteria
Risk	Increased serum creatinine × 1.5 or GFR decrease >25%	UO<0.5 ml/kg/h × 6 h
Injury	Increased serum creatinine × 2 or GFR decrease >50%	UO<0.5 ml/kg/h × 12 h
Failure	Increased serum creatinine × 3 or GFR decrease >75% or a serum creatinine >4 mg/dL	UO<0.3 ml/kg/h × 24 h or anuria × 12 h
Loss	Complete loss of kidney function >4 weeks	
ESKD	Complete loss of kidney function >3 months	

Source: Adapted from Bellomo et al. [3]

- Key procedure-specific risk factors are as follows:
  - Emergency surgery
  - High-risk surgery (i.e., intraperitoneal, intrathoracic, or suprainguinal vascular procedures)

40.3 Common Causes of Postoperative Renal Failure

- In evaluating a patient with postoperative AKI, it is important to consider what the most common causes of AKI are in this population, as the common causes dictate the initial workup. Among hospitalized patients, the most common causes of AKI are – in addition to postoperative status – renal hypoperfusion, nephrotoxic medications, contrast-induced nephropathy, and sepsis.[1,7]
- Table 40.2 shows some of the important elements of the workup for AKI in the postoperative patient.

Table 40.2 Approach to AKI in the postoperative patient

	Reason/examples
Clinical assessment	
Review the medication list for any nephrotoxic medications.	For instance, in patients with AKI, ACE inhibitors should usually be stopped. If the patient is on an aminoglycoside, use an alternative antibiotic if at all possible.
Review the chart and radiology test list to see if the patient received IV contrast.[a]	If the AKI is due to contrast-induced nephropathy, then supportive care is needed, and further nephrotoxic insults need to be carefully avoided.
Examine the chart and vitals sheets for any sign of hypotension.[b]	If hypotension appears to be the cause of the AKI, any medications that could lower the blood pressure should be adjusted or stopped. If hypovolemia was contributing, this can be corrected.

(continued)

Table 40.2 (continued)

	Reason/examples
Examine the patient to see if hypovolemia appears to be present.	Even in the absence of hypotension detected upon chart review, the patient may still be hypovolemic, which can lead to AKI. Data like orthostasis or dry mucous membranes suggest hypovolemia. Considering laboratory data, such as the fractional excretion of sodium, is also helpful (see below).
Laboratory assessment	
Urine sodium and urine creatinine	Allows for calculation of the fractional excretion of sodium (FE_{Na}).[c] A $FE_{Na}<1\%$ suggests the kidney is sodium avid, as in hypovolemia. A $FE_{Na}>2\%$ suggests the kidney is not sodium avid, which can occur when the kidney is well perfused, or when the kidney tubules are damaged, as in acute tubular necrosis.
Urine urea and urine creatinine	Allows for calculation of the fractional excretion of urea (FE_{urea}).[d] An $FE_{urea}<35\%$ is analogous to a $FE_{Na}<1\%$ and an $FE_{urea}>50\%$ is analogous to a $FE_{Na}>2\%$. The main role of the FE_{urea} is in patients who have received diuretics, although its advantages over the FE_{Na} in this setting are debated.
Urinalysis	A high specific gravity indicates concentrated urine, which can be seen in hypovolemia. Heme positive urine can be seen with hematuria and myoglobinuria (as with rhabdomyolysis). High-level proteinuria (>3.5 g) suggests glomerular disease, though this is a rare cause of postoperative AKI.
Urine microscopy	Muddy brown casts are suggestive of acute tubular necrosis. The absence of red blood cells in the urine in a patient with a heme positive urinalysis raises the possibility of rhabdomyolysis.
Urine eosinophils	Urine eosinophils classically have been associated with acute interstitial nephritis (AIN). However, recent data by Fletcher showed urine eosinophils have a sensitivity of only 25% in diagnosing AIN.[11]
Renal ultrasound	Looks for hydronephrosis, which suggests urinary obstruction.

[a]Radiology studies can get mislabeled regarding the use of IV contrast in the study. If in doubt, review the study yourself to see if IV contrast was used. Some surgical procedures, such as endovascular repair of abdominal aortic aneurysms, involve the use of IV contrast

[b]It is easy to miss hypotensive episodes when reviewing a chart. For instance, hypotension may be documented in the nurse's note but not the vital signs flow sheet. Also, vitals signs during procedures, where hypotension is common, are often kept separate from the main vital signs flowsheet

[c]The FE_{Na} is calculated as (urine sodium x plasma creatinine)/(plasma sodium x urine creatinine). Multiply by 100 to convert to a percent

[d]The FE_{urea} is calculated in the same way as the FE_{Na}, except urine urea substitutes for urine sodium and blood urea nitrogen substitutes for serum sodium

- Medications that are common causes of AKI in hospitalized patients include antibiotics such as aminoglycosides, NSAIDs, ACE inhibitors and angiotensin receptor blockers, diuretics, amphotericin B, and platinum-containing chemotherapies.[1,7]
- AKI can occur in sepsis even when the sepsis is not severe enough to result in hypotension.[8] In a patient who has progressed to septic shock, the rate of AKI is greater than 50%.[8] Preexisting CKD increases the risk of AKI in sepsis and the mortality rate.
- Atheroembolic renal disease (AERD) occurs when atherosclerotic plaques break off and cause arterial occlusion and inflammation. Especially when the atherosclerotic plaque that fragments is in the aorta, the kidneys can be affected.[9]
  - Typical clinical manifestations of AERD are kidney injury, which can be acute or subacute, as well as the results of atheroemboli affecting other organs, such as ischemic toes, livedo reticularis, or abdominal pain.
  - Although AERD can occur spontaneously, it commonly occurs after vascular procedures, such as angiography, PTCA, cardiovascular surgery, and anticoagulation or fibrinolysis.
  - Laboratory findings that support the diagnosis of AERD are eosinophilia and hypocomplementemia.[9]
- Acute interstitial nephritis (AIN) is an immune-mediated cause of AKI, which most commonly is drug induced.
  - The classic signs of AIN are fever, rash, arthralgias, eosinophilia, and eosinophiluria. However, it is uncommon to see these classic signs together, and so this diagnosis can be challenging.[10] In a patient who has postoperative AKI in whom no alternative diagnosis is apparent, AIN should be a consideration, especially if any of the associated signs are present. Recent data show eosinophiluria is of limited diagnostic utility for AIN, having a sensitivity of only 25%. Kidney biopsy is the diagnostic gold standard.[11]
  - Drugs that are common causes of AIN are beta-lactams, cephalosporins, sulfonamides, and NSAIDs. A class of medications that has recently been appreciated as a cause of AIN is proton pump inhibitors.
  - Treatment is withdrawal of the offending medications, and, under some circumstances, glucocorticoids.
- Although uncommon, abdominal compartment syndrome is a cause of AKI that can be seen in the postoperative population. Abdominal compartment syndrome occurs, usually after complicated abdominal surgery or trauma, when the intra-abdominal pressure increases to >20 mmHg, accompanied by organ dysfunction.[12] This elevated intra-abdominal pressure impairs renal perfusion, leading to AKI and decreased urine output.
  - Diagnosis is assisted by transduction of intravesicular (bladder) pressure, which estimates intra-abdominal pressure.
  - Treatment consists of sedation, optimizing the patient's hemodynamic status, and, if necessary, surgical decompression.[12,13]

40.4 Treatment of Postoperative AKI

- Identifying the cause of postoperative AKI is important because one of the key interventions is to correct the underlying cause of the AKI (e.g., give isotonic IV fluids to a patient who is hypovolemic and hypotensive) or stop the identified nephrotoxin (e.g., an aminoglycoside). After this, it is crucial to provide good supportive care, which includes avoiding further nephrotoxins (e.g., no IV contrast studies) and maintaining a normal blood pressure.
- Beyond the above measures, there are not proven specific pharmacologic or other therapies to treat postoperative AKI.[14] Various interventions to treat postoperative AKI have been tried, including furosemide for forced diuresis, dopamine, fenoldopam, statins, N-acetylcysteine (NAC), and erythropoietin. However, despite preliminary promising data for some of these treatments, none has been clearly proven to be beneficial such that widespread use is recommended. Some of these treatments, such as furosemide for forced diuresis and low-dose dopamine to maintain renal perfusion, have been shown to be ineffective.
- While using furosemide to treat AKI is theoretically appealing since nonoliguric AKI has better outcomes than oliguric AKI, studies have shown this approach to be ineffective. Meta-analyses found that there was no clinical or mortality benefit to using furosemide to either treat or prevent AKI.[15]
- The practice of using low-dose (so-called renal-dose) dopamine is common to protect renal function in patients at risk of AKI. However, the practice is not supported by the data and should be stopped.[16]
- Studies of fenoldopam, a selective dopamine-1 agonist, have yielded mixed results. Studies have involved different patient populations (ICU, all surgery, cardiovascular surgery), and some have reported a benefit in reducing overall AKI, with a few reporting a mortality benefit. Overall, the results with fenoldopam are encouraging, but the data are not sufficient to recommend its widespread use.
- The effect of statins in preventing AKI is also mixed. The clinical data are not convincing enough to recommend the use of statins perioperatively to prevent AKI. Moreover, clinical data is lacking on the use of statins to prevent AKI in noncardiac surgery patients.
- The data regarding the use of N-acetylcysteine (NAC) to prevent postoperative AKI is limited to cardiac surgery patients and has not shown a significant benefit. Moreover, it may increase blood loss.
- Erythropoietin has also been tested as a medication to prevent postoperative AKI, but the clinical data are very limited.
- In summary, no specific pharmacologic treatment has been convincingly shown to prevent or treat AKI in postoperative patients.[14] In the case of some medications, such as fenoldopam and statins, there are some promising data regarding their effect in reducing postoperative AKI. However, the data are too limited to recommend their widespread use in this setting.
- Given the absence of medications that are clearly beneficial in preventing postoperative AKI, it is important to provide patients good supportive care postoperatively to try to prevent AKI. This means maintaining euvolemia, avoiding hypotension, avoiding

nephrotoxic medications, dosing medications appropriately for the patients' renal function to help limit toxicity, and avoiding IV contrast. When IV contrast is absolutely necessary, appropriate prophylactic measures should be taken.

40.5 Contrast-Induced Nephropathy

- Contrast-induced nephropathy (CIN) is an important cause of AKI in the postoperative setting.
- Significant patient-specific risk factors for CIN include hypotension, CHF, age >75 years, anemia, diabetes, and preexisting CKD.[17]
- In addition to the patient-specific risk factors, the volume of IV contrast used and the type of contrast used also affects the risk of CIN. Lower contrast volumes are safer, and using less then 30 ml of contrast appears to reduce the risk of CIN.[18] Regarding the type of contrast used, lower osmolality appears to be safer.
  - The terminology in this area is confusing, because so-called low-osmolality contrast agents (600–900 mOsm/L) have higher osmolality than the iso-osmolar contrast agent iodixanol (which is approximately iso-osmolar to plasma at about 300 mOsm/L). Both of these types of agents are lower osmolality than high osmolality contrast, which is about 2,000 mOsm/L. It is not clear whether iso-osmolar contrast is safer than the low-osmolality contrast. However, both appear to be safer than high-osmolality contrast.[19]
- Among the pharmacologic approaches to CIN prophylaxis, N-acetylcysteine (NAC) is among the most studied. It has been found to be effective in preventing CIN, is inexpensive, has low toxicity, but is dose dependent.[20,21]
  - Therefore, a common NAC protocol is 1,200 mg po bid the day before the procedure and the day of the procedure.[22]
  - Administration of NAC should be strongly considered in patients with eGFR < 60 ml/min/1.73 m^2, a serum creatinine >1.5 mg/dl, or with risk factors for CIN, especially diabetes.[17,22]
- Along with NAC, the other common measure to prevent CIN is IV hydration with isotonic fluids. Intravenous hydration with isotonic fluids appears to be superior to hydration with hypotonic fluids.[23] Isotonic sodium bicarbonate may be more effective than normal saline.[24] For patients with CKD or other risk factors for CIN, if hydration can be safely given, IV hydration with isotonic fluids is appropriate.
  - Among the protocols recommended are ≥1 ml/kg/h for 12 h before and 12 h after the procedure. Another recommended protocol is 3 ml/kg/h for 1 h before the procedure and 1 ml/kg/h for 6 h after the procedure.[22] The overriding principle is that patients receiving IV contrast should be well hydrated.
- Statins have a small amount of data suggesting they may be beneficial in preventing CIN. Various nonrandomized studies on statin use to prevent CIN have reached conflicting conclusions.[25]

- Additional medications that have shown early promise in reducing the risk of CIN include theophylline/aminophylline and ascorbic acid.[26]
- In light of the data supporting the use of NAC and IV hydration with isotonic fluids, these prophylactic measures are recommended for patients at elevated risk for CIN but are not needed in patients with normal renal function and no risk factors for CIN.
- Even when pharmacologic measures are used to reduce the risk of CIN, supportive measures are still important. Among the supportive measures that should be taken in at-risk patients receiving IV contrast are avoiding dehydration and cumulative exposure to nephrotoxins.
  - This means considering stopping diuretics, ACE inhibitors, angiotensin blockers, and NSAIDs.[22] The risk and benefits of stopping these medications need to be carefully weighed, especially in CHF patients.
  - Multiple IV contrast studies, especially within 48 h of each other, should be avoided. Also, metformin should be stopped in patients receiving IV contrast due to the small risk of potentially catastrophic lactic acidosis.[27]

40.6 Hemodialysis

- Among the standard indications for hemodialysis (HD), the ones that are most likely to apply in the postoperative setting include volume overload, hyperkalemia, uremia with symptoms (e.g., pericarditis), and metabolic acidosis. HD will generally only be considered for treatment of these conditions if they are refractory to medical therapy.
- Based on studies of cardiac surgery patients and ICU patients, it appears that there may be a benefit to early initiation of HD and other renal replacement therapies.[28] Early consultation with a nephrologist in a patient who is heading toward needing renal replacement therapy is advisable.
- In addition to HD, other modalities of renal replacement therapy exist, such as continuous renal replacement therapy (CRRT). In CRRT, there is less intensive fluid removal and clearance as compared to HD, but CRRT is carried out for longer periods of time, with the goal of this modality being more physiologic. CRRT has the theoretical benefit of less hemodynamic stress than HD, and is used in hemodynamically unstable patients. However, it has not, in general, been shown to be superior to HD.[29,30]

40.7 Conclusions

- Postoperative AKI is an important problem and is associated with an increase in patient mortality.
- A limited number of causes account for a large proportion of cases of postoperative AKI. These causes include renal hypoperfusion, nephrotoxic medications, contrast induced

nephropathy, and sepsis. The workup in patients with postoperative AKI should be undertaken with these common causes in mind.

- Management of postoperative AKI consists of trying to identify the cause, so that it can be removed or corrected. Beyond this, supportive treatment is necessary, including avoiding further nephrotoxic insults, such as IV contrast, and avoiding hypotension. Outside of CIN, no specific pharmacologic treatment has been clearly shown to be useful in decreasing the risk of postoperative AKI. NAC and hydration with IV isotonic fluids appear to be helpful in patients at risk for CIN, though this is still debated.

References

1. Hou SH, Bushinsky DA, Wish JB, Cohen JJ, Harrington JT. Hospital-acquired renal insufficiency: a prospective study. *Am J Med.* 1983;74(2):243-248.
2. Abelha FJ, Botelho M, Fernandes V, Barros H. Determinants of postoperative acute kidney injury. *Crit Care.* 2009;13(3):R79.
3. Bellomo R, Ronco C, Kellum JA, Mehta RL, Palevsky P, Acute Dialysis Quality Initiative workgroup. Acute renal failure – definition, outcome measures, animal models, fluid therapy and information technology needs: the Second International Consensus Conference of the Acute Dialysis Quality Initiative (ADQI) Group. *Crit Care.* 2004;8(4):R204-R212.
4. Ricci Z, Cruz D, Ronco C. The RIFLE criteria and mortality in acute kidney injury: a systematic review. *Kidney Int.* 2008;73(5):538-546.
5. Kheterpal S, Tremper KK, Heung M, et al. Development and validation of an acute kidney injury risk index for patients undergoing general surgery: results from a national data set. *Anesthesiology.* 2009;110(3):505-515.
6. Josephs SA, Thakar CV. Perioperative risk assessment, prevention, and treatment of acute kidney injury. *Int Anesthesiol Clin.* 2009;47(4):89-105.
7. Nash K, Hafeez A, Hou S. Hospital-acquired renal insufficiency. *Am J Kidney Dis.* 2002;39(5):930-936.
8. Schrier RW, Wang W. Acute renal failure and sepsis. *N Engl J Med.* 2004;351(2):159-169.
9. Modi KS, Rao VK. Atheroembolic renal disease. *J Am Soc Nephrol.* 2001;12(8):1781-1787.
10. Clarkson MR, Giblin L, O'Connell FP, et al. Acute interstitial nephritis: clinical features and response to corticosteroid therapy. *Nephrol Dial Transplant.* 2004;19(11):2778-2783.
11. Fletcher A. Eosinophiluria and acute interstitial nephritis. *N Engl J Med.* 2008;358(16):1760-1761.
12. Malbrain MLNG, Cheatham ML, Kirkpatrick A, et al. Results from the international conference of experts on intra-abdominal hypertension and abdominal compartment syndrome. I. Definitions. *Intensive Care Med.* 2006;32(11):1722-1732.
13. Cheatham ML, Malbrain MLNG, Kirkpatrick A, et al. Results from the international conference of experts on intra-abdominal hypertension and abdominal compartment syndrome. II. Recommendations. *Intensive Care Med.* 2007;33(6):951-962.
14. Zacharias M, Conlon NP, Herbison GP, Sivalingam P, Walker RJ, Hovhannisyan K. Interventions for protecting renal function in the perioperative period. *Cochrane Database Syst Rev.* 2008;(4):CD003590.
15. Ho KM, Sheridan DJ. Meta-analysis of frusemide to prevent or treat acute renal failure. *BMJ.* 2006;333(7565):420.
16. Kellum JA, Decker JM. Use of dopamine in acute renal failure: a meta-analysis. *Crit Care Med.* 2001;29(8):1526-1531.

17. Mehran R, Aymong ED, Nikolsky E, et al. A simple risk score for prediction of contrast-induced nephropathy after percutaneous coronary intervention: development and initial validation. *J Am Coll Cardiol.* 2004;44(7):1393-1399.
18. Manske CL, Sprafka JM, Strony JT, Wang Y. Contrast nephropathy in azotemic diabetic patients undergoing coronary angiography. *Am J Med.* 1990;89(5):615-620.
19. Solomon R. The role of osmolality in the incidence of contrast-induced nephropathy: a systematic review of angiographic contrast media in high risk patients. *Kidney Int.* 2005;68(5): 2256-2263.
20. Marenzi G, Assanelli E, Marana I, et al. *N*-acetylcysteine and contrast-induced nephropathy in primary angioplasty. *N Engl J Med.* 2006;354(26):2773-2782.
21. Kelly AM, Dwamena B, Cronin P, et al. Meta-analysis: effectiveness of drugs for preventing contrast-induced nephropathy. *Ann Intern Med.* 2008;148(4):284-294.
22. Goldfarb S, McCullough PA, McDermott J, Gay SB. Contrast-induced acute kidney injury: specialty-specific protocols for interventional radiology, diagnostic computed tomography radiology, and interventional cardiology. *Mayo Clin Proc.* 2009;84(2):170-179.
23. Mueller C, Buerkle G, Buettner HJ, et al. Prevention of contrast media-associated nephropathy: randomized comparison of 2 hydration regimens in 1620 patients undergoing coronary angioplasty. *Arch Intern Med.* 2002;162(3):329-336.
24. Merten GJ, Burgess WP, Gray LV, et al. Prevention of contrast-induced nephropathy with sodium bicarbonate: a randomized controlled trial. *JAMA.* 2004;291(19):2328-2334.
25. Patti G, Nusca A, Chello M, et al. Usefulness of statin pretreatment to prevent contrast-induced nephropathy and to improve long-term outcome in patients undergoing percutaneous coronary intervention. *Am J Cardiol.* 2008;101(3):279-285.
26. Stacul F, Adam A, Becker CR, et al. Strategies to reduce the risk of contrast-induced nephropathy. *Am J Cardiol.* 2006;98(6A):59K-77K.
27. Benko A, Fraser-Hill M, Magner P, et al. Canadian Association of Radiologists: consensus guidelines for the prevention of contrast-induced nephropathy. *Can Assoc Radiol J.* 2007;58(2):79-87.
28. Palevsky PM. Indications and timing of renal replacement therapy in acute kidney injury. *Crit Care Med.* 2008;36(4 Suppl):S224-S228.
29. Dennen P, Douglas IS, Anderson R. Acute kidney injury in the intensive care unit: an update and primer for the intensivist. *Crit Care Med.* 2010;38(1):261-275.
30. Pannu N, Klarenbach S, Wiebe N, Manns B, Tonelli M, Alberta Kidney Disease N. Renal replacement therapy in patients with acute renal failure: a systematic review. *JAMA.* 2008;299(7):793-805.

Anemia and Bleeding

41

Kurt Pfeifer and Barbara Slawski

41.1 Introduction

- Postoperative anemia is common, and most often due to surgical blood loss.
- Perioperative anticoagulant and antiplatelet medication administration is one of the most common reasons for postoperative bleeding. However, anemia and bleeding may result from a variety of other postoperative care-related and patient-specific factors.
- Prompt evaluation is necessary to determine potential causes and appropriate treatment.

41.1.1 Incidence

- Anemia affects up to one-half of patients preoperatively and up to 90% postoperatively.[1]
- All patients sustain some degree of blood loss with surgery (Table 41.1).
  - Reported estimates of intraoperative hemorrhage can be up to 3-times lower than calculated or measured surgical blood loss.[2]
  - Approximately 2% of patients undergoing laparoscopic procedures experience postoperative hemorrhage.[3]
  - Excessive bleeding after open surgeries is highly variable, occurring anywhere from <1% to 90% of the time.

K. Pfeifer (✉)
General Internal Medicine, Medical College of Wisconsin,
9200 W. Wisconsin Ave., Milwaukee, WI 53226, USA
e-mail: kpfeifer@mcw.edu

S.L. Cohn (ed.), *Perioperative Medicine*,
DOI: 10.1007/978-0-85729-498-2_41, © Springer-Verlag London Limited 2011

Table 41.1 Typical intraoperative blood loss for common surgeries

Procedure	Blood loss (ml)
Coronary artery bypass grafting	500
Gastric bypass, open	250
Hip and knee arthroplasty	2,000
Hip fracture repair	750
Lumbar spine fusion	500–1,000
Radical prostatectomy	400–750
Transurethral resection of prostate	500

41.1.2 Timing

41.1.2.1 Immediate Postoperative Period

- Anemia in this period is usually due to surgical blood loss and hemodilution from intravenous (IV) fluids.
- Bleeding immediately after surgery is usually caused by inadequate intraoperative hemostasis.
- Medication-induced hemostasis inhibition and inherited or acquired bleeding disorders may also contribute to bleeding in this time frame.

41.1.2.2 Days to Weeks Following Surgery

- Anemia developing after the immediate postoperative period may be due to surgical site bleeding.
- Nonoperative site hemorrhage, inadequate red blood cell (RBC) synthesis, and hemolysis are also important considerations in this period.
- Bleeding occurring several days after surgery is most often related to anticoagulants or antiplatelet agents.

41.1.3 Causes

41.1.3.1 Anemia

- Anemia causes fall into three main categories:

  1. RBC loss

2. RBC destruction
3. Reduced RBC production

- Table 41.2 lists potential causes by category.

41.1.3.2 Bleeding

- Postoperative bleeding can be divided into two main categories: procedure-related and non-procedure-related.
- Procedure-related hemorrhage is caused by the surgery itself or complications or therapies related to the operation.
  - Inadequate surgical site hemostasis is the most common cause of operative site hemorrhage.
  - Postoperative administration of anticoagulants (venous thromboembolism prophylaxis or treatment) or antiplatelet agents (aspirin or clopidogrel for ischemic event prevention or nonsteroidal anti-inflammatory drugs (NSAIDs) for analgesia) is also a common etiology.

Table 41.2 Common causes of anemia

Category of anemia	Cause of anemia	Clinical features/pathophysiology
RBC loss	Surgical blood loss	Most common cause
	Phlebotomy	May decrease hematocrit 1.9% for every 100 ml of blood withdrawn (~10–20 specimen tubes)[4]
	Nonoperative site hemorrhage	GI bleeding most common
RBC destruction	Hemolysis – intrinsic RBC defects	Enzyme deficiencies (G6PD), hemoglobinopathies (sickle cell, thalassemia), membrane defects (spherocytosis)
	Hemolysis – extrinsic	Systemic infections, microangiopathy (DIC, TTP), autoimmune hemolytic anemia, hypersplenism
Reduced RBC production	Nutritional	Iron, B12 and folate deficiency
	Bone marrow failure	Myelodysplasia, aplastic anemia, drug-induced suppression, tumor/infection infiltration
	Low levels of erythropoiesis-stimulating hormones	EPO deficiency (chronic renal failure), hypothyroidism, hypogonadism

RBC red blood cell, *GI* gastrointestinal, *G6PD* glucose-6-phosphate dehydrogenase, *DIC* disseminated intravascular coagulation, *TTP* thrombotic thrombocytopenic purpura, *EPO* erythropoietin

- Some surgical procedures, including cardiopulmonary bypass and prostate surgery, may also cause complex abnormalities of hemostasis.

- Non-procedure-related bleeding can be caused by either acquired or inherited bleeding diatheses.
  - Severe liver disease, chronic renal failure and certain cancers may cause acquired abnormalities of hemostasis.
  - Inherited bleeding disorders (i.e., von Willebrand disease [vWD], hemophilia) may be previously unknown and manifest in the postoperative setting.

41.2 Diagnosis

41.2.1 Anemia

- Evaluation of postoperative anemia should begin with a detailed history looking for previous anemia or bleeding; operative blood loss and hemostasis (found in operative and anesthesia reports); and anticoagulant and antiplatelet use.
- Physical examination should look for evidence of hemodynamic consequences of anemia (tachycardia, hypotension) and hemorrhage, including operative site drainage, flank hematomas, and GI or vaginal blood.
- Serial hemoglobin and hematocrit provide information on the rate of blood loss and the likelihood that operative loss is the cause; both should stabilize within 2 days of surgery in patients with expected surgical blood loss.
- If no site of hemorrhage is found and the hemoglobin level continues to fall, perform a complete blood count (CBC), reticulocyte count, peripheral smear examination, LDH and haptoglobin to evaluate for hemolysis.
- Acute blood loss anemia should recover within 5–7 weeks of the precipitating event (i.e., surgery).[5] If this does not occur, perform a reticulocyte count and evaluation for nutritional deficiencies (iron, vitamin B12, folate.)

41.2.2 Bleeding

- A thorough history should seek previous episodes of bleeding (especially surgical or spontaneous), antiplatelet/anticoagulant use, easy bruisability, family history of bleeding, and history of liver or renal disease.
- The physical examination may provide a clue regarding the type of hemostatic defect causing bleeding.
  - Mucosal or skin petechiae often indicate abnormal primary hemostasis due to thrombocytopenia or platelet function defects.

- Purpuric skin lesions and oozing from wounds and vascular access sites is more suggestive of deficient secondary hemostasis due to coagulation cascade abnormalities.

- Laboratory evaluation of patients with postoperative bleeding begins with a platelet count, prothrombin time (PT) and activated partial thromboplastin time (PTT). If these tests fail to identify a cause, or a platelet function defect is highly suspected based on history, in vitro platelet function screening tests (i.e., Platelet Function Analyzer [PFA]-100©) should be performed.
- CT angiography may help identify arterial bleeds at the surgical site if not obvious on exam.
- The potential causes of a postoperative bleeding disorder are numerous, and more than one may contribute at the same time.
- Table 41.3 summarizes the clinical features of several common causes of postoperative bleeding.

41.3 Treatment

41.3.1 Anemia

- Minimize iatrogenic causes by limiting phlebotomy for blood tests and reducing IV fluids to prevent dilutional anemia.
- Treat nutritional deficiencies with appropriate oral or IV supplementation.
- Identify and treat nonoperative site bleeding.
- Blood transfusion remains the mainstay of treatment for critical anemia, but until recently much controversy existed regarding the indications for blood transfusion in the surgical setting.
  - Data from critical care patients indicate that a transfusion threshold of a hemoglobin of 7 g/dL is as safe as 10 g/dL.[6]
  - Carson et al. demonstrated that in hip fracture repair patients with cardiovascular disease, restricting transfusion to symptomatic anemia or a hemoglobin of <8 g/dl led to significantly less blood product use and no change in mortality compared to a transfusion trigger of 10 g/dl.[7]
  - Therefore, transfusion should be reserved for patients with symptoms attributed to anemia or with a hemoglobin <7–8 g/dl.

- Erythropoiesis-stimulating agents (ESAs) (i.e., erythropoietin) have a limited role in the perioperative period.
  - They have been approved for preoperative treatment of anemia in noncardiovascular surgery patients with a hemoglobin count of 10–13 g/dl, but the benefit must be weighed against the considerable risks of cardiovascular events and thrombosis.

Table 41.3 Clinical features of common causes of postoperative bleeding

Cause of postoperative bleeding		Clinical features		
		Pathophysiology	History/exam findings	Laboratory findings
Procedure-related	Inadequate local hemostasis	Insufficient intraoperative cauterization	Persistent bleeding from operative site	None specific
	Anticoagulant or antiplatelet use	Medication-induced hemostasis inhibition	None specific	Elevated PT, PTT or abnormal PFA depending on agent
	Post-prostatectomy hemorrhage	Hyperfibrinolysis from urokinase in genital tract epithelium	Excessive hematuria	None specific
	Cardiopulmonary bypass syndrome	Reduction of coagulation and fibrinolytic factors and inhibition of platelet function	Operative and vascular access site bleeding	Elevated PT, PTT and abnormal PFA
	Dilutional coagulopathy	Large volume fluid resuscitation or blood transfusion leads to thrombocytopenia and/or coagulation factor deficiency	Operative site and vascular access site bleeding	Thrombocytopenia and/or elevated PT/PTT
Non-procedure-related	ITP	Autoantibody-mediated platelet destruction	History of bleeding; petechiae and failure to achieve hemostasis during surgery	Thrombocytopenia with no response to platelet transfusions
	DIC	Consumption of coagulation factors and microangiopathic hemolytic anemia by indiscriminate activation of coagulation pathways	Operative and vascular access site bleeding	Thrombocytopenia, elevated PT/PTT and schistocytes on peripheral smear

von Willebrand disease	Dysfunctional or inadequate levels of von Willebrand factor causing abnormal platelet aggregation	Family and personal history of bleeding; failure to achieve hemostasis during surgery	Abnormal PFA and elevated PTT (~60% of patients)
Hemophilia	Inadequate levels of factor VIII (hemophilia A) or IX (hemophilia B).	Family and personal history of bleeding; spontaneous deep tissue/joint bleeding and delayed oozing from surgical sites	Elevated PTT
Liver disease	Inadequate synthesis of coagulation factors and plasmin inhibitors; thrombocytopenia due to splenic sequestration	History and exam evidence of liver disease	Thrombocytopenia and elevated PT
Renal disease	Uremia-induced platelet dysfunction	Evidence of uremia	Abnormal PFA; severely elevated BUN
Vitamin K deficiency	Inadequate synthesis of vitamin K-dependent coagulation factors	History of poor nutrition; operative and vascular access site bleeding	Elevated PT

PFA platelet function assay, *ITP* immune thrombocytopenic purpura, *DIC* disseminated intravascular coagulation *BUN* blood urea nitrogen

- In pre- or postoperative patients with critical anemia who refuse transfusion, ESAs may be used to rapidly correct hemoglobin concentrations.

  The dose of erythropoietin alpha is 300 units per kg per day for 15 days.
  Concurrent iron supplementation is necessary to prevent relative iron deficiency.
  VTE prophylaxis should be provided to prevent thrombotic complications from ESAs.

41.3.2 Bleeding

- Collaborate with surgical colleagues to determine the possibility of surgery-related bleeding and need for exploration of the operative site to achieve hemostasis.
- If the source of bleeding is not related to inadequate surgical hemostasis, focus treatment on the identified non-procedure-related cause.
- Closely examine the need for any anticoagulant or antiplatelet therapy, and when complications related to thrombosis are not considered more imminently dangerous than those from bleeding, stop these medications.
  - Give vitamin K and fresh frozen plasma (FFP) to rapidly reverse the effects of warfarin. Goal of therapy is INR<1.5.
  - Consider using protamine to rapidly reverse anticoagulation from heparins, but reversal with low-molecular-weight heparins may be incomplete.
  - If bleeding is critical, recombinant factor VIIa may be used.
- When coagulation abnormalities are identified, direct treatment is given to the specific hemostatic problem.
  - Thrombocytopenia:

    Discontinue medications, including heparins and H_2-antagonists, which may be causative.
    Administer platelet transfusions to maintain a platelet count of ≥50,000/uL for patients with bleeding. Exceptions to this recommendation:

      For patients who have or will undergo surgery on the brain or eyes, a platelet count of ≥100,000/uL should be maintained.
      Platelet transfusions are contraindicated in patients with heparin-induced thrombocytopenia (HIT) and ITP.

        HIT patients should be started on an anticoagulant other than heparins or vitamin K antagonists.
        ITP patients can be given intravenous immunoglobulin (IVIG) 0.5–1.0 g/kg or methylprednisolone 1 g IV to rapidly improve platelet counts.

  - Platelet Dysfunction (abnormal PFA):

    VWD patients should receive prophylactic desmopressin or factor VIII concentrates prior to most surgical procedures, and treatment should continue to maintain factor

VIII levels ≥50% until healing is complete. Care of VWD patient should be coordinated with a hematologist.
Consider either desmopressin 0.3 mcg/kg subcutaneously (SC)/IV or cryoprecipitate 10 units IV for patients with uremia and evidence of bleeding.
Platelet transfusions, tranexamic acid, aminocaproic acid (ACA) or recombinant factor VIIa may be used if other therapies fail.

- Coagulopathy (elevated PT and/or PTT):

Reverse vitamin K antagonists or deficiency with vitamin K and FFP to achieve INR < 1.5.
Hemophilia patients should receive recombinant factor VIII (hemophilia A) or factor IX (hemophilia B) preoperatively to achieve factor levels near 100% until at least 72 h after surgery and then levels of 50% until healing is complete. Care of hemophilia patients should be coordinated with a hematologist.

- Complex Bleeding Disorders:

DIC:

Identify and treat the underlying cause.
Give platelet transfusions to maintain a platelet count ≥50,000/uL in the presence of significant bleeding.
Transfuse cryoprecipitate to maintain fibrinogen >100 mg/dl.
Transfuse FFP to achieve a target INR of <1.5 in the presence of bleeding.

Postprostatectomy hemorrhage: administer ACA IV or orally for excessive urinary bleeding.
Cardiopulmonary bypass syndrome:

Platelet dysfunction is usually self-limited and requires no specific treatment.
Coagulation factor depletion causing elevated PT/PTT should be treated with FFP to achieve INR < 1.5.
Excessive fibrinolysis can be treated with ACA, tranexamic acid and aprotinin. These medications are part of standard cardiopulmonary bypass protocols at many institutions.

References

1. Dunne JR, Malone D, Tracy JK, et al. Perioperative anemia: an independent risk factor for infection, mortality, and resource utilization in surgery. *J Surg Res*. 2002;102(2):237-244.
2. Rosencher N, Kerkkamp HE, Macheras G, et al. OSTHEO Investigation. Orthopedic Surgery Transfusion Hemoglobin European Overview (OSTHEO) study: blood management in elective knee and hip arthroplasty in Europe. *Transfusion*. 2003;43(4):459-469.
3. Schafer M, Lauper M, Krahenbuhl L. A nation's experience of bleeding complications during laparoscopy. *Am J Surg*. 2000;180(1):73-77.
4. Thavendiranathan P, Bagai A, Ebidia A, et al. Do blood tests cause anemia in hospitalized patients? The effect of diagnostic phlebotomy on hemoglobin and hematocrit levels. *J Gen Intern Med*. 2005;20(6):520-554.

5. Pottgiesser T, Specker W, Umhau M, et al. Recovery of hemoglobin mass after blood donation. *Transfusion*. 2008;48(7):1390-1397.
6. Hebert PC, Wells G, Blajchman MA, et al. A multicenter, randomized, controlled clinical trial of transfusion requirements in critical care. Transfusion Requirements in Critical Care Investigators, Canadian Critical Care Trials Group. *N Engl J Med*. 1999;340:409-417.
7. Carson JL, et al. Transfusion trigger trial for functional outcomes in cardiovascular patients undergoing surgical hip fracture repair (FOCUS): the principle results. American Society of Hematology Meeting 2009, New Orleans; Abstract LBA-6.

Postoperative Jaundice

42

Richard B. Brooks and Nomi L. Traub

42.1 Introduction

- Postoperative increases in liver function tests are common, ranging in incidence from 25% to 75% of patients.
- Overall, clinically significant increases in bilirubin levels are uncommon in patients without underlying liver disease, but occur in almost half of the patients with a known history of cirrhosis.
- Postoperative jaundice has also been reported to occur in over 25–35% of patients undergoing certain cardiac operations and conferred a higher mortality rate in those cases.[1,2]

42.2 Causes

- The etiology of postoperative jaundice is often multi-factorial. It can be worsened or exaggerated by concomitant renal failure, which results in decreased clearance of serum bilirubin.
- Patient-specific and surgery-specific risk factors are listed in Table 42.1.
- The differential diagnosis can be broken down into three broad categories:
  - Disordered bilirubin metabolism
  - Hepatocellular damage
  - Intrahepatic and extrahepatic cholestasis

R.B. Brooks (✉)
Department of Medicine, University of California,
San Francisco General Hospital, San Francisco, CA, USA
e-mail: richard.brooks@ucsf.edu

S.L. Cohn (ed.), *Perioperative Medicine*,
DOI: 10.1007/978-0-85729-498-2_42, © Springer-Verlag London Limited 2011

Table 42.1 Risk factors for postoperative jaundice

Patient-specific risks	Surgery-specific risks
History of liver disease	Cardiac surgery (valve>CABG)
Alcohol abuse	Upper abdominal surgery (GI/liver/GB)
Cardiac disease/CHF	Intraoperative hypotension
Infection	Transfusions
Perioperative TPN	Anesthesia
Sickle-cell disease	Medications

- Etiologies caused by disordered bilirubin metabolism include those causing increased production of bilirubin, as well as impaired uptake or storage of bilirubin:
  - Hemolysis and subsequent breakdown of hemoglobin, which may be caused by
    - Transfusion reactions
    - Toxins (e.g., sulfa drugs in patients with G-6-PDH deficiency)
    - Mechanical heart valves (traumatic)
    - Sickle-cell disease
    - Cardiopulmonary bypass
    - Aortic cross-clamping
  - Resorption of hematomas
  - Multiple red blood cell transfusions
  - Underlying Gilbert's syndrome (glucuronyl transferase deficiency)
  - Medications (e.g., atazanavir, ethinyl estradiol, gentamicin, probenecid, and ceftriaxone)
  - Bile leak after bile duct surgery
- Etiologies caused by hepatocellular injury include:
  - Hepatic ischemia, usually due to intraoperative or postoperative hypotension
  - Toxic injury from anesthetic agents or other medications
  - Congestive hepatopathy due to hypervolemia, often seen as a consequence of congestive heart failure
  - Acute rejection after liver transplant
  - Viral hepatitis, including flares of chronic hepatitis B infection
  - Nonalcoholic steatohepatitis (NASH), also known as fatty liver disease
  - Alcoholic hepatitis
  - Budd–Chiari syndrome
- Etiologies caused by intrahepatic or extrahepatic cholestasis include the following:
  - Intrahepatic

    Hyperbilirubinemia of sepsis
    Benign postoperative cholestasis

TPN administration
Medications (e.g., carbamazepine, estrogens, methimazole, niacin, benzodiazepines)

– Extrahepatic

Bile duct gallstones (choledocholithiasis)
Biliary stricture
Obstructing mass in the biliary system, e.g., pancreatic cancer or cholangiocarcinoma
Sphincter of Oddi dysfunction
Calculous or acalculous cholecystitis

– Infiltrative liver diseases (e.g., sarcoidosis, lymphoma, amyloidosis) can contribute to both intrahepatic and extrahepatic cholestasis

42.3 Diagnosis

- Careful review of the medical record, analysis of the pattern and timing of liver test abnormalities, and knowledge of the most common etiologies of postoperative jaundice, help narrow the differential diagnosis.
- Figure 42.1 demonstrates a diagnostic approach to the patient with postoperative jaundice.
- The most common etiologies of postoperative jaundice are:
  - Decompensation of preexisting liver disease
  - Hepatic ischemia
  - Hemolysis
  - Benign postoperative cholestasis
  - Infections/sepsis
  - Toxic injury from medications (haloalkane anesthetic toxicity is currently rare)

42.3.1 History

- Review preoperative data seeking clues to unrecognized underlying liver disease, such as parenteral drug use, alcohol use, use of therapeutic or illegal drugs, transfusions prior to 1992, and metabolic syndrome. Preoperative elevated aminotransferases suggest chronic hepatitis, such as viral hepatitis, alcoholic liver disease, or nonalcoholic fatty liver disease.
- Preoperative thrombocytopenia, decreased albumin, or prolonged PT may suggest the presence of cirrhosis. Normal aminotransferases do not rule out cirrhosis. Cirrhotic patients have an increased risk of hepatic decompensation postoperatively and increased susceptibility to hepatic ischemia due to reliance on hepatic artery flow.

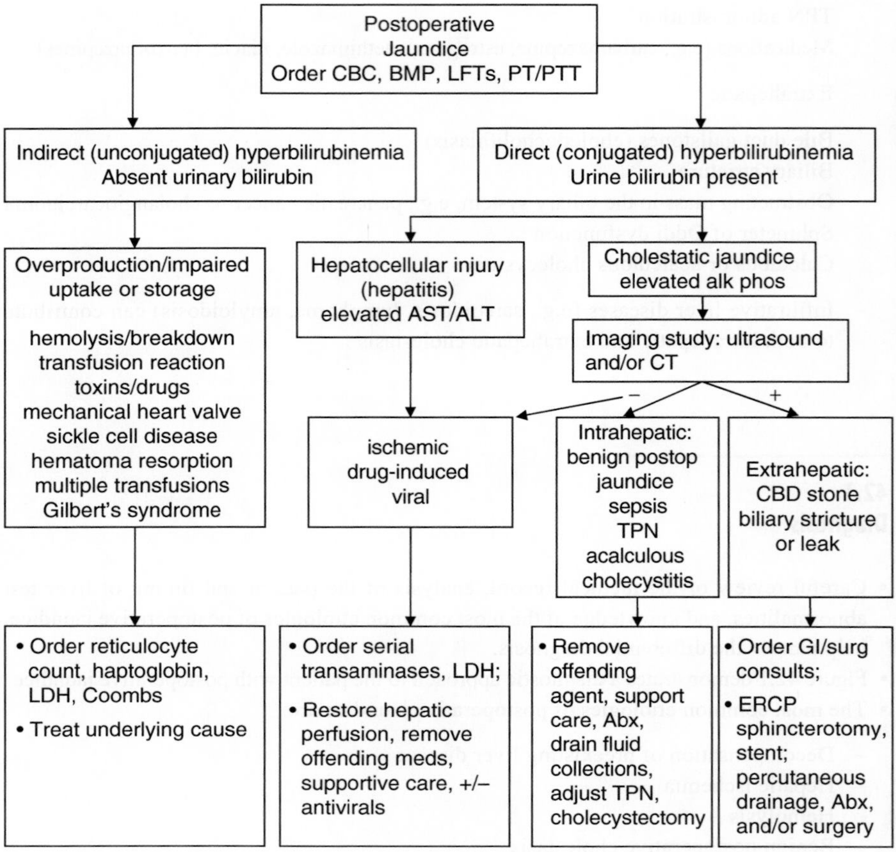

Fig. 42.1 Approach to the patient with postoperative jaundice

- Preoperative or prior episodes of unconjugated hyperbilirubinemia suggest Gilbert's syndrome.
- Review anesthesia and operative records for anesthetic agents, and evidence of transient hypotension or hypoxemia.
- Review recent medication use, especially any recent changes in medications.
- Review any history of perioperative blood product transfusions.
- Timing:
  - Problems that usually occur within 1–2 weeks of surgery:
    - Decompensation of preexisting liver disease
    - Unconjugated hyperbilirubinemia related to transfusions, hematomas, hemolysis, and Gilbert's syndrome (within 2 weeks)
    - Hepatic ischemia (within 24 h)
    - Benign postoperative intrahepatic cholestasis (within a few days)

    - Biliary obstruction related to surgery, such as retained stones, bile duct injury
    - Toxic injury from medications (anesthetic toxicity 2–15 days)
- Problems that occur after 3 weeks:
    - Toxic injury from medications
    - Total parenteral nutrition
    - Viral hepatitis (likely acquired preoperatively), including flare of chronic HBV

42.3.2 Physical Exam

- Look for stigmata of chronic liver disease – spider telangiectasias, gynecomastia, palmar erythema, caput medusa, Dupuytren's contractures, hepatomegaly (in patients without cirrhosis), splenomegaly, encephalopathy, ascites.
- Check carefully for hematomas as a source of unconjugated bilirubin elevation.
- Fever and skin rash can be seen in toxic injury from medications or anesthesia.

42.3.3 Laboratory

Patterns of liver test abnormalities may be helpful in diagnosis.

- Predominantly elevated unconjugated (indirect) bilirubin points to bilirubin overproduction or a genetic disorder of bilirubin metabolism. Etiologies include hemolysis of transfused red blood cells, resorption of hematomas, underlying hemolytic diseases (sickle-cell disease, thalassemias, G6PD deficiency, and autoimmune hemolytic anemia), mechanical heart valves, and Gilbert's syndrome.
- Additional clues to hemolysis are elevated reticulocyte count, reduced haptoglobin, elevated LDH and AST, and schistocytes on peripheral smear. ALT and alkaline phosphatase should be normal.
- Marked elevations of aminotransferases (5–200× the upper limit of normal) associated with markedly elevated LDH levels occur in hepatic ischemia, which usually occurs within the first few days postoperatively. Levels decline at a rapid rate once hypoperfusion is corrected. Hyperbilirubinemia and coagulopathy can occur in severe cases. Alkaline phosphatase remains normal or mildly elevated.
- Similar or somewhat less marked aminotransferase elevation is seen with toxic injury, viral hepatitis, congestive hepatopathy, and hepatocellular necrosis after liver transplantation.
- Benign postoperative cholestasis is a poorly understood condition in which there is usually a progressive rise in conjugated (direct) bilirubin within the first 2–10 days of surgery. Total bilirubin may reach 10–40 mg/dL and is usually associated with milder alkaline phosphatase elevation (2–4× upper limit normal), and normal aminotransferase levels (<5× the upper limit of normal). This occurs after complicated abdominal or thoracic surgery and is variably associated with multiple transfusions, postoperative infections, and in the setting of burns or trauma. Diagnosis is based on exclusion of other causes of jaundice, particularly obstruction.

- Marked alkaline phosphatase elevation, associated with moderate bilirubin elevation, and only mild to moderate aminotransferase elevation, suggests biliary obstruction. Obstruction may be related to strictures, retained stones, pancreatitis, or less commonly mass effect. Obstruction most often occurs after major upper abdominal surgery or surgery of the biliary tract. If obstruction is ruled out, this pattern may occur with medication-induced cholestasis, infections, TPN administration, and intrahepatic cholestasis after liver transplant.

42.3.4 Imaging and Biopsy

- If biliary obstruction is suspected due to elevated alkaline phosphatase and conjugated hyperbilirubinemia, abdominal ultrasonography (US) or CT scanning should be performed, looking for ductal dilatation or any evidence of choledocholithiasis.
- In patients who have had upper abdominal surgery, US or CT can evaluate for bile leaks, biloma, or abscess.
- Magnetic resonance cholangiopancreatography (MRCP) is helpful to investigate biliary leaks or biloma, and to exclude extrahepatic obstruction when the index of suspicion for biliary obstruction is low.
- Endoscopic retrograde cholangiopancreatography (ERCP) should be considered when the index of suspicion of biliary pathology is high, and for therapeutic intervention such as sphincterotomy, or placement of an internal biliary stent.
- Rarely, when the clinical picture is obscure, liver biopsy may be necessary to confirm hepatic ischemia, benign postoperative cholestasis, and particularly to evaluate liver biochemical abnormalities in transplant patients.

42.4 Treatment

- Treatment should be targeted to the suspected underlying cause of the jaundice.
- Most often, treatment is supportive in nature, with efforts made to correct volume overload, prevent hypotension, avoid hepatotoxic medications, and treat any underlying infections.
- Any medications thought to be causing or contributing to hemolysis should be avoided.
- Any resulting coagulopathy should be treated with vitamin K, 5–10 mg PO daily × 3 days.
- Hepatic encephalopathy can be treated with lactulose 30 g PO given several times a day, titrated to 3–4 bowel movements per 24 h. If the patient cannot tolerate PO medications, lactulose retention enemas can also be used.
- If a toxic etiology is suspected, all attempts should be made to remove the offending agent.
- Treatment of acute viral hepatitis is largely supportive. Studies have not shown benefit to using antiviral medications to treat acute hepatitis B; however, it might be reasonable to use antiviral medications in patients with fulminant hepatitis, including coagulopathy and encephalopathy, as the risks are relatively low despite the unclear benefits. Furthermore, reduction of the HBV DNA level prior to liver transplant would be an important benefit of treatment.[3]

- If acetaminophen overdose is suspected, *N*-acetylcysteine administration should begin immediately and serial acetaminophen levels checked. Oral dosing of *N*-acetylcysteine begins with a loading dose of 140 mg/kg followed 4 h later by a dose of 70 mg/kg every 4 h for a total of 17 doses. IV dosing begins with a loading dose of 150 mg/kg over 15–60 min, followed by a 4-h infusion at 12.5 mg/kg/h, and then a 16-h infusion at 6.25 mg/kg/h. The local Poison Control Center should be notified. A thorough medication assessment should be completed and all products containing acetaminophen stopped.
- Acute cholecystitis should be treated with appropriate antibiotics and potentially cholecystectomy or cholecystostomy.
- Obstructive bile duct stones (choledocholithiasis) may necessitate ERCP with stone removal and/or sphincterotomy. Biliary strictures can be ballooned using ERCP.
- In the majority of cases, bile leaks can be treated via endoscopically placed biliary stents or nasobiliary drainage with or without sphincterotomy. In refractory cases, surgical intervention to repair the leak may be necessary.[4,5]
- The diagnosis of Budd–Chiari Syndrome should result in discussion with a radiologist to help determine the acuity of the thrombus. Prompt consultation with a gastrointestinal specialist is recommended, as decisions regarding anticoagulation, thrombolysis, radiologic interventions, shunt placement, and potential transplant are not straightforward and are largely based on availability and experience at each individual institution.[6]

References

1. Mastoraki A, Karatzis E, Mastoraki S, et al. Postoperative jaundice after cardiac surgery. *Hepatobiliary Pancreat Dis Int*. 2007;6:383-387.
2. Wang MJ, Chao A, Huang CH, et al. Hyperbilirubinemia after cardiac operation. Incidence, risk factors, and clinical significance. *J Thorac Cardiovasc Surg*. 1994;107:429-436.
3. Kumar M, Satapathy S, Monga R, et al. A randomized controlled trial of lamivudine to treat acute hepatitis B. *Hepatology*. 2007;45:97-101.
4. Bergman JJ, van den Brink GR, Rauws EA, et al. Treatment of bile duct lesions after laparoscopic cholecystectomy. *Gut*. 1996;38:141-147.
5. Sandha GS, Bourke MJ, Haber GB, et al. Endoscopic therapy for bile leak based on a new classification: results in 207 patients. *Gastrointest Endosc*. 2004;60:567-574.
6. Murad SD, Plessier A, Herenandez-Guerra M, et al. Etiology, management, and outcome of the Budd-Chiari syndrome. *Ann Intern Med*. 2009;151:167-175.

Suggested Reading

Faust TW, Reddy KR. Postoperative jaundice. *Clin Liver Dis*. 2004;8:151-166.

LaMont JT. Postoperative jaundice. *Surg Clin North Am*. 1974;54(3):637-645.

LaMont JT, Isselbacher KJ. Current concepts of postoperative hepatic dysfunction. *Conn Med*. 1975;39(8):461-464.

Munoz SJ, Killackey MT. Postoperative jaundice. In: Schiff ER, Sorrell MF, Maddrey WC, eds. *Schiff's diseases of the liver*. 10th ed. Philadelphia, Pennsylvania: Lippincott, Williams and Wilkins; 2007:697-705.

Postoperative Stroke and Seizures

43

Lane K. Jacobs and Benjamin L. Sapers

43.1 Cerebrovascular Accident (Stroke)

43.1.1 Introduction

Perioperative cerebrovascular accident (CVA) is associated with both high mortality and prolonged and severe morbidity. General medical illness, poor physiological reserve, and the stress of surgery are all important risk factors for this potentially devastating complication.

43.1.2 Incidence, Timing, and Risk Factors (See Chap. 29)

- A retrospective review of 1,455 patients with stroke revealed that the odds ratio (OR) for CVA in the month following surgery can be as high as 2.9–3.9 – even excluding procedures high risk for stroke.
  - Incidence after routine surgical procedures is 0.02–0.07.
  - Events are rarely hemorrhagic.
  - Most new events are diagnosed, on the average, at 7 days after surgery but can be delayed up to 3–4 weeks.

L.K. Jacobs (✉)
Section of General Internal Medicine, Carolinas Medical Center,
1000 Blythe Blvd, 5th Floor MEB, Charlotte, NC 28203, USA
e-mail: ljacobs@carolinas.org

S.L. Cohn (ed.), *Perioperative Medicine*,
DOI: 10.1007/978-0-85729-498-2_43, © Springer-Verlag London Limited 2011

Intraoperative strokes are very rare: approximately one in 40,000 ambulatory surgical procedures.
Forty-five percent of embolic strokes are diagnosed on the first postoperative day.
Hypoperfusion watershed CVAs are usually identified on the first postoperative day and are associated with postoperative events rather than intraoperative hypotension.

  - In the patient with a prior history of CVA or transient ischemic attack (TIA), the risk of surgery-associated recurrent stroke is greatest in the 2 weeks following the initial event.

- Risk varies with type and site of surgical intervention.
  - General surgery <0.2% (0.08–0.7%)
  - Vascular surgery 0.8–3%
  - Head and neck surgery 4.8%
  - Heart valve surgery and/or aortic arch repair 8–10%
- Risk varies with the age of the patient undergoing surgery.
  - Risk at age 55: 2.2/100,000 cases
  - Ages 75–84: 10–24/100,000
- Perioperative stroke is deadly and debilitating
  - Mortality is 30% without a history of previous stroke, and up to 60% with such a history
  - Thirty percent of survivors will need assisted living postoperatively after a stroke.
  - Annual cost of this problem is estimated at $6 billion in the United States alone.

43.1.3 Diagnosis

43.1.3.1 Initial Approach to Postoperative CVA

1. CAB (Circulation (chest compressions), Airway, Breathing) assessment and blood glucose assessment.
2. Determine if this is a stroke or stroke mimic.
3. Determine location/vascular distribution.
4. Rule-out hemorrhagic event (rare).
5. Is the patient a candidate for intravascular intervention or thrombolysis?
6. Identify etiology of stroke.
7. Begin secondary preventive therapy.

   - Determine whether the neurological deficit represents a new event or merely an exaggeration of previous symptoms in the setting of surgical stress. Physical examination and imaging will help distinguish between these two possibilities.
   - Localize the lesion through careful physical examination.
   - Check blood glucose as well as the patient's vital signs.

- Review the intraoperative anesthesia notes for evidence of fluctuating blood pressure, blood glucose abnormalities, and prolonged operative time.
- Imaging with computer tomography (CT) can differentiate between a hemorrhagic and ischemic infarction. Computer assisted angiography (CTA) is useful if intravenous or intra-arterial thrombolysis is being considered. Magnetic resonance imaging (MRI) with diffusion imaging or angiography may also be of value for more precise localization of the lesion.
- Electroencephalography (EEG) applied in the comatose patient helps differentiate between status seizure and catastrophic CVA, but its sensitivity for diagnosing acute CVA is poor.

43.1.4 Treatment

The risk of surgical bleeding needs to be taken into account when considering treatment of perioperative CVA.

43.1.4.1 Antiplatelet Agents

- Aspirin
  - 160–300 mg within 48 h of stroke onset improves mortality and reduces recurrent stroke within the first 2 weeks of the initial event.

- Other antiplatelet agents (clopidogrel, aspirin/extended-release dipyridamole) either have not been studied in acute stroke or have not been shown to be beneficial.
- Clopidogrel
  - Daily dosing of 75 mg a day has a delay of 5 days before robust platelet inhibition.
  - An oral loading dose of 300 mg causes immediate platelet inhibition and has increased the effectiveness of this drug in acute coronary syndromes.
  - Neither strategy has been studied in acute stroke.
  - Starting clopidogrel for prophylaxis of secondary events after an acute CVA is reasonable.

- Aspirin with extended release dipyridamole
  - No evidence exists for the utility of this combination agent in acute CVA.
  - Starting after an acute event for prophylaxis of secondary events is reasonable.
  - Combination of aspirin and clopidogrel.
  - No added benefit in acute stroke.
  - Increase in hemorrhagic events in long-term concomitant use for secondary prevention.

- The recent PRoFESS (Prevention Regimen For Effectively Avoiding Second Strokes) trial demonstrated equivalent safety and outcomes between combination aspirin/dipyridamole and clopidogrel started within 72 h after mild ischemic stroke for secondary prevention.

43.1.4.2 Anticoagulation

- Systemic anticoagulation after major surgery is generally not a therapeutic alternative. Moreover, its use after acute stroke offers no clear advantage over treatment with antiplatelet agents alone, and it increases hemorrhagic complications.
- If anticoagulation is deemed necessary because of the presence of a mechanical heart valve or atrial fibrillation, short acting agents such as unfractionated heparin (UFH) are preferred over longer acting less easily reversible agents like low molecular weight heparin (LMWH) or a direct thrombin inhibitor.

43.1.4.3 Thrombolysis

- Systemic thrombolysis is contraindicated after major surgery.
- Intra-arterial intracranial thrombolysis may be considered in an advanced center where such expertise is available, **but it is not considered the standard of care at this time.**

43.1.4.4 HMG Co-A Reductase Inhibitors (Statins)

- Interrupting statin therapy in the setting of acute stroke appears to worsen outcome and is not recommended.
- Initiating statin therapy in the setting of acute stroke may improve overall outcomes at the expense of a small increase in risk of hemorrhagic stroke.

43.1.4.5 Blood Pressure

- Blood pressure (BP) management in acute stroke has been well defined in published guidelines. Briefly stated, normalization of blood pressure is not recommended, but systolic BP should be maintained at <180 mmHg. Target ranges are:

  – Less than 180/100–105 for patients with known hypertension
  – Less than 160–180/90–105 for patients without history of hypertension

- Angiotensin converting enzyme inhibitors (ACEI) or angiotensin receptor blockers (ARB) may reduce morbidity and mortality.

43.1.4.6
Glycemic Control

- Hyperglycemia is associated with a higher likelihood of stroke in certain clinical settings (e.g., carotid endarterectomy) and with poorer outcome after acute stroke.
- A target glucose ≤140 for the first 24 h after a stroke may be of benefit regarding morbidity and mortality.

43.1.4.7
Venous Thromboembolism (VTE) Prophylaxis

- Appropriate VTE prophylaxis should be implemented in the perioperative setting, especially if the patient has suffered an acute neurological deficit. In such cases, chemoprophylaxis with any of a variety of drugs as well as concomitant mechanical prophylaxis is indicated. For acute ischemic stroke, LMWH may be preferable to UFH based on results from the PREVAIL (Prevention of VTE after Acute Ischemic Stroke with LMWH Enoxaparin) trial.

43.1.4.8
Aftercare

- After the patient's neurologic condition is stabilized, the focus turns to nutritional support, and to planning for both acute and chronic rehabilitation.
  - Consultation with physical therapy, occupational therapy, speech therapy is indicated as soon as is reasonable.
  - Aggressive pulmonary toilet is warranted to prevent atelectasis, aspiration, and pneumonia.
  - Temporary percutaneous gastrostomy tube should be considered in patients with nutritional deficiencies and adequate recovery potential.
  - Early aggressive rehabilitation in an acute or sub-acute setting is advised.
  - Long-term skilled home care or nursing facility placement may need to be considered.
  - Ample communication with the patient's family is essential to guide discharge planning.

43.2 Postoperative Seizure

43.2.1 Incidence, Timing, and Risk Factors

- Postoperative seizures are infrequent (0.03%). When they do occur they are most commonly the result of a known underlying seizure disorder (with an incidence of approximately 2% in postoperative patients with epilepsy), and/or immediate postsurgical physiological derangements.
- The risk of seizure varies by type and location of surgery.
  - Craniotomy and subarachnoid hemorrhage with aneurysm repair carry a seizure risk of 13–40% (average 20%), while the risk associated with coronary artery bypass or liver transplant is 5–7%.
  - In general, neurosurgery patients carry the highest risk of postsurgical seizure with a broad range of incidence (17–92%) in patients with brain abscess as the primary diagnosis.
- Subtherapeutic anti-epileptic drugs (AED) levels are a common cause of breakthrough seizures in the perioperative setting. Medication noncompliance, drug–drug interactions with anesthesia and other medications, and impaired oral bioavailability – due to altered gastrointestinal motility – all may contribute to subtherapeutic levels.
- Seizures occurring immediately postoperatively are more often due to metabolic derangements; those occurring several weeks later often suggest the development of a true seizure disorder.
  - Late epilepsy occurs in the range of 41% for neurosurgical patients experiencing early postoperative seizure.

43.2.2 Diagnosis

- Evaluation begins with a thorough history and physical exam.
  - Assess if the patient has a history of epilepsy and if so, is s/he on anti-epileptic drugs (AED) and compliant with them.
  - Obtain recent AED levels if available.
  - A good description of the current seizure including its duration and type (partial versus generalized, seizure versus pseudoseizure) is crucial. In epileptic patients any resemblance of perioperative seizure to prior events can be useful.
  - Physical examination may demonstrate post-ictal motor or sensory residua.

43.2.2.1
Differential Diagnosis

- True epilepsy – new or breakthrough
  - Partial or generalized
- Toxin effect
  - Substance abuse: cocaine, methamphetamine
  - Perioperative medication: anesthetic agents, opiates
- Substance withdrawal
  - Alcohol, benzodiazepines, Selective Sertonin Reuptake Inhibitor (SSRI) antidepressants
- Metabolic derangement: hypoglycemia, hyponatremia, hypocalcemia
- Acute intracranial event: CVA or intracerebral hemorrhage
- Acute perioperative complication: VTE, hemorrhage
- Pseudoseizure

43.2.2.2
Status Epilepticus

The longer a seizure continues, the harder it is to suppress it.

  - Most seizures last no more than 1–2 min. Seizures lasting 5 min or more are considered status epilepticus.

- The state of persistent epilepsy, status epilepticus, is divided into three subtypes: generalized convulsive, focal motor, and non-convulsive. Complications can be both neuronal and systemic (Table 43.1).
- Seizures lasting over 10 min usually do not resolve spontaneously.
- Mortality of status epilepticus is 20–25%.

Table 43.1 Complications from status epilepticus

Neurological complications	Systemic complications
Depletion of energy stores and subsequent inhibition of protein synthesis	Hyperthermia
Direct excitotoxic injury	Rhabdomyolysis
Generation of additional epileptogenic foci	Aspiration with pneumonia
Synaptic disorganization	Metabolic acidosis Arrhythmia

43.2.3
Treatment (Table 43.2)

"Time is Brain"

- The longer a patient remains in status epilepticus, the more dismal the prognosis becomes. Each minute the patient spends in status increases the potential for seizure-related brain damage and the likelihood of a perioperative complication such as myocardial infarction (MI) or stroke. Even in a paralyzed patient, 20 min or more of uncontrolled seizure activity is associated with brain damage. Moreover, in the perioperative brain whose reserve is already depleted by surgical stress, the further demands on oxygen and blood flow from the disorganized electrical activity of a seizure can be devastating.
- The goal of intervention should be to terminate the seizure as soon as possible and certainly within 30 min.
- An EEG should always be used to confirm successful termination of seizure activity.

43.2.3.1
Treatment for Non-status Seizure

- Dependent on etiology
  - Known **epilepsy: check AED levels and correct accordingly**
  - New seizure: discern etiology and treat accordingly.

Table 43.2 Treatment for status epilepticus

Time (min)	Intervention
0	Circulation, airway, breathing, blood glucose, oxygenation as needed Confirm IV access History
5	Send blood sample for lab tests: specifically potassium, sodium, bicarbonate, calcium, creatinine, and blood urea nitrogen (BUN). Thiamine 100 mg IV with 50 ml of 50% dextrose
10	Begin first line agents: benzodiazepines. Lorazepam 0.05–0.1 mg/kg Diazepam 0.1 mg–0.4 mg/kg
15	Second line agents. Phenytoin or fosphenytoin 15–20 mg/kg. Valproate 15–20 mg/kg. Phenobarbital 10–20 mg/kg
20	EEG monitoring (if not yet begun) then intubate. Third line agents: general anesthetics. Pentobarbital coma 10–20 mg/kg and titrate to burst suppression on EEG. Midazolam 0.2 mg/kg load to maximum of 20 mg then titrate as above. Propofol 1–2 mg/kg load then titrate as above

– Neurosurgery or recent stroke: load AED
– Toxic-metabolic: treat accordingly.

- Consult with surgical team about integrity of surgical site, especially for tonic-clonic seizure.
- Take into account functional free drug levels in patients with malnutrition or other causes of hypoalbuminemia.

Suggested Reading

Adams HP, Soppo G, Alberts MJ, et al. Guidelines for the early management of adults with ischemic stroke. A guideline from the American Heart Association/American Stroke Association Stroke Council, Clinical Cardiology Council, Cardiovascular Radiology and Intervention Council, and the Atherosclerotic Peripheral Vascular Disease and Quality of Care Outcomes in Research Interdisciplinary Working Groups. *Stroke*. 2007;38:1655-1711.

Bateman BT, Schumacher HC, Wang S, Shaefi S, Berman MF. Perioperative acute ischemic stroke in noncardiac and nonvascular surgery incidence, risk factors, and outcomes. *Anesthesiology*. 2009;110(2):231-238.

Christopher MJ, Bhatt DL. The efficacy and safety of perioperative antiplatelet therapy. *J Thromb Thrombolysis*. 2004;12(1):21-27.

Emmanuel T, Trinquart L, Chatiellier G, Mas JL. Systematic review of the perioperative risks of stroke or death after carotid angioplasty and stenting. *Stroke*. 2009;40(12):e683-e693.

Larsen SF, Zaric D, Boysen G. Postoperative cerebrovascular accidents in general surgery. *Acta Anaesthesiol Scand*. 1988;32:698-701.

Magdy S. Perioperative stroke. *N Engl J Med*. 2007;356:706-713.

Niesen AD, Jacob AK, Aho LE, et al. Perioperative seizures in patients with a history of seizure disorder. *Anesth Analg*. 2010;111:729-735.

Pasternak JJ, Lanier WL. Neuroanesthesiology review 2005. *J Neurosurg Anesthesiol*. 2006;18: 93-105.

Szeder V, Torbey MT. Prevention and treatment of perioperative stroke. *Neurologist*. 2008;14: 30-36.

Voss LJ, Sleigh JW, Barnard JPM, Kirsch HE. The howling cortex: seizures and general anesthetic drugs. *Anesth Analg*. 2008;107:1689-1702.

Postoperative Delirium

44

Alok Kapoor and Joleen Elizabeth Fixley

44.1 Introduction

- Postoperative Delirium (PD) is common, costly, and often fatal. Although populations as young as 40 years old have been included, the disease mainly afflicts adults aged 65 or older. It is the most common cause of morbidity postoperatively in the elderly.[1]
- PD is on a continuum with preexisting dementia, new postoperative cognitive dysfunction, and new or deepening dementia.
- The average cost of a delirium episode is estimated at upward of $2,900 (adjusted to 2,010 USD)[1] and has been found to be 2.5-fold higher in the year following delirium diagnosis for the patient developing recurrent delirium.
- Delirium has been shown to have an independent association with poor outcomes.
  - Short-term outcomes of increased length of stay, increased hospital mortality rates, and increased nursing home dispositions have been reported.[2] Delirium has also been associated with poor functional outcomes, measured by poorer walking ability on discharge.[3]
  - Long-term outcomes are also affected. Symptoms of delirium and cognitive decline may persist for 6–12 months.[2] In 40% of hip fracture patients, cognitive declines may persist up to a year.[4]
  - One-year mortality rates associated with delirium in hospitalized older adults are 35–40%.[1] The estimates for PD in the elective surgery population are generally lower, although firm estimates are not available.

A. Kapoor (✉)
Hospital Medicine Unit, Section of General Internal Medicine,
Boston University School of Medicine, Boston, MA 02118, USA
e-mail: alok.kapoor@bmc.org

S.L. Cohn (ed.), *Perioperative Medicine*,
DOI: 10.1007/978-0-85729-498-2_44, © Springer-Verlag London Limited 2011

44.2 Incidence

- The incidence of PD varies widely depending upon population studied and surgery performed.
  - The incidence in a population of age>50 ranges from 2% without any risk factors present to more than 50% with multiple risk factors present.[5]
  - Cardiac surgery, aortic aneurysm repair, and hip fracture repair represent three of the highest risk settings with incidence ranging from 40–60%.[5,6]

44.3 Timing

- PD can begin in the hours after surgery and can linger for several days afterward.
- Peak period of onset is within the first 72 h.

44.4 Etiologies

- The etiology of PD is multifactorial and may be subcategorized into predisposing and precipitating factors. Predisposing factors are preoperative and may not be modifiable, but serve to increase the index of suspicion for diagnosis. Precipitating factors are often iatrogenic.
- The pneumonic DELIRIUMS SPAC; includes the most common underlying causes:
  - **D**rugs, **E**motional/**D**epression, **L**ow PO2 states, **I**nfection, **R**etention of urine or feces, **I**mmobile/**I**ctal states, **U**ndernourished/or dehydrated states, **M**etabolic, **S**urgery specific, **S**ensory/Sleep deprivation, **P**ain, **A**ge, **C**ognitively impaired baseline.

44.5 Predisposing/Preoperative Risk Factors (See Table 44.1)

- Age has a modest effect on predisposing delirium but associated comorbidities and preexisting conditions contribute substantially.
- Preexisting cognitive impairment is probably the most important preoperative risk factor for the development of PD. Underlying dementia was present in 28–66% of hospitalized and/or postoperative delirious patients.[1]
- Psychiatric disease (psychosis, depression, anxiety) and non-compliance with psychiatric medications increases risk.

Table 44.1 Diagnostic guide including etiologies and risk factors with their corresponding manifestations and suggested labs and interventions

	Etiologies and predisposing/precipitating factors	History	Physical	Labs	Interventions
D	**D**rugs (intoxications/withdrawals)	≥3 new meds, accurate preop. medicine dose and schedule	Lethargy, somnolence, agitation, emotional lability	Drug levels	Discontinue/Reinstitute/Treat
E	**E**motional (depression)	Current state of	≥5 on GDS	–	Psych. Consult
L	**L**ow **P**02 states: MI, CHF, PE, Anemia, CVA, Subdural	Chest pain, sob, orthopnea, PND vs. no symptoms	Diaphoretic, Low-grade fever tachypneic, tachycardic, hematoma, lateralizing defects	Sa02, EKG, cardiac enzymes, Hgb, ABG, spiral chest CT, Head CT	See corresponding chapters
I	**I**nfection	Wound: pain/purulent d/c Wind: cough/sob Water: Foley Encephalitis	Check under bandage, breath sounds, tachypnea, fever	CBC w/diff., blood culture, UA, CXR, CSF	See corresponding chapters Remove Foley
R	**R**etention of Urine or Feces	I/O's	PVR, Rectal	BUN/creatinine	Consider drug-related causes, catheterize, bowel protocol
I	**I**mmobile/**I**ctal States	In bed/absence vs. atypical vs. tonic-clonic	Foley/restraints, clonus, + Babinski	EEG	D/C Foley and restraints-mobilize, antiepileptics
U	**U**ndernourished/**D**ehydrated states	I/O's, NPO status	Hypotension, tachycardia, dry mucous membranes	BUN/creatinine, albumin	Nourish/hydrate
M	**M**etabolic	Myriad	Myriad	CMP, Mg, PO4, TSH, B12, Folate	Correct abnormalities

(continued)

Table 44.1 (continued)

	Etiologies and predisposing/precipitating factors	History	Physical	Labs	Interventions
S	**S**urgery specific: hip, cardiac, vascular, thoracic	–	–	–	–
S	**S**ensory/**S**leep deprivation	Wears glasses/hearing aids	Poor hearing/visual acuity	–	Glasses/hearing aids, sleep hygiene
P	**P**ain	At rest > predictive than with activity	Withdrawn	–	Treat accordingly
A	**A**ge	≥65	–	–	Prophylactic
C	**C**ognitively impaired baseline	Preoperative evaluation vs. family members	MMSE < 27 and MMSE < 24 further increases	–	Prophylactic

Adapted from "DELIRIUMSP" mnemonic[7] and "DELIRIUMS" mnemonic[8]

MI myocardial infarction, *CHF* congestive heart failure, *CVA* cerebrovascular accident, *PE* pulmonary embolism, *GDS* geriatric depression scale, *MMSE* Folstein's mini mental status examination, *PND* paroxysmal nocturnal dyspnea, *d/c* discharge, *UA* urine analysis, *CXR* chest xray, *CSF* cerebrospinal fluid, *PVR* post void residual, *I/O's* ins and outs, *EEG* electroencephalogram, *D/C* discharge, *NPO* nothing by mouth, *BUN* blood urea nitrogen, *CMP* complete metabolic profile, *Pysch.* pyschiatric

- Poor functional status measured by dependence in activities of daily living is another major predictor of PD.
- Sensory impairments, visual or hearing also predict increase rates of PD.
- Other factors associated with increased rates of PD include preexisting stroke or transient ischemic episode, lower educational level, substance use (including alcohol use as little as four times per week), and poor nutritional status.

44.6 Precipitating/Postoperative/Iatrogenic Risk Factors (See Table 44.1)

- Medications are implicated in up to 40% of PD episodes (See Table 44.2)
  - The addition of >3 new medications in the perioperative period predicts increased PD rates.[9]
  - Anticholinergics, sedative-hypnotics, and opioids are commonly implicated.
- Pain is another precipitating factor. A subgroup of cognitively intact hip fracture patients was nine-fold more likely to develop PD if they experienced severe pain at rest.[10]
- Consider environmental causes: postoperative immobilization and sleep deprivation.
- Postoperative factors include hypoxia, pain, and anemia. Medical complications including myocardial infarction, congestive heart failure, pulmonary embolism, cerebrovascular accident, infection, and urinary retention are also factors for PD.

Table 44.2 Medications associated with postoperative delirium

Sedative-hypnotics Benzodiazepines (especially longer acting agents flurazepam, diazepam) Barbiturates, sleeping medications (chloral hydrate)
Narcotics and analgesic agents All narcotics especially meperidine Epidural anesthesia
Other Anticholinergics Neuroleptics (chlorpromazine, haloperidol, thioridizine) Heterocyclic antidepressants (amitryptyline, imiprazine, doxepin) Antispasmodics (oxybutynin, cyclobenzaprine) Antihistamines (H1 – diphenhydramine, hydroxyzine; H2 blockers – ranitidine)
Miscellaneous Lithium

44.7 Surgery-Specific Risk Factors

- The hip fracture repair population tends to represent a population of urgently scheduled surgery with poor nutritional status and frailty.
- Emergency surgery has a 54% PD incidence compared with elective surgery 18% in a cohort of elderly hip-surgery patients.[11]
- Cardiac surgery, especially procedures using a heart bypass machine, increases risk.
- Other procedures associated with increased risk of PD include ophthalmic surgery, transplants, transurethral prostatectomy (TURP), and hysterectomy.

44.8 Screening and Risk Assessment for PD

- Although there is no formal recommendation from a professional society, screening seems prudent in certain age populations (e.g., age>65) and types of surgery.
- The goal of screening is to identify a high-risk group who may be candidates for augmented measures aimed at preventing and minimizing the severity of PD; the exact threshold for triggering such measures has not been established.
- Screening should combine multiple domains including physical, cognitive, sensory impairment, substance and medication use.
- Identifying cognitive impairment is an important component of screening. One instrument available is the MiniCog, a combination of a 3-item, 5-min recall and a clock drawing test. Other instruments including a Folstein Mini Mental Status Exam (MMSE) are available but may not be feasible to administer in the course of a typical preoperative visit.
- The clinical prediction rule developed by Marcantonio et al.[5] remains the mainstay of preoperative risk assessment in the noncardiac surgery population. (Table 44.3).

Table 44.3 Postoperative delirium prediction rule for patient undergoing elective noncardiac surgery

Risk factor	# of points	Delirium risk
Age ≥ 70	1	0 points = 2% risk
Alcohol abuse	1	1–2 points = 11% risk
Cognitive impairment	1	≥3 points = 50% risk
Severe physical impairment	1	
Markedly abnormal preoperative Na, K, or glucose	1	
Aortic aneurysm repair	2	
Noncardiac thoracic surgery	1	

From Marcantonio et al.,[5] with permission.

- The study measured the association of a common set of predisposing and precipitating causes in a group of patients aged>50 undergoing major surgery – i.e., general surgery, orthopedic surgery, and thoracic noncardiac surgery. Patients with zero factors developed PD only 2% of the time, whereas those with 3 or more develop PD 50% of the time. Limitation to use of the rule include that its component items such as blood sodium, potassium, and glucose may not always be available at the time of a preoperative encounter.

- Other preoperative assessment tools are available for more specialized surgical populations such as the Delirium in the Elderly at Risk (DEAR) tool[12] for the total hip or knee replacement population.

  - Results of the analysis using DEAR suggest that the presence of two of five risk domains (age >80, cognitive impairment, physical impairment, sensory impairment, or substance or psychoactive medication use) conferred an eight-fold increase in the odds of PD. Rudolph et al. conducted a derivation and validation study in the cardiac surgery population and found that prior cerebrovascular disease, abnormal Mini Mental State Examination score, low serum albumin, and elevated Geriatric Depression Scale score all independently predicted PD.[6]

44.9 Diagnosis

- Delirium is an altered state of consciousness whose main hallmark is deficiency of attention. These changes are accompanied by a change in cognition. Cognitive changes will present as memory deficit, disorientation, or change in speech patterns.
- Onset is acute (hours to days).
- Fluctuation throughout the day is the norm, with symptoms being more severe in the evening hours.
- Patients may have memory of these events and report the disturbing episode the next day. Perceptual disturbances including illusions, hallucinations or delusions may be present.
- Psychomotor activity may be increased, decreased, or shift unpredictably. The hyperactive form is characterized by agitation. The hypoactive delirious patient may be lethargic or somnolent.

44.10 Differential Diagnosis

- Onset of cognitive change in dementia is insidious rather than acute. Although patients with dementia have "good days and bad days," the fluctuations are not typically as extreme or as rapid. Attention is preserved in dementia except in very severe disease.

Depression is often diagnosed inaccurately in the hypoactive form of delirium. Failure to diagnose delirium by clinicians has been reported at a rate of 33–66% in observational cohorts. Hypoactive delirium, age>80, vision impairment, and preexisting dementia all predict under-recognition. A patient with ≥3 of these risk factors had a 20-fold increase in risk of having delirium signs be missed by nursing staff.[13]

- Diagnostic Tools – Confusion Assessment Method (**CAM**)
  - Considering ease of use, test performance, and clinical importance of heterogeneity, authors of a recent systematic review[14] found CAM to have the best supportive data as a bedside delirium instrument with a positive LR 9.6 and negative LR 0.16.
  - The accuracy of the CAM has been estimated at 94–100% sensitivity and 90–95% specificity compared to a comprehensive evaluation.[15]
  - Diagnosis requires acute onset with a fluctuating course and presence of inattention AND either presence of disorganized thinking OR altered level of consciousness.

44.11 History

- PD occurs typically with acute onset with relapsing and remitting course.
- Since the patient may be unable to provide adequate history, question family members for additional information.
- Ask about pain and baseline status.
- Obtain an accurate medication list and confirm dosing and frequency.

44.12 Physical Examination

- Orientation to time, place, and person will fluctuate. Cognitive changes of memory can be shown by poor performance of three-item recall. Inattention makes it difficult for a patient to complete serial 7s or spell "world" backward.
- Agitation, emotional lability, lethargy, somnolence, rambling, or incoherent language with illogical flow of ideas may all be present.
- Signs of delirium itself may be the only notable changes in the patient, regardless of etiology – e.g., acute myocardial infarction presenting without chest pain.
- Although physical findings are usually nonspecific, the presence of fever, hypotension, focal neurologic defects, respiratory distress, etc., may suggest an underlying etiology.

44.13 Laboratory Testing and Neuroimaging (See Table 44.1)

- Baseline blood tests should include a complete blood count (CBC) and basic metabolic panel (with electrolytes, glucose, and renal function). Additional testing will depend on specific findings.
- Neuroimaging is generally not indicated for the management of delirium unless there is a new, focal neurological deficit in sensory or motor exam or persistent delirium without an obvious cause.

44.14 Treatment

- Prevention is the best treatment.
- Currently there have been only two interventions in the perioperative period which have proven in randomized controlled trials to be efficacious in preventing delirium. Because of the importance of a multicomponent intervention reported by Inouye et al.[16] in hospitalized older adults, we also discuss that intervention. The absence of benefit related to most, single-component interventions suggests that a multicomponent intervention aimed at the multifactorial etiology of PD is the most viable approach to preventing PD.
  - Preemptive geriatric consultation: Consultation performed preoperatively or within 24 h from the time of hip fracture repair was reported in one trial[17] to reduce the rate of PD from 50% (in controls) to 32% (in the intervention group) ($p=0.04$). Key recommendations were to maintain blood hematocrit>30% (although preliminary results from an ongoing trial[18] suggest this may not be efficacious), decrease or discontinue psychoactive medications, remove urinary catheters, prescribe a bowel protocol to prevent constipation and ileus, mobilize patients early, encourage use of glasses and hearing aids, recommend a family member or other sitter to stay at the bedside, and add low-dose haloperidol 0.25–0.5mg as necessary. Subsets with pre-fracture dementia or ADL impairment did not appear to benefit from consultation and invariably developed PD.
  - Environmental/supportive therapy: In the randomized controlled trial by Inouye, frequent orientation, adherence to sleep hygiene, early mobilization, use of visual and hearing aids, and early recognition and treatment of dehydration was shown to reduce incidence of delirium in elderly general medicine hospitalized patients from 15% in controls to 10% in the intervention group. Relative benefits may be greater in the perioperative setting, but absolute risk reductions may be more modest given the overall better health of surgical patients.

Table 44.4 Treatment of postoperative delirium

Treatment strategy	Recommendation
Maintain quiet environment	Reassurance 1:1 supervision as needed Have family member stay with patient
Control pain	Try to use non-narcotic analgesics
Minimize medications with CNS toxicity	Try to avoid or use low-dose opioids, anticholinergics, steroids
Control agitation/anxiety	Use neuroleptics such as haloperidol or risperidone
Treat alcohol withdrawal	Use lorazepam and thiamine

  - Pharmacological Prophylaxis: Low-dose haloperidol (in addition to preemptive geriatric consultation) beginning 1–3 days before hip fracture repair or hip replacement and continued for 3 days postoperatively decreased the duration of delirium by 6.4 days and the delirium severity by 25%; the actual incidence was decreased from 16.5% to 15.1%, but the difference was not statistically significant.[19]
- Once PD has developed, the goal of therapy is to identify and correct the underlying causes. Various treatment strategies are summarized in Table 44.4.
- Symptom control for cases of extreme agitation or risk of danger with low-dose haloperidol 0.25–0.5 mg po/IM/IV q4 h or risperidone 0.25–1 mg po q12 h in the elderly.

44.15 Emerging Pharmacological Preventive Therapies

- Dexmedetomidine: A new generation drug for sedation in critically ill patients, Dexmedetomidine is part of an ongoing trial[20] aimed at reducing the incidence of PD and subsequent cognitive impairment. In addition to its sedative properties, dexmedetomidine provides some pain relief and controls the body's response to stress.
- Cholinesterase inhibitor: There is a pilot study[21] to test the tolerability and efficacy of donepezil, a cholinesterase inhibitor medication used commonly in persons with dementia, for the prevention of new or worsening delirium in patients with hip or long-bone fracture.
- Gabapentin: A pilot study[22] examined prophylactic use of gabapentin (900 mg daily preoperatively through postoperative day 3) to both reduce the need for narcotics postoperatively and reduce pain. The patient population included subjects as young as 45 years old, so this intervention may be applicable in younger populations. Although the sample was small, the results were encouraging: delirium did not occur in the treated group (0/9) but occurred in 5 of 12 patients in the placebo group.

44.16 Conclusion

- PD is a very prevalent postoperative complication with widespread health and financial implications. PD occurs between 2% and 50% frequency depending on the type of surgery and the presence of associated predisposing and precipitating conditions.
- Although a subset of postoperative patients without other risk factors for dementia will only experience transient delirium, developing theories of PD describe it as being on a continuum with preexisting dementia, postoperative cognitive dysfunction, and new or deepening dementia.[1]
- Preoperative cognitive impairment, age, nutritional status, cerebrovascular disease, and substance/psychoactive medication use are among the most significant predictors of PD. Combinations have also been evaluated in the form of a clinical prediction rule and patients with multiple risk factors represent potential targets for augmented preventive measures.
- Prevention is the best cure for PD. Although there are multiple emerging single-component therapies for both preventing and minimizing the severity of PD, multicomponent interventions such as a preemptive geriatric or medical consultation, which are geared to addressing the multifactorial nature of PD, are likely to translate into improved postoperative outcomes.

References

1. Inouye SK, Inouye SK. Delirium in older persons. *N Engl J Med.* 2006;354(11):1157-1165.
2. Inouye SK, Schlesinger MJ, Lydon TJ. Delirium: a symptom of how hospital care is failing older persons and a window to improve quality of hospital care. *Am J Med.* 1999;106(5): 565-573.
3. Olofsson B, Lundstrom M, Borssen B, et al. Delirium is associated with poor rehabilitation outcome in elderly patients treated for femoral neck fractures. *Scand J Caring Sci.* 2005; 19(2):119-127.
4. Gruber-Baldini AL, Zimmerman S, Morrison RS, et al. Cognitive impairment in hip fracture patients: timing of detection and longitudinal follow-up. *J Am Geriatr Soc.* 2003;51(9): 1227-1236.
5. Marcantonio ER, Goldman L, Mangione CM, et al. A clinical prediction rule for delirium after elective noncardiac surgery. *JAMA.* 1994;271(2):134-139.
6. Rudolph JL, Jones RN, Levkoff SE, et al. Derivation and validation of a preoperative prediction rule for delirium after cardiac surgery. *Circulation.* 2009;119(2):229-236.
7. Edward Vandenberg M.D. Geriatric pearls at geriatrics.unmc.edu.
8. Flaherty JH, Morley JE. Delirium: a call to improve current standards of care. *J Gerontol A Biol Sci Med Sci.* 2004;59(4):341-343.
9. Inouye SK, Charpentier PA. Precipitating factors for delirium in hospitalized elderly persons. Predictive model and interrelationship with baseline vulnerability. *JAMA.* 1996;275(11): 852-857.

10. Morrison RS, Magaziner J, Gilbert M, et al. Relationship between pain and opioid analgesics on the development of delirium following hip fracture. *J Gerontol A Biol Sci Med Sci*. 2003;58(1):76-81.
11. Kalisvaart KJ, Vreeswijk R, de Jonghe JF, et al. Risk factors and prediction of postoperative delirium in elderly hip-surgery patients: implementation and validation of a medical risk factor model. *J Am Geriatr Soc*. 2006;54(5):817-822.
12. Freter SH, Dunbar MJ, MacLeod H, Morrison M, MacKnight C, Rockwood K. Predicting post-operative delirium in elective orthopaedic patients: the Delirium Elderly At-Risk (DEAR) instrument. *Age Ageing*. 2005;34(2):169-171.
13. Inouye SK, Foreman MD, Mion LC, Katz KH, Cooney LM Jr. Nurses' recognition of delirium and its symptoms: comparison of nurse and researcher ratings. *Arch Intern Med*. 2001;161(20):2467-2473.
14. Wong CL, Holroyd-Leduc J, Simel DL, et al. Does this patient have delirium?: value of bedside instruments. *JAMA*. 2010;304(7):779-786.
15. Inouye SK, van Dyck CH, Alessi CA, Balkin S, Siegal AP, Horwitz RI. Clarifying confusion: the confusion assessment method. A new method for detection of delirium. *Ann Intern Med*. 1990;113(12):941-948.
16. Inouye SK, Bogardus ST Jr, Charpentier PA, et al. A multicomponent intervention to prevent delirium in hospitalized older patients. *N Engl J Med*. 1999;340(9):669-676.
17. Marcantonio ER, Flacker JM, Wright RJ, Resnick NM. Reducing delirium after hip fracture: a randomized trial. *J Am Geriatr Soc*. 2001;49(5):516-522.
18. Robert Wood Johnson Medical School. Focus transfusion trigger trial. http://www.focustrial.org/. Accessed May 22, 2010.
19. Kalisvaart KJ, de Jonghe JF, Bogaards MJ, et al. Haloperidol prophylaxis for elderly hip-surgery patients at risk for delirium: a randomized placebo-controlled study. *J Am Geriatr Soc*. 2005;53(10):1658-1666.
20. ClinicalTrials.gov. Perioperative Cognitive Function – Dexmedetomidine and Cognitive Reserve http://clinicaltrials.gov/ct2/results?term=NCT00561678. Accessed May 22, 2010.
21. ClinicalTrials.gov. Supporting the Health of Adults Undergoing Orthopedic Surgery During the Recovery Period (SHARP). http://clinicaltrials.gov/ct2/show/NCT00586196. Accessed May 22, 2010.
22. Leung JM, Sands LP, Rico M, et al. Pilot clinical trial of gabapentin to decrease postoperative delirium in older patients. *Neurology*. 2006;67(7):1251-1253.

Pain Management 45

Darin J. Correll

45.1 Background

- Pain is often the most common presenting or associated symptom in hospitalized patients, and patients are frequently more concerned about being in pain than they are about the primary reason for being in the hospital.
- Outcome benefits from improved pain control vary depending on the patient population and modality used. Epidural anesthesia and analgesia can lead to benefits in terms of cardiovascular and respiratory complications in high-risk patients as well as benefits in terms of gastrointestinal and hematological outcomes. Other modalities, such as intravenous patient-controlled analgesia, may improve pulmonary complications.
- Improved pain control in the acute setting, not related to a specific modality, can lead to a decreased chance of delirium, improved wound healing, increased patient satisfaction and quality of life, and a quicker return to normal functioning. Also, acute pain can develop into chronic, persistent pain if it is not treated properly.

45.2 Pain Management Guidelines

- Listen to and believe the patient – pain is a subjective experience, thus providers must accept the patient's own report of pain.
- The fact that pain is a subjective experience allows for the placebo response to be beneficial. Use of a placebo should never include being deceitful to a patient or giving them an inactive substance to ascertain if they are lying or to punish them. The legitimate use of the placebo effect is that if a patient believes that a particular therapy is

D.J. Correll
Department of Anesthesiology, Preoperative and Pain Medicine, Brigham and Women's Hospital/Harvard Medical School, Boston, MA, USA
e-mail: dcorrell@partners.org

S.L. Cohn (ed.), *Perioperative Medicine*,

DOI: 10.1007/978-0-85729-498-2_45, © Springer-Verlag London Limited 2011

going to work then it is more likely to do so. So truthfully "talking up" a genuine attempt at analgesia is the proper use. This also happens in the reverse; when a patient tells you a particular therapy "never works for them," more likely than not it is not going to work.
- Assess and reassess the level of pain and degree of pain relief on a regular basis, given the specific situation.
- Treat pain promptly – do not withhold therapy while seeking a diagnosis. Pain treatment will not impair the ability to diagnose a disease.
- Discuss the analgesic plan with the patient and, if appropriate, the family, be aware of the patient's expectations for pain management, and propose reasonable goals from the intended therapy.
- The best way to achieve the greatest possible analgesia with the lowest incidence of side effects is to use a multimodal approach for managing pain as opposed to using a single modality to its "limit." The method can include both pharmacologic and non-pharmacologic measures.
- Pain management must be part of an overall plan for improving postoperative care.
- If pain is present most of the time or if it is expected to last for an extended period of time (e.g., greater than a few weeks), use around-the-clock dosing or long-acting agents. In these cases, as-needed (i.e., prn) doses of immediate release agents will also be needed if breakthrough pain exists. If pain is intermittent and/or only expected to last a short time (e.g., less than a couple weeks) then as-needed therapy with immediate release agents can be used effectively.
- Contacting the patient's primary care provider to inform them of the discharge analgesic plan is essential if there has been a significant alteration to a prior analgesic regimen. Make certain that the patient has someone to contact if there is a lack of effectiveness of the analgesic regimen or if side effects develop after discharge from the hospital. In addition, either have a plan for a taper off of analgesics (or back to their baseline if they were on analgesics prior to admission) or ensure the patient can follow-up with someone as an outpatient.

45.3 Pain Assessment

- Location – where the patient is having pain and any radiation from the major area.
- Intensity – use scales appropriate to the patient and situation.
- Character – the quality of the pain, best assessed having the patient use adjectives.
- Aggravating and alleviating factors – what makes the pain worse or better.
- Impact on functional ability – in the inpatient setting, does the pain affect the patient's ability to cough, get out of bed, ambulate, etc.
- Prior analgesic history – what agents have either worked or not worked in the past.
- Ongoing analgesics – if the patient is taking any analgesics presently, and if so the exact doses.

45.4 Pain Intensity

- The most common measurement tool for intensity of pain in an acute setting is the single-dimension verbal numeric scale where patients are asked to verbally state a number between 0 and 10 to correspond to their present pain intensity. Some patients prefer to use words (e.g., none, mild, moderate, severe) to describe the intensity of their pain; this is termed a verbal descriptor scale.
- Variations of the single-dimension scales that may be of benefit in the elderly or cognitively impaired are ones that use drawn faces ranging from content-looking smiling faces to distressed-looking faces (e.g., Faces Pain Scale or Wong-Baker Faces Scale) instead of asking the patient to choose a number or word to rate their pain.
- Pain assessments are estimates; one cannot assume that they represent a specific "quantity" of pain and base specific treatment decisions on them.

45.5 Determine Mechanism of Pain (Table 45.1)

- To choose the correct therapy for the pain, the physiologic generator needs to be determined.
- The way to determine this is to have the patient describe the character of the pain using adjectives (e.g., aching, burning, dull, electric-like, sharp, shooting, stabbing, throbbing).

Table 45.1 Determine mechanism of pain

Mechanism	Characteristics	Examples	Treatment options
Somatic	Well localized; constant; sharp, aching	Cut, fracture, burn, abrasion, localized inflammation	Heat/cold, acetaminophen, NSAIDs, opioids, local anesthetics (topical or infiltrate)
Visceral	Not well localized; constant or intermittent; achy, cramping or pressure, sometimes sharp	Muscle spasm, GI or renal colic, sickle cell crisis, inflamed internal organ	NSAIDs, opioids, muscle relaxants, local anesthetic nerve-block
Neuropathic	Dermatomal and/or radiating, can be diffuse; burning, tingling, electric shock, lancinating	Trigeminal, post-herpetic, post-amputation, peripheral neuropathy, nerve infiltration	Anticonvulsants, antidepressants, NMDA antagonists, neural blockade

Modified from Correll[1], with permission. Copyright © 2008 The McGraw Hill Companies, Inc.

45.6 Analgesic Modalities

- Non-pharmacologic measures (e.g., hypnosis, Transcutaneous Electrical Nerve Stimulation (TENS), relaxation, guided imagery, acupuncture) – scientific data on the use of these measures is either limited or equivocal; however, since they have little risk, if the patient believes that a particular therapy is going to help then it is likely to be of at least some benefit due to the subjective nature of pain.
- Pharmacologic measures – fall into three general categories:
  - (1) Non-opioid analgesics, (2) opioids, and (3) adjuvant analgesics
- There are no standard protocols to treat pain. Therapy must be individualized for each patient using a multimodal approach, adding or altering agents when pain control is inadequate and the altering or diminishing agents as pain resolves.

45.7 Non-opioid Analgesics (Table 45.2)

- Unless contraindicated, all patients in pain should be prescribed a non-opioid analgesic of some sort. They are primary analgesics for low-intensity pain associated with headache or musculoskeletal disorders and are used as adjuncts for moderate to severe pain.
- Acetaminophen: No negative gastrointestinal or platelet effects. No clinically significant anti-inflammatory actions.
- Nonselective Nonsteroidal Anti-inflammatory Drugs (NSAIDs): Negative effects on platelets, gastrointestinal and renal systems. Increased risk of major cardiovascular events with certain NSAIDs. No NSAID is more effective as an analgesic than any other, but there is inter-patient variability in response – thus changing agents may be of benefit if one does not seem to be effective.
- COX-2 Selective NSAID: No effect on platelet aggregation, lesser effect on the gastrointestinal mucosa, but equivalent effect on the renal system compared to nonselective NSAIDs. Should not be used as first-line agent because of higher cost and should not be used long-term, especially at high doses, given the data that it increases the risk of major cardiovascular events.

45.8 Opioid Therapy Basics

- Use the pure opioid agonists, especially for treating moderate to severe pain, as opposed to the agonist/antagonists.
- Be familiar with the characteristics of several opioids (Table 45.3).
- The optimal dose varies widely among patients, even if they are naïve to opioids.

Table 45.2 Non-opioid analgesic examples

Agent	Adult dosing suggestions	Maximum 24-hour dose	Select comments
Acetaminophen	650–1,000 mg q 6 h	4,000 mg	Single doses above 1,000 mg do not improve analgesia
Etodalac	200–400 mg q 6–8 h	1,000 mg	Low GI and renal effect incidence, safest NSAID in liver disease
Ibuprofen	400–600 mg q 4–6 h	3,000 mg	<1,500 mg QD has low risk of GI effects, possible increased renal effects, inhibits CV benefits of aspirin when given concomitantly
Ketorolac	30 mg q 6 h	120 mg	High risk of renal and GI complications; use for no more than 5 days; 15 mg q 6 h in renal impairment, age>65 year, weight<50 kg
Naproxen	250–500 mg q 6–12 h	1,500 mg	Possible increased liver and renal effects, probably least negative CV effects
Celecoxib	100–200 mg QD	200 mg	Use 100 mg dose if possible; long-term use has increased negative CV effects

Modified from Correll[1], with permission. Copyright © 2008 The McGraw Hill Companies, Inc.
GI gastrointestinal, CV cardiovascular

Table 45.3 Opioid characteristics

Agonist	Route	Equianalgesic dose (mg)	Onset (min)	Peak effect (min)	Duration of effect (h)
Morphine	Parenteral Oral	10 30	5–10 15–60	10–30 60–120	3–5 4–6
Codeine	Parenteral Oral	120 200	10–30 30–45	90–120 60	4–6 3–4
Hydromorphone	Parenteral Oral	1.5 7.5	5–20 15–30	15–30 90–120	3–4 4–6
Oxycodone	Oral	20	15–30	30–60	4–6
Fentanyl	Parenteral	0.1	<1	5–7	0.75–2+
Oxymorphone	Parenteral Oral	1 10	5–10 Meaningful relief=60	30–60	3–6 4–6

Modified from Correll[1], with permission. Copyright © 2008 The McGraw Hill Companies, Inc.

- The analgesic effect and side effects from opioids vary widely between patients. Thus it is always best to ask the patient which agents have either worked or not worked in the past and/or have given them intolerable side effects.
- Monitor patients carefully for efficiency and side effects whenever there is a change of agent and/or route or if there is the addition of another analgesic to the regimen.

45.9 Opioid Choices

- Codeine, a prodrug, is not an appropriate first choice since approximately 10–20% of the population does not have an active form of cytochrome P450 2D6 that is necessary to convert it into an active drug (i.e., morphine).
- All opioids must be used with caution in patients with renal or hepatic insufficiency, where lower doses and/or longer dosing intervals may be appropriate. Morphine is relatively contraindicated in patients with severe renal insufficiency (and the elderly) due to the accumulation of one of its active metabolites, morphine-6-glucuronide, which could lead to sedation and respiratory depression.
- *Meperidine is not recommended for pain management* for a number of reasons. Its metabolite, normeperidine, can accumulate in a couple days to levels that can cause nervous system excitation (tremors, twitching, convulsions). It causes strong euphoric feelings especially when given as an intravenous (IV) push. It is a weak agonist and often causes more nausea than other agents.
- Hydrocodone use needs to be monitored closely because of the acetaminophen component in all the available preparations.

45.10 Opioid Administration

- Whenever possible, the enteral route is best due to its ease of use and the fact that it offers the most stable pharmacokinetics.
- If the enteral route cannot be used or if adequate analgesia cannot be achieved in a timely manner then the IV route should be used.
- Intramuscular administration is not recommended (IT HURTS, and it has unpredictable pharmacokinetics).
- With a competent patient, the use of an IV patient-controlled analgesia (PCA) is usually the best overall pain management option.

45.11 Opioid Dosing

- The recommended starting doses for moderate to severe pain in the opioid naïve are shown in Table 45.4.

Table 45.4 Recommended starting doses of select opioids in adults

Agonist	Oral	Intravenous
Tramadol	50–100 mg q 4–6 h[a]	n/a
Oxycodone	5–10 mg q 3–4 h	n/a
Morphine	10–30 mg q 3–4 h	5–10 mg q 2–4 h
Hydromorphone	2–6 mg q 3–4 h	1–1.5 mg q 3–4 h
Oxymorphone	10–20 mg q 4–6 h	1 mg q 3–4 h

Modified from Correll[1], with permission. Copyright © 2008 The McGraw Hill Companies, Inc.
[a]Maximum recommended 24-h dose: 400 mg in adults <75 years old; 300 mg in adults >75 years old

- If a patient is not receiving adequate relief at a given dose, increase the dose by 25–50%.
- If a patient is having an unacceptable level of pain before the next dose is due, reduce the interval and/or increase the dose.
- Rotation from one opioid to another may be needed in several situations:
  – If the dose of an opioid needs to be increased a few times and the patient is still not receiving any pain relief, changing opioids may provide better analgesia.
  – If a patient is having intolerable side effects not easily treated with appropriate agents, changing to a different opioid may offer a better side effect profile.
  – If a particular opioid is not available by the necessary or preferred route of administration in a given patient.
  – If a patient has been on a particular opioid for an extended period of time and they have an acutely painful event (e.g., surgery) or otherwise have tolerance to the analgesic effects of their chronic opioid; changing to a different opioid may provide better analgesia.

45.12 Equianalgesic-Dosing Charts (See Table 45.3)

- Several different versions exist, so the calculations must be seen as estimates only and clinical judgment is required.
- Incomplete cross-tolerance exists between the various opioids. This means that patients will not be "as tolerant" to a new opioid as they are to the one they were on previously. Thus, when converting between opioids, the calculated equianalgesic dose of the new agent must be reduced by 25–75% in order to prevent over-sedation and/or respiratory depression. The exact percentage to reduce by in any given individual is unfortunately not able to be determined. So, clinical judgment/impression must be used and close follow-up for over- or under-dosing is needed.

45.13
Sustained-Release or Long-Acting Opioids

- Sustained release formulations should only be initiated in the acute setting if pain is present almost all of the time and it is assumed that the pain will last for a while (e.g., >2weeks). If the pain is more incident-related or expected to be of a brief duration then immediate release agents should be used.
- If initiating or increasing a sustained-release opioid (e.g., if >4 rescue doses are needed in 24 h while on a sustained-release agent already), start or go up on the sustained-release agent by 50–100% of the total 24-hour breakthrough dose used.
- When using a sustained-release opioid, also provide an immediate release opioid in doses equivalent to 10–15% of the 24-hour total, available every few hours on a prn basis.
- Transdermal fentanyl is not appropriate for acute pain, especially in the opioid naïve. There is a black box warning against its use in the acute setting due to the risk of severe respiratory depression from the delayed peak effect of the drug as the pain level decreases. It is intended for use in patients who are already tolerant to opioids of comparable potency.
- Methadone is not appropriate as the first-line agent in the acute setting, especially in the opioid naïve. Its use requires an understanding of the unique pharmacology of the drug and is best left to prescribing by those with experience with its use.

45.14
Weaning Opioids

- If the reason for the pain is effectively eliminated, discontinuation of opioids will be necessary while avoiding the development of withdrawal symptoms.
- When weaning a patient from immediate-release agents, reduce the opioid dose by 50% for 2 days and then reduce the daily dose by 25% every 2 days thereafter until the total dose is 30 mg/day (in oral morphine equivalents). The drug may be discontinued after 2 days on the 30 mg/day dose.
- To wean off of long-acting agents, decrease the dose by 25–50% every 2 days. If they are also using immediate-release agents it is often best to start to wean the long-acting agent when the patient is not requiring many or any immediate-release doses. The patient may need to occasionally re-start some immediate-release agents back after the long-acting agent is reduced.

45.15
Patient-Controlled Analgesia (PCA) Basics

- A PCA is a maintenance therapy. If the patient is in moderate to severe pain when it is to be started, IV loading doses must be used to achieve comfort first because incremental dosing with the PCA will not achieve comfort in a reasonable period of time. This

Table 45.5 Suggested initial PCA demand doses and dose changes

	Morphine (mg)	Hydromorphone (mg)	Fentanyl (mcg)
Initial demand dose	1.0–1.5	0.2	20–25
Dose change	0.5	0.1	5–10

Modified from Correll[1], with permission. Copyright © 2008 The McGraw Hill Companies, Inc.

modality helps overcome the wide inter-patient variation in opioid requirements by allowing the patient to control the dosing regimen.

- PCA – Opioid Choice, Dose, and Lockout Interval
  - Morphine: most common first choice agent.
  - Fentanyl: quicker onset and shorter duration than morphine. Good if there is concern about accumulating effects, but bad in that patients must "constantly" activate the PCA – can be difficult for some patients to get sleep at night.
  - Hydromorphone: excellent choice due to its pharmacokinetics.
  - In the opioid naïve patient, the recommended starting doses and suggestions for how to change the dose if the patient does not receive adequate pain relief are shown in Table 45.5.
  - Commonly used lockout intervals range from 5 to 10 min. Even though time to peak effect is longer than this for morphine and hydromorphone, in practice no major differences are seen with longer lockouts for specific opioids. There have also been no good studies to suggest that a particular lockout interval is better than any other.
- PCA – Basal Rates
  - May be needed in opioid-tolerant patients or if fentanyl is used.
  - Not recommended in opioid naïve, elderly, obstructive sleep apnea or morbidly obese patients.
  - Decrease or discontinue the basal rate if a patient is not activating the PCA (i.e., they do not need to self-administer a dose) or if side effects increase, in order to maintain the inherent safety of this method of pain management and not increase the chance of severe events (i.e., respiratory depression).

45.16 Opioid-Induced Side Effects

- Nausea, vomiting, pruritus, constipation, sedation, and respiratory depression are the most common opioid-related side effects. The opioid naïve patient is more likely to develop these effects in the acute setting than a patient who chronically takes opioids as an outpatient. Tolerance will develop to all of these effects, except constipation.
- Treatment of these side effects can be accomplished by:
  - Changing the dose or schedule of the agent.

  - Changing to a different agent (side effects vary widely among patients to the different opioids),
  - Therapy to counteract the side effect,
  - Addition of another analgesic and/or adjuvant to decrease the required dose of the opioid (i.e., opioid-sparing effect).
- Constipation should be expected with the use of opioids, and the prophylactic use of stool softeners (e.g., docusate) and stimulant laxatives (e.g., senna preparations) is recommended.
- Nausea/vomiting can be treated with any of the various agents available (e.g., prochlorperazine, ondansetron, metoclopramide, promethazine) as none has proven more or less effective.
  - Metoclopramide is a pro-motility agent with limited anti-nausea effects and thus is most effective for treating vomiting.
  - Promethazine or prophylactic use of a scopolamine patch may be more effective if the patient has a history of motion sickness or if movement induces the nausea, as opioids sensitize the inner ear labyrinthine system.
- Pruritus is a very common side effect and, in the absence of a rash or true allergic reaction, it is a central mu-related phenomenon.

Table 45.6 Treatment of respiratory depression assumed to be opioid-induced

<u>Initial, non-pharmacologic treatment of respiratory depression:</u> • If patient is taking effective breaths but the rate is <8min: – Use tactile and verbal stimulation to improve respiratory rate. • If patient is taking ineffective breaths and/or with a respiratory rate<4/minute: – Ventilatory assistance with mask and supplemental oxygen is required. This should be instituted while diluting and administering naloxone.
<u>Naloxone should only be considered:</u> • If patient is unarousable or minimally arousable to tactile/verbal stimulation OR • If patient requires ventilatory assistance.
<u>Proper naloxone dilution and dosing:</u> • The 1 ml vial (0.4 mg) of naloxone must be diluted with 9 ml of saline to yield 0.04 mg/ml. • Administer intravenously in 1–2 ml increments (0.04–0.08 mg) at 2–3 min intervals until response. • If NO change in respiratory depression after 0.4 mg naloxone has been titrated, consider another etiology other than opioid-induced. • If there is some, but not sufficient, improvement after 0.4 mg of naloxone has been titrated, continue titration. • Naloxone's half-life is less than most of the opioid agonists, so respiratory depression may recur. Therefore, be prepared for the need to re-administer naloxone boluses or consider use of a naloxone infusion.

Modified from Correll[1], with permission. Copyright © 2008 The McGraw Hill Companies, Inc.

- Diphenhydramine is only effective if the etiology is definitely due to histamine release, which is usually only the case for large doses of morphine given quickly or a true allergic reaction.
- Nalbuphine 5 mg IV q 4 h prn is more effective in that it treats the cause by antagonism of the central mu receptors.

• The proper treatment of respiratory depression from opioids is described in Table 45.6.

45.17 Adjuvant Analgesics (Table 45.7)

• Adjuvant agents are needed when pain is not well controlled with just "standard" therapies, particularly in opioid-tolerant patients. Certain adjuvants produce opioid-sparing leading to a reduction in side effects. Adjuncts are also used to treat or prevent

Table 45.7 Adjuvant analgesic examples

Class	Agent	Adult dosing	Side effects/ comments
Antiepileptics	Gabapentin Pregabalin	Start with 300 mg po q 8 h, increase by 300 mg QD after a few days to a max of 3,600 mg/day in divided doses Start with 50 mg po q 8 h or 75 mg po q 12 h; in 1 week increase to max of 300 mg/day in divided doses	Dizziness and somnolence; do not stop suddenly – must be weaned off
Tricyclic antidepressants	Amitriptyline	25 mg po qhs; increase to max of 150 mg/day in a single or divided doses	Anticholinergic symptoms (e.g., dry mouth, confusion), sedation, and hypotension
Skeletal muscle relaxants	Tizanidine Orphenadrine	4–8 mg po q 6–24 h 100 mg po q 12 h 60 mg IV q 12 h	Long-term use can lead to dependence
Antispasmotic	Baclofen	10 mg po q 8 h, titrate slowly to max of 80 mg/day in divided doses	Drowsiness; may impair renal function; sudden D/C may cause seizures
Alfa-2 Agonist	Clonidine	0.2 mg/day via a transdermal patch, left on for 1 week	Hypotension and sedation; monitor for rebound hypertension on D/C if used for >1 week

Modified from Correll[1], with permission. Copyright © 2008 The McGraw Hill Companies, Inc.

neuropathic symptoms (e.g., hyperalgesia or allodynia) and potentially the development of chronic pain. In addition, not all pain is well treated with opioids (e.g., muscle spasm), and other appropriate agents are available.

- Antiepileptics: Effective for treatment of neuropathic pain. May have analgesic effects in the acute setting as well.
- Tricyclic Antidepressants: Effective for treatment of neuropathic pain. Doses used are lower than for depression and onset of analgesia is faster (i.e., days) than antidepressant effects.
- Skeletal Muscle Relaxants: Useful for relief of muscle injury/spasms.
- Antispasmodics: Treatment of pain with a spastic component (including muscles) or in neuropathic pain states.
- Alpha-2 agonist: Analgesic and opioid-sparing effects.
- Benzodiazepines: Treatment of anxiety or insomnia. Be aware of the development of dependence with long-term use.
  - These agents do not have any analgesic properties.
  - May be useful to help patients sleep, making it easier to "deal" with pain.
  - Anxiety can play a role in pain states, especially acute pain; when this is added to persistent pain, an anti-anxiety medication may be useful.
  - Use with caution in acute pain, especially when high doses of opioids are required, as significant sedation and respiratory depression can occur in the benzodiazepine-naïve patient.
  - In anxious patients with pain, adequate titration with analgesics should occur before the addition of a benzodiazepine.

45.18 Acute Pain in the Opioid Tolerant

- If a patient who has chronic pain and takes opioids experiences an episode that increases their pain (e.g., surgery), opioid use will be higher than just replacement of what they were on before the insult, and it is most often SIGNIFICANTLY higher than in an opioid-naïve patient.
- More pain complaints and higher pain scores will likely occur.
- It is of utmost importance to discuss reasonable goals and expectations of analgesic therapy with the patient.
- The use of multimodal therapy in this patient population is particularly helpful.

Reference

1. Correll DJ. Pain Management. In: McKean SC, Bennett A, Halasyamani L, eds. *Hospital Medicine – Just the Facts*. New York: McGraw Hill; 2008:530.

Suggested Reading

American Pain Society. *Principles of Analgesic Use in the Treatment of Acute Pain and Cancer Pain*. 6th ed. Glenview: American Pain Society; 2008.

American Society of Anesthesiologists Task Force on Acute Pain Management. Practice guidelines for acute pain management in the perioperative setting: an updated report. *Anesthesiology*. 2004;100:1573-1581.

Galvagno SM, Correll DJ, Narang S. Safe oral equianalgesic opioid dosing for patients with moderate-to-severe pain. *Res Staff Phys*. 2007;53(4):17-23.

Gordon DB, Dahl JL, Miaskowski C, et al. American Pain Society recommendations for improving the quality of acute and cancer pain management. *Arch Intern Med*. 2005;165:1574-1580.

Pereira J, Lawlor P, Vigano A, Dorgan M, Bruera E. Equianalgesic dose ratios for opioids: a critical review and proposals for long-term dosing. *J Pain Symptom Manage*. 2001;22:672-687.

United States Food and Drug Administration/Center for Drug Evaluation and Research website http://www.accessdata.fda.gov/scripts/cder/drugsatfda/index.cfm. Accessed 9/15/2010.

Walder B, Schafer M, Henzi I, Tramèr MR. Efficacy and safety of patient-controlled opioid analgesia for acute postoperative pain. A quantitative systematic review. *Acta Anaesthesiol Scand*. 2001;45:795-804.

White PF, Kehlet H. Improving postoperative pain management: what are the unresolved issues? *Anesthesiology*. 2010;112:220-225.

Index

S.L Cohn (ed.), *Perioperative Medicine*,
DOI: 10.1007/978-0-85729-498-2, © Springer-Verlag London Limited 2011

H